6200582019

D0364559

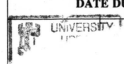

FETAL AND INFANT ORIGINS OF ADULT DISEASE

FETAL AND INFANT ORIGINS OF ADULT DISEASE

Papers written by

The Medical Research Council Environmental Epidemiology Unit
University of Southampton

Edited by

D J P Barker

Director, MRC Environmental Epidemiology Unit, and
Professor of Clinical Epidemiology
University of Southampton

With an introduction by

Roger J Robinson

Emeritus Professor of Paediatrics,
United Medical and Dental Schools of Guy's and St Thomas' Hospitals,
University of London and
Associate Editor, *British Medical Journal*

Published by the British Medical Journal
Tavistock Square, London WC1H 9JR

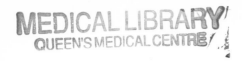
© British Medical Journal 1992

ISBN 0 7279 0743 3

Printed in Great Britain by
Latimer Trend & Company Ltd, Plymouth

Contents

V Blood pressure

VI Haemostatic factors

VII Review

VIII Glucose tolerance

IX Cholesterol

X Body fat distribution

XI Fetal growth

XII   The future

List of contributors

Medical Research Council Environmental Epidemiology Unit, University of Southampton, Southampton General Hospital, Southampton SO9 4XY

D J P Barker MD PhD FRCP	Director
A R Bull MFPHM	Epidemiologist
J E Cade PhD	Nutritionist
D Coggon PhD MRCP	Epidemiologist
A M Cruddas PhD	Statistician
C Fall MRCP	Paediatrician
K M Godfrey MRCP	Epidemiologist
C M Law MD MRCP MFPHM	Epidemiologist
A Lee BN	Research assistant
B M Margetts PhD	Nutritionist
C N Martyn DPhil MRCP	Epidemiologist
J A Morris MSc	Statistician
C Osmond PhD	Statistician
K Phipps MRCGP	General practitioner
S M Robinson PhD	Nutritionist
S O Shaheen MRCP	Epidemiologist
S J Simmonds BSc	Research assistant
J M Slattery MSc	Statistician
C Wickham MSc	Statistician
P D Winter MSc	Computing manager

MRC National Survey of Health and Development, Department of Community Medicine, University College London and the Middlesex Hospital Medical School, London

D Kuh MA	Scientist
M E J Wadsworth PhD	Director

MRC Dunn Nutrition Unit, Cambridge

T J Cole PhD	Statistician
F A Foord BSc SRN	Nurse midwife
M G M Rowland FRCP MPHM	Consultant in public health medicine

MRC Epidemiology and Medical Care Unit, Northwick Park Hospital, Harrow, Middlesex

T W Meade FRCP	Director
Y Stirling FIMLS	Senior scientific officer

University of Bristol, Department of Child Health, Bristol
J Golding PhD — Professor of paediatric and perinatal epidemiology

University of Cambridge, Department of Clinical Biochemistry, Addenbrooke's Hospital, Cambridge
P M S Clark PhD — Principal biochemist
L J Cox MSc — Research assistant
C N Hales FRS — Professor of clinical biochemistry

University of London, United Medical and Dental Schools of Guy's and St Thomas' Hospitals, London
R J Robinson BM DPhil FRCP — Emeritus professor of paediatrics

University of Oxford, Department of Obstetrics and Gynaecology, John Radcliffe Hospital, Oxford
C W G Redman FRCP — Clinical reader

University of Southampton, Department of Human Reproduction, Southampton
T Wheeler DM FRCOG — Senior lecturer
M C Hayes — Research assistant

Shirley Health Centre, Southampton
R J Walton MRCP MRCGP — General practitioner

City General Hospital, Stoke-on-Trent
P H M Carson FRCP
J S Mann MRCP
K G Oldroyd MRCP

Acknowledgements

We thank our colleagues in the MRC Environmental Epidemiology Unit. The following were fieldworkers: in Preston—Julia Hart, Margaret Kelly, Margaret Livesey, Janet Peace, and Marie Ward; in Hertford—Peggy Harwood, Susan Haynes, Pauline Howell, Rochelle Rosenthal, and Susan Wolfe; in Stoke-on-Trent—Sylvia Kirham and Julie Veitch; in Ipswich—Jane Whitehead; in Wakefield—Lesley Raper; in Salisbury—Helen Howes and Patricia Zwartouw; and in Southampton—Maire Dudleston and Millicent Mitchell.

Jackie Ariouat and Brian Pannett discovered the records in Preston and Hertford. Sue Forster and Eric Gordon were the MRC Environmental Epidemiology Unit administrators. Rosemarie Kirby, Carol Mincher, and Graham Wield helped with the computing and analysis. Jill Anthony, Julie Coleman, Joann Matthews, Sunita Parhar, and Lesley Theobold computerised the data. Hilary Brenan, Linda Fairley, Gill Strange, and Bridget Wilde typed the manuscripts.

We also thank the staff at the NHS Central Register, Southport; at the Office of Population Censuses and Surveys, London; at Hertfordshire Family Health Services Authority; and at Lancashire Family Health Services Authority who traced the men and women in Hertfordshire and Preston.

The studies were funded by the Medical Research Council, the Wellcome Trust, the British Heart Foundation, the Dunhill Medical Trust, the Wessex Medical Trust, the British Diabetic Association, and Lilly Research Laboratories.

The editor of the *British Medical Journal*, Richard Smith, suggested compiling a book from the articles listed below and allowed the articles published in the *BMJ* (chs 2, 3, 5, 8, 14–16, 20, 22, and 25) and in *Archives of Diseases in Childhood* (chs 9 and 18) and *Journal of Epidemiology and Community Health* (chs 4, 6, 10, 26, 29, and 30) to be reprinted.

We also thank the following publishers for permission to reprint the papers indicated: Blackwell Scientific Publications Ltd for: (ch 12) Coggon D, Margetts B, Barker DJP, Carson PHM, Mann JS, Oldroyd KG, Wickham C. Childhood risk factors for ischaemic heart disease and stroke. *Paediatric and Perinatal Epidemiology* 1990;4:464–9, (ch 17) Barker DJP, Godfrey KM, Osmond C, Bull A. The relation of fetal length, ponderal index and head circumference to blood pressure and the risk of hypertension in adult life. *Paediatric and Perinatal Epidemiology* 1992;6:35–44,

ACKNOWLEDGEMENTS

(ch 27) Godfrey KM, Redman CWG, Barker DJP, Osmond C. The effect of maternal anaemia and iron deficiency on the ratio of fetal weight to placental weight. *British Journal of Obstetrics and Gynaecology* 1991;**98**:886–91, and (ch 28) Robinson SM, Wheeler T, Hayes MC, Barker DJP, Osmond C. Fetal heart rate and intrauterine growth. *British Journal of Obstetrics and Gynaecology* 1991;**98**:1223–7; The Lancet Ltd for: (ch 1) Barker DJP, Osmond C. Infant mortality, childhood nutrition, and ischaemic heart disease in England and Wales. *Lancet* 1986;i:1077–81 and (ch 13) Barker DJP, Winter PD, Osmond C, Margetts B, Simmonds SJ. Weight in infancy and death from ischaemic heart disease. *Lancet* 1989;ii:577–80; Macmillan Magazines Ltd for: (ch 31) Barker DJP. Rise and fall of Western diseases. *Nature* 1989;**338**:371–2. Reprinted by permission from *Nature* vol **338**, pp 371–2. © 1989 Macmillan Magazines Ltd; The Medical Research Council for: (ch 11) Osmond C. *Time trends in infant mortality, ischaemic heart disease and stroke in England and Wales.* Medical Research Council Environmental Epidemiology Unit, 1987:28–34. (Scientific report No 8); Oxford University Press for: (ch 19) Margetts BM, Rowland MGM, Foord FA, Cruddas AM, Cole TJ, Barker DJP. The relation of maternal weight to the blood pressures of Gambian children. *International Journal of Epidemiology* 1991; **20**:938–43. © 1991 International Epidemiological Association; the Royal College of Physicians of London for: (ch 21) Barker DJP. The intrauterine origins of cardiovascular and obstructive lung disease in adult life: the Marc Daniels lecture 1990. *Journal of the Royal College of Physicians of London* 1991;**25**:129–33; Springer-Verlag for: (ch 23) Robinson S, Walton RJ, Clark PM, Barker DJP, Hales CN, Osmond C. The relation of fetal growth to plasma glucose in young men. *Diabetologia* 1992; vol **35**:444–6 and (ch 24) Hales CN, Barker DJP. Type 2 (non-insulin-dependent) diabetes mellitus: the thrifty phenotype hypothesis. *Diabetologia* (in press); and Taylor & Francis Ltd for: (ch 7) Barker DJP, Osmond C, Golding J. Height and mortality in the counties of England and Wales. *Annals of Human Biology* 1990; **17**:1–6.

LIST OF ALL ORIGINAL PUBLICATIONS, BY CHAPTER NUMBER

1 Barker DJP, Osmond C. Infant mortality, childhood nutrition, and ischaemic heart disease in England and Wales. *Lancet* 1986;i:1077–81.
2 Barker DJP, Osmond C. Death rates from stroke in England and Wales predicted from past maternal mortality. *BMJ* 1987;**295**:83–6.
3 Barker DJP, Osmond C. Childhood respiratory infection and adult chronic bronchitis in England and Wales. *BMJ* 1986;**293**:1271–5.
4 Barker DJP, Osmond C, Law CM. The intrauterine and early postnatal origins of cardiovascular disease and chronic bronchitis. *J Epidemiol Community Health* 1989;**43**:237–40.
5 Barker DJP, Osmond C. Inequalities in health in Britain: specific explanations in three Lancashire towns. *BMJ* 1987;**294**:749–52.
6 Osmond C, Barker DJP, Slattery JM. Risk of death from cardiovascular disease and chronic bronchitis determined by place of birth in England and Wales. *J Epidemiol Community Health* 1990;**44**:139–41.

7 Barker DJP, Osmond C, Golding J. Height and mortality in the counties of England and Wales. *Ann Hum Biol* 1990;**17**:1–6.

8 Cade JE, Barker DJP, Margetts BM, Morris JA. Diet and inequalities in health in three English towns. *BMJ* 1988;**296**:1359–62.

9 Barker DJP. Childhood causes of adult diseases. *Arch Dis Child* 1988;**63**:867–9.

10 Barker DJP, Osmond C. Diet and coronary heart disease in England and Wales during and after the second world war. *J Epidemiol Community Health* 1986;**40**:37–44.

11 Osmond C. *Time trends in infant mortality, ischaemic heart disease and stroke in England and Wales*. Southampton: Medical Research Council Environmental Epidemiology Unit, 1987:28–34. (Scientific report No 8.)

12 Coggon D, Margetts B, Barker DJP, Carson PHM, Mann JS, Oldroyd KG, Wickham C. Childhood risk factors for ischaemic heart disease and stroke. *Paediatr Perinat Epidemiol* 1990;**4**:464–9.

13 Barker DJP, Winter PD, Osmond C, Margetts B, Simmonds SJ. Weight in infancy and death from ischaemic heat disease. *Lancet* 1989;ii:577–80.

14 Barker DJP, Godfrey KM, Fall C, Osmond C, Winter PD, Shaheen SO. Relation of birth weight and childhood respiratory infection to adult lung function and death from chronic obstructive airways disease. *BMJ* 1991;**303**:671–5.

15 Barker DJP, Osmond C, Golding J, Kuh D, Wadsworth MEJ. Growth in utero, blood pressure in childhood and adult life, and mortality from cardiovascular disease. *BMJ* 1989;**298**:564–7.

16 Barker DJP, Bull AR, Osmond C, Simmonds SJ. Fetal and placental size and risk of hypertension in adult life. *BMJ* 1990;**301**:259–62.

17 Barker DJP, Godfrey KM, Osmond C, Bull A. The relation of fetal length, ponderal index and head circumference to blood pressure and the risk of hypertension in adult life. *Peadiatr Perinat Epidemiol* 1992;**6**:35–44.

18 Law CM, Barker DJP, Bull AR, Osmond C. Maternal and fetal influences on blood pressure. *Arch Dis Child* 1991;**66**:1291–5.

19 Margetts BM, Rowland MGM, Foord FA, Cruddas AM, Cole TJ, Barker DJP. The relation of maternal weight to the blood pressures of Gambian children. *Int J Epidemiol* 1991;**20**:938–43.

20 Barker DJP, Meade TW, Fall CHD, Lee A, Osmond C, Phipps K, Stirling Y. Relation of fetal and infant growth to plasma fibrinogen and factor VII concentrations in adult life. *BMJ* 1992;**304**:148–52.

21 Barker DJP. The intrauterine origins of cardiovascular and obstructive lung disease in adult life: the Marc Daniels Lecture 1990. *J Roy Coll Physicians Lond* 1991;**25**:129–33.

22 Hales CN, Barker DJP, Clark PMS, Cox LJ, Fall C, Osmond C, Winter PD. Fetal and infant growth and impaired glucose tolerance at age 64. *BMJ* 1991;**303**:1019–22.

23 Robinson S, Walton RJ, Clark PM, Barker DJP, Hales CN, Osmond C. The relation of fetal growth to plasma glucose in young men. *Diabetologia* 1992; vol **35**:444–6.

24 Hales CN, Barker DJP. Type 2 (non-insulin-dependent) diabetes mellitus: the thrifty phenotype hypothesis. *Diabetologia* (in press).

25 Fall CHD, Barker DJP, Osmond C, Winter PD, Clark PMS, Hales CN. Relation of infant feeding to adult serum cholesterol concentration and death from ischaemic heart disease. *BMJ* 1992;**304**:801–5.

26 Law CM, Barker DJP, Osmond C, Fall CHD, Simmonds SJ. Early growth and abdominal fatness in adult life. *J Epidemiol Community Health* (in press).

27 Godfrey KM, Redman CWG, Barker DJP, Osmond C. The effect of maternal anaemia and iron deficiency on the ratio of fetal weight to placental weight. *Br J Obstet Gynaecol* 1991;**98**:886–91.

28 Robinson SM, Wheeler T, Hayes MC, Barker DJP, Osmond C. Fetal heart rate and intrauterine growth. *Br J Obstet Gynaecol* 1991;**98**:1223–7.

29 Barker DJP, Martyn CN. The maternal and fetal origins of cardiovascular disease. *J Epidemiol Community Health* 1992;**46**:8–11.

30 Osmond C, Barker DJP. Ischaemic heart disease in England and Wales around the year 2000. *J Epidemiol Community Health* 1991;**45**:71–2.

31 Barker DJP. Rise and fall of Western diseases. *Nature* 1989;**338**:371–2.

Introduction

ROGER J ROBINSON

"The child is father of the man". Wordsworth neatly summarised the argument of the papers collected in this book. Their general theme is that factors affecting the fetus and the young have long lasting effects and are important causes of later diseases, such as ischaemic heart disease, stroke, and chronic bronchitis.

It is natural to ask what has led to such a major research effort, with such important conceptual and biological implications. The original question was about the causes of ischaemic heart disease. Current views emphasised factors in lifestyle, such as diet, exercise, and smoking. However, there are features of the epidemiology of ischaemic heart disease which cannot be explained by these factors, and which in some respects—for example, the geographical and social class differences in death rates from this disease in Britain—are the opposite of what the accepted paradigm would predict. The Barker group took up the observation that areas in Britain which now had high rates of death from cardiovascular diseases—ischaemic heart disease and stroke—used to have high infant death rates. Factors which were unfavourable for health in infancy might, therefore, also cause later disease in adult life. A detailed geographical comparison of infant mortality in the earlier part of this century with more recent adult mortality suggested that particular periods in pregnancy and infancy might have specific importance for the later development of particular diseases—ischaemic heart disease, stroke, and chronic bronchitis.

These mortality studies suggested possible relations between early influences and later diseases, but to find what structural and functional changes in early life led to later proneness to disease, the focus needed to move to studies of individuals. The later chapters in the book show how the problems of such studies—(which at first sight need to cover a whole life span)—were tackled, and how the original idea evolved and changed. It embraced the concepts of "sensitive" or "critical" periods—with the sensitive period extending back to fetal life as well as infancy—and of "programming"—meaning that an early stimulus or insult, operating at a critical or sensitive period, results in a long term change in the structure or function of the organism.[1] These concepts are not new to biology, nor is the idea that adverse influences or factors can have effects which are long delayed, and which become apparent after a latent period. Rheumatic heart disease and herpes zoster infection are two examples from classical medicine.

Three features of this research seem to be particularly notable. Firstly, the thoroughness, detail, and specificity of the comparisons of mortality data led to hypotheses about the particular periods in early life during which events may predispose to particular diseases. Secondly, the extension of the studies to individuals has shown some of the physical, biochemical, and physiological changes which underlie programming of later diseases, and has led to new ideas about conditions which were not the original subject of study—hypertension and diabetes. Thirdly, there has been a logical development of the strategy of research, with new methods and new populations being found to answer questions raised by earlier phases of the inquiry.

The best way to assess this body of work is to read the original presentations of the evidence, and it is not easy for the ordinary reader to assemble, at the same time, all the journals to do this in a logical order. For this reason, the 31 papers are reprinted in substantially the form in which they first appeared in many different journals. The only changes are that, for the convenience of the reader, some duplication between the "Methods" sections of some of the papers has been removed, and cross references between the different papers use the chapter numbers of the book.

This introduction is intended as a guide to the reader, and a more detailed summary of the development of this research and of the content of the book follows. Two brief words of explanation are necessary. Firstly, the non-epidemiological reader may like a reminder about the definitions of categories of mortality which recur so often throughout this introduction and the chapters of the book. Infant mortality is the number of deaths before the age of 1 year per 1000 live births in the same period. Infant mortality is subdivided into neonatal mortality—deaths in the first 28 days after birth—and postneonatal mortality—deaths between 28 days and 1 year. Neonatal deaths are strongly dependent on problems occurring during pregnancy, birth, and the period immediately after birth, whereas postneonatal deaths are particularly dependent on environmental factors in infancy. Maternal mortality is the number of women dying of causes related to pregnancy and childbirth per 1000 total births in the same period. Maternal deaths are now very rare in developed countries, but they were more common in the historical period to which some of these papers refer, and an important distinction was between those due to puerperal fever (streptococcal infection) and those from other causes. Finally, when death rates from adult diseases such as ischaemic heart disease are compared, it is necessary to allow for the fact that areas differ in the age structure of their populations. Epidemiologists correct for this by using a "standardised mortality ratio", and it is usually standardised mortality ratios which are compared in these papers. For simplicity, however, I use the terms "death rate" or "mortality".

The second point concerns two shorthand terms which I use often, again for simplicity. These papers represent the work of a team of people from many disciplines, some based in the MRC Environmental Epidemiology Unit at the University of Southampton, and some elsewhere. Their names appear at the front of the book and in the headings of the papers, but I will refer to "the Barker group" to mean the authors collectively or severally, and to "the programming hypothesis" to mean the main argument of the book.

Summary of contents

GEOGRAPHICAL STUDIES

The first group of studies relates recent death rates from ischaemic heart disease, chronic bronchitis, or stroke to infant or maternal death rates at a much earlier period. The infant deaths occurred around the time of birth or infancy of the people who died in the more recent period. All these studies are geographically based—they take mortality data from areas throughout England and Wales and look for a tendency for later adult death rates to vary from area to area according to earlier infant death rates in the same areas. It is therefore the experience of areas rather than the experience of individuals which is being compared.

Death rates from ischaemic heart disease, chronic bronchitis, and stroke in all the 212 administrative areas in England and Wales in the period 1966–78 were the first compared with infant mortality rates in 1921–5 (chapter 1). Deaths from stroke related to earlier neonatal mortality, those from chronic bronchitis to postneonatal mortality, and those from ischaemic heart disease were related to both neonatal and postneonatal mortality. Certain other diseases such as stomach cancer and rheumatic heart disease also showed a relation, but a less strong one, with infant mortality. The suggested explanation is that stroke is related to adverse maternal factors operating both before and during pregnancy (these were the factors which then made the greatest contribution to neonatal mortality); that chronic bronchitis relates to adverse living conditions, including risk of infection, in the first year of life; whereas ischaemic heart disease has its roots in both maternal factors and those of infancy. It is fundamental to this and the subsequent geographical studies that infant death rates are used as markers of adverse circumstances. Obviously the people dying of, say, stroke in 1966 did not die in the neonatal period in 1921! However, the argument is that they will have been exposed to the same risk of adverse maternal or perinatal factors which determined the neonatal death rate in 1921.

Another theme is introduced in chapter 1. Ischaemic heart disease, chronic bronchitis, and stroke are all more common in areas which used to have the highest infant mortality. The secular trends in these diseases differ, however, with a contrast between chronic bronchitis and stroke, which have both become less common, and ischaemic heart disease, which has become more common. Some factors in addition to those which determine infant mortality must therefore contribute to the cause of ischaemic heart disease, otherwise its incidence should have declined like that of the other two diseases. Ischaemic heart disease may be caused by a combination of factors, first those associated with early adversity, then followed by other factors associated with later affluence.

Deaths from stroke in 1968–78 were related not only to earlier neonatal mortality but also, and even more closely, to maternal mortality in 1911–14, other than that caused by puerperal fever—again using a nationwide geographical comparison (chapter 2). Non-streptococcal maternal mortality at the time was largely caused by poor maternal health and physique (in turn related to poor nutrition and rickets in childhood). Mortality from stroke has fallen steadily over the past 40 years, which may reflect gradual improvement in maternal health.

Chapter 3 looks in more detail at mortality in the same 212 areas in relation to the cause of chronic bronchitis. The areas with the highest death rates from chronic bronchitis were those which, in the earlier period, had had the highest infant mortality from "bronchitis and pneumonia". Though there were other correlations, both between other causes of infant death and adult deaths from bronchitis, and between other causes of adult death, such as rheumatic heart disease, and adult deaths from chronic bronchitis, the strongest correlation was between 1921–5 *infant* deaths from bronchitis and pneumonia and 1959–78 *adult* deaths from chronic bronchitis. Only deaths from measles in infancy (then an important cause of pneumonia) showed nearly as strong a correlation with later deaths from bronchitis. The authors suggest that lung infection in early infancy has a deleterious effect on lung function, and this persists into adult life and predisposes to later chronic bronchitis. The high rates of respiratory infection in infancy which used to occur in certain areas are attributed to poor living conditions including poor housing, overcrowding, and early stopping of breast feeding. The Barker group argues that experience in infancy is a stronger determinant than smoking of later chronic bronchitis, and that a predisposition to atopy and asthma is not the link between early respiratory infection and later chronic bronchitis.

The relations found in these first chapters are further developed and explained in chapter 4, and a fascinating 'tale of three cities' follows in chapter 5. Burnley, Nelson, and Colne are three Lancashire towns, which are very close to each other and which all depended on cotton weaving as their main industry. In the early part of the century, however, they had very different infant death rates, with that of Burnley nearly twice that of Nelson, and Colne having an intermediate rate. Among "those dark satanic mills" some had much darker living conditions than others, and housing in Burnley was much damper, darker, and more crowded than that in Nelson. Furthermore, Nelson women were healthier than those in Burnley, many being first generation migrants from rural areas, whereas those in Burnley and Colne were mostly third generation town dwellers. The three towns are now very similar in socioeconomic conditions, with Nelson if anything slightly less favoured than the other two. Current adult mortality, however, follows the same pattern as infant mortality earlier in the century, with much higher death rates in Burnley than in Nelson, Colne again occupying the middle position. Enough people have spent their lives in the town of their birth for the comparison to be meaningful. The excess of deaths in

5

Burnley is largely caused by ischaemic heart disease, chronic bronchitis, and stroke. The findings therefore mirror those seen in the much larger scale studies of all the areas in England and Wales. They give a vivid picture of the kind of adverse living conditions which led to the appallingly high infant mortality in poor urban areas and which, according to the arguments in this book, also led to recent cardiovascular and respiratory disease.

All the geographical studies summarised so far compare death rates in different areas at two widely separated times. It is important in such studies that the population in an area remains reasonably stable and is not greatly affected by migration into and out of the area—or at least that enough people who are born in an area remain there for the comparison of death rates to have some meaning. If there really is an effect of maternal and early infantile factors on much later mortality, it also follows that that mortality should be related to the place and circumstances of birth and early childhood, even for those who later move to a different place to live. This question is addressed in chapter 6, which analyses the cause of death in nearly 2 million people dying in England and Wales in 1969–72 for whom the death certificate recorded place of birth as well as place of death. Even among those who had moved, people born in the north and in industrial towns had an increased risk of dying of ischaemic heart disease or stroke, and people born in and around London had a low risk. This study is more difficult than the others for the average reader to understand, because it cannot be based on actual death rates for the different groups (the denominators—the total numbers of those who had and had not moved—were unknown), but rather on the relative incidences of the different causes of death. Migration studies seem at first sight to be an ideal way to test the programming hypothesis, but they are both difficult to do and difficult to interpret—people who move out of an area differ in other important ways from those who stay.

Geographical variations in height and in adult mortality are examined in chapter 7, using data from three British cohort studies. The heights of people born over the 50 year period 1920–70 were available, as maternal and paternal heights, as well as heights of the children born into the cohort, were known. There was a secular trend for height to increase, but the differences between counties remained, and those with the shortest people had the highest rates of death from ischaemic heart disease, stroke, chronic bronchitis, and other diseases in 1968–78. As height is largely determined by growth in childhood, this is further evidence of a link between childhood factors and death from these diseases.

Two studies show that dietary differences between populations at different times and in different places do not account for their patterns of death from ischaemic heart disease. Chapter 8 is another tale of three cities, comparing the diets of middle aged men and women in Ipswich, Wakefield, and Stoke-on-Trent. People in Stoke had the highest death rates but the lowest consumption of fat and other nutrients. The implication is that present day diet does not explain the disease differences, and though smoking may play some part, better child health in Ipswich in the past is the likelier explanation. Likewise, chapter 10 shows that trends in mortality from ischaemic heart disease in England and Wales do not appear to have been much affected—as the dietary hypothesis would predict—by the fall in fat consumption during the second world war.

STUDIES IN INDIVIDUALS—THE HERTFORDSHIRE LONGITUDINAL STUDY

The geographical studies relate mortality from cardiovascular and chronic lung disease to the previous health experience of populations rather than of individuals. It might seem that the ideal way to test the hypothesis that fetal and infantile factors cause or contribute to these diseases would be to follow a cohort of people throughout their lives, with good information on the gestation and infancy, and to record their experience of illness and their cause of death. There are obvious difficulties in mounting a study which would last most of a century and produce few results for a generation. (In any case, the "ideal" cohort study is an unrealistic idea for another reason—that, even over a much shorter period than the one suggested, a hypothesis will develop and change so much in the light of progress in knowledge that the kinds of information eventually wanted will include many items that were not originally recorded.)

Instead, the Barker group took a different approach. If they could find accurate records of the gestation and infancy of people who were now in late adult life, or who had died of one of the diseases being studied, this might provide some of the information which could have been obtained from the "ideal" but impracticable longitudinal study. The group therefore systematically searched throughout the country for old maternity and infant welfare records. It was not an easy task—old medical records have a high chance of having been lost or destroyed. Furthermore, these particular records were often kept by the old local authority medical services, and after the 1974 reorganisation of the health services they were deposited in county archives, where they were often not catalogued. Members of the MRC unit, including an historian, toured county archives and hospital records departments to search for such records; former medical officers of health were asked if they knew of any records which had been deposited in county archives; and every obstetrician in the country was asked for information on old obstetric records. Two of the collections of records discovered, those from Hertfordshire and Preston, have so far been used for longitudinal studies.

From 1911 onwards, children born in Hertfordshire (mostly at home) were weighed by the midwife, and records of infant feeding, childhood illnesses, and weight at one year were kept by the health visitor. These records were found, and, astonishingly, in 71% of the males it was possible to find out if they were now alive or dead, and if dead, from what cause. Chapters 13, 14, 20, 22, 25, and 26 give the results.

There is something both touching and fascinating about these Hertfordshire studies. The infant data were collected by a devoted body of health visitors, most of whom must now be dead, and none of whom can have had any idea of the use which 70 or more years later would be made of their observations, to reach conclusions about the diseases not of infancy but of middle and old age. Then there is the use of scanty data to make deductions of huge importance to health. Most of us have marvelled at the way archaeologists can work out the way of life of a past civilisation, or the structure of a forgotten language, from a fragment of a pot or of an inscription on a stone. It needed a search of archaeological thoroughness to find these original Hertfordshire data, and they are of almost archaeological meagreness, and yet they have been used, particularly in the detailed studies on those still living, to make deductions of archaeological elegance and significance.

Among the Hertfordshire men, the death rate from ischaemic heart disease fell with increasing birth weight, and particularly with increasing weight at 1 year (chapter 13). The death rate from obstructive lung disease fell with increasing weight at 1 year. These findings, referring to individuals, support the conclusions from the geographical studies, suggesting that maternal factors (which determine birth weight) and health and nutrition in infancy (which influence growth in the first year) are both, and independently, related to the later risk of ischaemic heart disease.

The study has been extended by detailed examination and observations of a smaller number of men aged 59 to 70, whose infant data were available and who still lived in Hertfordshire.

Adult lung function was impaired if either birth weight or weight gain in infancy had been low, or if there had been respiratory infection in infancy (chapter 14). This helps to clarify the relation between early growth and adult death from obstructive lung disease.

The relation of fetal and infant growth to ischaemic heart disease has been explored further by looking at certain risk factors in these surviving men. Those with lower birth weight and lower weight at 1 year were more likely as adults to have higher blood pressure and impaired glucose tolerance or frank diabetes (chapter 22). Those with lower weight at 1 year also had, in adult life, higher plasma concentrations of apolipoprotein B (chapter 25) and of the clotting factors, fibrinogen and factor VII (chapter 20)—all of which are associated with an increased risk of ischaemic heart disease. Lower birth weight and lower weight at 1 year also increased the tendency for men to store fat abdominally—as indicated by an increased ratio of waist to hip circumference (chapter 26). This pattern of fat storage increases the risk of cardiovascular disease and diabetes. The general message from these Hertfordshire studies is clear and straightforward—not only death rates from ischaemic heart disease but also many of the physiological variables which increase the risk of heart disease are adversely affected by impaired growth of the fetus or infant.

Detailed analysis of the results from this longitudinal study, and another done at Preston, shows complex relations between these physiological variables and the *time* of early growth impairment. Study of these relations makes more demands on the reader, but takes the argument beyond the straightforward and important general message and into the possible mechanisms which underlie the "programming". At this point I will mention the findings concerning cholesterol, and then deal under separate headings with those concerning blood pressure, glucose tolerance, and diabetes.

Low density lipoprotein cholesterol concentrations in the men in their 60s were higher in those who had been breast fed who had not been weaned at 1 year and in the small number who had been exclusively bottle fed (chapter 25). In these two feeding groups, the adult low density lipoprotein cholesterol concentrations were inversely related to weight at 1 year. These results suggest that nutrition in the first year or so of life has an important effect on later cholesterol metabolism. Animal studies have also shown a programming effect of nutrition in infancy on cholesterol concentrations in adult life.[1][2]

EARLY INFLUENCES ON BLOOD PRESSURE

Another valuable collection of records from the maternity department at a Preston hospital was found, which enabled the group to do another longitudinal study. This particular hospital kept unusually detailed anthropometric measurements of women and their newborn infants during the period 1935–43. Compared with the Hertfordshire data, these are less informative in that they relate to only the minority of babies who at that time were born in hospital, and there is no information on the infants after the time of their birth. The value of these data lies in the greater detail concerning placental weights and body measurements of newborn infants, including lengths and head circumferences. These people are younger than those in the Hertfordshire study, being now around the age of 50, so no mortality figures have been published, but their blood pressure and fibrinogen concentrations have been studied.

Chapters 16 and 17 show how blood pressure in these men and women relates to measurements made at birth 50 years earlier. Adult blood pressure was inversely related to birth weight, and positively related to placental weight. As raised blood pressure is associated with increased risks of stroke and ischaemic heart disease, there is again a concordance between these findings, those of the geographical studies, and those from Hertfordshire. Further study of the interrelation between newborn body measure-

9

ments, placental weight, and later blood pressure showed complex but very interesting findings. Among infants with smaller placentas, later blood pressure was higher if the infant had been relatively long and thin at birth and the head circumference had been reduced. Among those with larger placentas, blood pressure was higher in those who had been short in relation to their head size. These Preston studies therefore show that a placental weight which is high in relation to the weight of the fetus, and a disproportionate body size of the newborn infant—both of which may indicate some compromise of fetal haemodynamics or fetal nutrition, or both—both predispose to raised blood pressure in adult life. (A high placental weight compared with infant birth weight was also associated with raised fibrinogen concentrations and with increased abdominal fatness in the adults—chapters 20 and 26).

Another approach has been to examine some of the relations which were found in the Hertfordshire and Preston studies, for example between blood pressure, birth weight, and placental weight, in more recently born children studied at younger ages.

There have been three major cohort studies in Great Britain, in which a sample, or all, of the children born in one week have been followed, with information about pregnancy, birth, development, and subsequent course. The cohorts born in 1946 and 1970 were aged 36 and 10, respectively, at the time of the study described in chapter 15. Systolic blood pressure, as in Hertfordshire, was found to be inversely related to birth weight, both at age 10 and more strongly at age 36.

Maternal and fetal influences on blood pressure were examined in a new group of 4 year old children in Salisbury (chapter 18). The relations of blood pressure to fetal growth and placental weight seen in adults in the Preston study were also present, through less strongly, in young children. Systolic pressure rose with decreasing birth weight and with increasing placental weight. It also rose with lower head circumference, increased body length, and lower ponderal index (that is, a thinner baby) at birth. Maternal anaemia increased the child's blood pressure, as did increased body weight at 4 years.

The puzzling significance of heavier placentas was investigated by a retrospective survey of over 8000 pregnancies in Oxford. Maternal anaemia was associated with increased placental size and with an increased ratio of placental weight to birth weight (chapter 27). It is suggested that increased placental size is a sign of maternal, and possibly fetal, malnutrition.

Further evidence of an effect of intrauterine nutrition on later blood pressure was found in Gambian children (chapter 19). Mothers who gained less weight in the last trimester of pregnancy tended to have children with higher blood pressures, but this effect only became apparent after the children reached the age of 8.

To summarise these important and detailed studies of the effects of early influences on later blood pressure: firstly, a lower birth weight leads to a higher blood pressure at ages 4, 10, 36, 50, and 65, with a tendency for the effect to become stronger with increasing age. Secondly, features which may indicate impaired fetal nutrition (differences in bodily proportions in the newborn infant and an increased size of the placenta relative to the fetus) predispose to higher blood pressure in childhood and in adult life.

EARLY INFLUENCES ON IMPAIRED GLUCOSE TOLERANCE AND DIABETES

In the Hertfordshire study both reduced birth weight and reduced weight at 1 year were associated (around age 65) with impaired glucose tolerance, increased plasma proinsulin concentrations, and an increased risk of diabetes. As expected, obesity, indicated by an increased body mass index, also predisposed to impaired glucose tolerance. Thus increased body weight at 1 year and increased body mass index in late adult life had opposite effects, the former protecting against, and the latter predisposing to, a diabetic tendency.

These relations were re-examined in a younger group of men, aged 18 to 25 (chapter 23). Glucose tolerance tests showed that men of lower birth weight had higher plasma glucose concentrations and lower plasma insulin concentrations when these were corrected for blood glucose. Higher plasma glucose was associated with higher blood pressure.

The original reason for these particular studies was that impaired glucose tolerance is a risk factor for cardiovascular disease. The relations found conform with the programming hypothesis, in that low birth weight and reduced growth in the first year predispose to abnormalities of glucose and insulin metabolism as well as to ischaemic heart disease. The results are, however, of wider interest in relation to two other issues of great current concern—the aetiology of non-insulin dependent diabetes and the association between insulin and hypertension. The Barker group proposes that men who had impaired body growth in fetal life or infancy may also have had early impairment of growth of the pancreatic islet cells, and hence a reduced capacity for insulin production. This predisposes to diabetes, particularly if nutritional deficiency in early life is followed by nutritional abundance, increased body mass, and insulin resistance in later life. This very radical idea about the cause of non-insulin dependent diabetes is fully explained in chapter 24.

The results also have a bearing on another topic which has been of great interest recently—the association between raised plasma insulin concentrations, insulin resistance, and hypertension.[3][4] The argument is that impaired fetal and infant growth independently predispose, as these studies show, both to hypertension and to a diabetic metabolic profile. The apparent contradiction that impaired fetal islet cell development would be expected to reduce insulin production, whereas hypertension is associated with raised plasma insulin concentrations, is partly explained on the grounds that defective islet cells release abnormal amounts of proinsulin into the circulation, and this may be assayed as active insulin. There is also some evidence from these studies that insulin resistance may be partly determined during fetal life and infancy. Increased abdominal fat storage, which was related to lower weight at birth and at 1 year (chapter 26), is associated with insulin resistance.

Comments and questions

It is not surprising that a concept of such a far reaching nature and with such wide implications should have been received with critical interest. This section does not attempt either a comprehensive critical assessment of the evidence for the programming hypothesis or a review of relevant publications. Instead, I will summarise some of the comments and questions of one ordinary reader with a paediatric background.

INDIRECTNESS OF THE MEASURES

The first concern is the indirectness of many of the measures used—they are proxies for something else which is the real subject of interest but which cannot be measured.

The geographical studies use past infant mortality as a proxy for adverse cirumstances affecting the fetus and infant, and maternal mortality as a proxy for poor maternal health and nutrition. It is also assumed that health experience depends on geographical location —that a baby born in an area of high infant mortality is likely to have experienced adverse circumstances in fetal life or infancy. There is a further assumption that the population in an area remains reasonably constant—that those living and dying in an area roughly correspond with those born there 50 years or so previously. All these assumptions may clearly be untrue for an individual, but it is central to epidemiology that applying such assumptions to whole populations can lead to reliable conclusions—that the individual deviations from the general pattern will come out in the epidemiological wash. The methodology is not fundamentally different from that which has led to some of the most important of medical discoveries, like the link between smoking and lung cancer.

Even the studies based on individuals measure things which are often proxies for what the investigators really want to know. For example, the original reason for the studies of blood pressure was that raised blood pressure increases the risk of ischaemic heart disease and stroke, and may therefore be a link between some adverse factors in infancy and the later development of cardiovascular disease. The same applies to measurement of other cardiovascular risk factors.

There are two answers to this criticism. Firstly, direct measures are often not possible in an inquiry which by its nature spans a lifetime for the individual patient. The use of proxy measurements is likely to weaken any association between the real changes or abnormalities in which we are interested, so if even proxy measures show very strong relations—as in these studies—the real underlying relation is probably even stronger. Secondly, the authors have shown great ingenuity in approaching the questions by several different routes, and in finding new populations and sets of data on which to test the hypothesis. The later studies, in chapters 13 to 29, approach much closer to the actual biological differences suggested by the proxy measurements.

CONFOUNDING FACTORS

When studies span such a long period of time, and the measures used are indirect, there will always be concern as to whether the associations found are the result of unrecognised or unmeasured factors, rather than of the ones believed to be most important. The most obvious of the possible confounding factors in these studies is continuing adversity. Can we be sure that a person born in adverse conditions for health, and continuing to live in the same community, is not simply showing the effects of continuing adverse circumstances rather than of those circumstances operating specifically at an early and particularly sensitive period? Several of the chapters address this question, for example by showing that effects occur independently of current socioeconomic status, and the migration study is one attempt to answer this. However, very often the data necessary to deal with this point are understandably simply not available. This issue is probably the one about which the sceptical reader will feel most doubt, and it is the one given most prominence in a recent pair of critical reviews of the concept that early life experience determines the risk of later cardiovascular disease.[5 6]

There are several reasons for believing that the effects described in this collection of papers really are the results of very early experience rather than of later and continuing adversity:

(1) The relations found in the individual studies—for example, between birth weight, placental weight, and blood pressure—are very strong. They are also graded—for example, impaired glucose tolerance became progressively more prevalent among men as their weight at 1 year became lower.

(2) The relations linking early experience with later disease or physiological change are also very specific in their times of operation. Even in the geographical studies, it is not a question of *all* indicators of early disadvantage correlating with *all* the diseases of interest. Thus stroke is linked with earlier maternal and neonatal mortality, chronic bronchitis with postneonatal mortality, and ischaemic heart disease with infant mortality of both kinds. If the early mortality indices were simply acting as markers of later adversity, we would not expect these specific relations. Similarly, the

studies on individuals show very specific relations between growth at a particular phase—for example in fetal life or infancy—and later measurements of blood pressure, concentrations of cholesterol and fibrinogen, and glucose tolerance. For example, blood pressure was related to birth weight but not weight at 1 year; the reverse was true of fibrinogen concentrations.

(3) Though the mortality studies could not control for the effects of continuing socioeconomic factors, because the information was not available, in studies of living people the relations found between early weight and later risk factors were independent of socioeconomic status, either currently or at birth.

(4) The programming hypothesis, that it is early rather than later adverse circumstances which have the major impact on later diseases, is biologically plausible and supported by animal studies.[7]

A possible confounding factor in the studies on chronic lung disease is atopy and asthma. Nowadays, lower respiratory illness in young children is usually associated with wheezing, and has a very close relation to asthma.[8] Debate continues as to whether children who wheeze in infancy and develop classic asthma in later childhood are simply showing the effects of an inherited asthmatic tendency at both ages, or whether viral respiratory infection may predispose to later asthma.[9] The Barker group (chapter 3) argues against an atopic explanation of the relation between early respiratory infection and later bronchitis. Here I was not wholly convinced by their argument. Chronic bronchitis has become much less common, however, whereas the trend in childhood asthma has, if anything, been upwards at least in recent years.[10 11] This suggests that the authors are right that asthma is not the cause of the relation they found.

LOW BIRTH WEIGHT AND PLACENTAL WEIGHT

The geographical studies did not have data on birth weight, but it was suggested that low birth weight might be the link between neonatal mortality and later mortality from cardiovascular disease, as low birth weight is a major contributory cause of neonatal mortality. It is the longitudinal studies which show a direct relation between birth weight and later cardiovascular mortality, blood pressure, and cardiovascular "risk factors".

Not all these studies have definite information on what type or cause of low birth weight is in question. Firstly, in the Hertfordshire studies it is uncertain whether low birth weight is the result of preterm birth or of intrauterine growth retardation, because information on length of gestation is not available. The authors argue, however, that intrauterine growth retardation is the main cause of low birth weight, and this was shown to be the case in the Preston study and the studies of people born more recently.

Secondly, current obstetric and paediatric opinion distinguishes between three different types of intrauterine growth retardation, depending on the cause and on the stage of gestation when growth was restricted. Growth restriction dating from early in pregnancy (from various causes that are usually intrinsic to the fetus) results in a "symmetrically" or proportionately growth retarded infant, who is uniformly small. Restriction in the third trimester (usually from maternal causes affecting placental function and fetal nutrition) causes "asymmetrical" or disproportionate growth restriction, affecting weight and body length more than head size. Fetal malnutrition at the very end of pregnancy results in a thin baby who is underweight, but whose length and head size are normal.[12–16]

In the Preston and Salisbury studies (chapters 17 and 18), measurements of infants at birth gave some indication of the type of fetal growth retardation which had occurred, but the patterns of fetal growth which related to later increase in blood pressure did not correspond exactly with those just outlined. For example in the Salisbury study, blood pressure at age 4 was increased if the baby's head size had been small (suggesting early intrauterine growth retardation), if the ponderal index was low (suggesting late growth retardation), or if body length was increased (suggesting neither).

Another surprising feature is that mostly the infants who later died of cardiovascular disease, or who had a higher incidence of "risk factors", had birth weights which were a little low rather than extremely so. Paediatricians constantly deal with infants of much lower birth weight than most of those in these studies. The implication is that small variations in fetal growth—much smaller than those recognised in everyday practice—lead to large variations in later cardiovascular mortality. Of course, we do not know the eventual outcome for the low birth weight infants being seen and followed up today. The more minor variations in birth weight in the Hertfordshire and Preston studies may be markers of more subtle but more important changes in organ structure and function which determine later disease. Indeed, the studies reported here may add to our understanding of variations in birth weight, in addition to their main purpose. Thus chapter 28 shows that alterations in fetal heart rate at 18 weeks may predict a pattern of disproportionate fetal growth—contrary to the current views on intrauterine growth retardation.

Finally, there is the puzzling issue of placental size. A large placenta, or a large ratio of placental weight to birth weight, is taken by the authors to be a sign of fetal malnutrition. However, it is not a generally recognised feature of intrauterine growth retardation, when a small placenta is the more expected finding.[14 15 17] At first I thought that the relation of a large placenta to raised adult blood pressure was simply an oddity of the Preston findings, and therefore best discounted. However, three other studies (chapters 18, 23, and 27) suggest that a large placenta has a pathophysiological significance, and the link may be that a large placenta is a sign of maternal anaemia and hence an indicator of suboptimal maternal nutrition. A large placenta may also be a non-specific sign of fetal anaemia (Wigglesworth JS, personal communication), which is another possible way to make sense of the findings. Maternal smoking (chapter 27) and intrauterine infection[18] are other factors associated with a relatively large placenta. I now believe that these epidemiological studies have uncovered something interesting and important about placental weight, which deserves further investigation.

Fetal malnutrition, or intrauterine growth retardation, has a central conceptual place in the programming hypothesis. It would be helpful to bring together more closely these ideas and current obstetric and paediatric ideas about the categories and consequences of intrauterine growth retardation, and to place the puzzling business of the apparently unfavourable significance of a large placenta in this context. Cohorts of small for dates babies—and many have been followed up in paediatric studies of the outcome for low birthweight infants—might be informative in future studies of the kind the Barker group has been doing more recently. Equally, neonatal and developmental paediatricians may find it worthwhile to study the effects of the less severe degrees of impaired or deviant fetal growth which the Barker group has found to be important.

THE HISTORICAL DIMENSION

The historial sweep of the geographical studies, and the historical nature of the data used in some of the longitudinal studies, are fascinating and attractive features of this research. It is natural to ask, however, whether the conclusions based on children born up to 80 years ago are applicable to those born today. Infant mortality in England and Wales in 1921–5 varied from 44 per 1000 in West Sussex to 114 in Burnley, the nationwide figure being 76. In 1990 infant mortality in England was 7·9 per 1000. If infant mortality can be taken as an indicator of early health experience or risk of later disease, the population now growing up is totally different in these respects from those who were the subjects of many of these studies.

There are, however, strong reasons to believe that the findings are relevant to the present day. There remain considerable variations in infant death rates between the English health districts, from 4·9 in Norwich to 14·8 in north Warwickshire (1989 figures, excluding districts with less than 20 deaths, for which rates are less meaningful).[19] In relative terms, the difference is comparable to that between the lowest and highest rates in the early 1920s. The studies on younger populations, including the children aged 4 in chapter 18, still indicate important effects of differences in fetal nutrition, and chapters 18 and 27 show that anaemia in pregnancy remains an appreciable problem.

My own abiding impression after reading this collection of papers was of the strength and coherence of the main message. The doubts raised mainly arise from the intrinsic difficulties of any direct and definitive test of the programming hypothesis. The Barker group has tested it using several different indirect approaches, applied to several different populations and age groups, and all have given results consistent with it. Furthermore, the findings from these later studies have suggested new ideas and hypotheses to explore, for example about the aetiology of non-insulin dependent diabetes.

Conclusions and implications

(1) THE PREVENTIVE POSSIBILITIES IN EARLY LIFE

This work strongly argues the value of a healthy environment during pregnancy and in early childhood as an investment likely to pay dividends in terms of preventing later disease. Winston Churchill's remark in 1943 that "there is no finer investment for any community than putting milk into babies" was even truer than he realised. (Of course, the case for good care and a good environment for pregnant women, infants, and children does not rest on the long term argument. There is more to childhood than just the potential for an old age free of ischaemic heart disease or chronic bronchitis, as we are reminded by Wordsworth's immortality ode, to which the first sentence of this introduction is the epigraph.)

The work is also a reminder of the amount at stake in the care of the fetus and infant. It is a matter of straightforward arithmetic that there are more QALYs (quality adjusted life years) to be gained by improving health in infancy than at any subsequent time. Furthermore, the effects of under-nutrition of the fetus and infant may be seen not only in the later life of the individuals affected, but even in their children and grandchildren, as studies of children born after the Dutch famine winter of 1944–5 suggest.[20]

Nevertheless, the argument that cardiovascular and chronic lung disease in adult life may have important causes early in life does not mean that later preventive efforts are without value. Even if early experience has a very major role, there would still be room for a good deal of modification of risk later. For example, the later development of obesity increased the risk of diabetes in those who had been predisposed to it by impaired growth in fetal life and infancy.

(2) THE LONG PERSPECTIVE NEEDED IN PAEDIATRICS

Paediatricians, particularly those caring for newborn babies, spend much of their time dealing with urgent and often life threatening day to day problems. It is important for us to remember, both in clinical work and research, that the consequences of childhood illness and health are on a very long time scale, extending far beyond the paediatric age range. This message is certainly not new to paediatrics,[21] but is worth repeating.

17

(3) THE LONG TERM VALUE OF MEDICAL RECORDS

The Hertfordshire and Preston studies were only possible because, as a result of major searches, some very old records relating to child health and obstetrics came to light. I have often listened to committees discussing which records should be destroyed because of storage problems and to the occasional lone voice protesting that such destruction is an act of clinical and academic vandalism, because we never know of what use the records might be in the future, for the individual patient or for research. With the availability of microfiche and other techniques there is now less reason to destroy records, but it still happens. The chapters also show the value of cohort studies. Much has been learnt, and much of it unforeseen, from the three major British postwar cohort studies of children followed up from pregnancy through childhood and into adult life. The current cohorts are an asset which should be fully used, and new cohort studies should be begun so that secular trends in the pattern of illness can be followed.

(4) THE UNITY OF MEDICINE

The studies reported in this book are the outcome of research by workers in several different disciplines within, or related to, medicine. They have implications for people in an even wider number of disciplines, and are a reminder of the continuity of human life, whose healthiness or health problems should not be separated into compartments which are the responsibility of isolated specialists.

(5) THE IMPORTANCE OF INEQUALITIES IN HEALTH

The studies are a further reminder of the persistence and importance of inequalities in health[22][23] and of their serious, and it now seems very long lasting, consequences. Chapter 5, though not the most important in the development of the programming hypothesis, is the one which will remain most vividly in my mind when details of some of the others have been forgotten. I happened to be reading Wordsworth's *The Excursion* at the time I was asked to read the papers that make up this book and to write its introduction, and I was struck by a common theme. Book VIII of *The Excursion*, written around 1812, describes the first impact on child health of the wave of the industrial revolution; the dismal living conditions 100 years later in Burnley, which are described in chapter 5, were its "melancholy long withdrawing roar". Wordsworth's and Barker's observations have a similar emotional effect on the reader and carry the same social message.

(6) THE NATURE AND AIMS OF RESEARCH

I find a more general message from this book about the nature and objects of research. One of the strongest influences, and a highly beneficial one, on scientific method in medicine in the latter half of this century must have been that of Sir Karl Popper. Popper's axiom that "the criterion of the scientific status of a theory is its falsifiability, or refutability or test-ability"[24][25] has become so deeply embedded in the design of research that it is now often used without conscious awareness of its origin. (It is also often used without awareness of what Popper actually said. I do not remember reading a research application which began "We have a good idea and we want funds to try to prove that it is wrong"). However, the requirement for readily testable hypotheses can have a narrowing influence on the subjects of inquiry. Hypotheses which can be easily tested in the short term, and which are therefore most readily funded, are not necessarily the most interesting or important. I admire the vision of the Barker group in undertaking a research programme where the hypothesis is less easy to test, but the long term implications are of such importance. They have shown that ingenuity and resource can find ways to study such a problem, and that the resulting conclusions and ideas may be even more interesting and challenging than the original far reaching hypothesis.

1 Lucas A. Programming by early nutrition in man. In: Bock GR, Whelan J, eds. *The childhood environment and adult disease*. Ciba Foundation Symposium 156. Chichester: Wiley, 1991:38–55.

2 Mott GE, Lewis DS, McGill HC. Programming of cholesterol metabolism by breast or formula feeding. In: Bock GR, Whelan J, eds. *The childhood environment and adult disease*. Ciba Foundation Symposium 156. Chichester: Wiley, 1991:56–76.

3 Reaven GM, Hoffman BB. A role for insulin in the aetiology and course of hypertension? *Lancet* 1987;**ii**:435–6.

4 Yudkin JS. Hypertension and non-insulin dependent diabetes. *BMJ* 1991;**303**:730–2.

5 Elford J, Shaper AG, Whincup P. Early life experience and cardiovascular disease—ecological studies. *J Epidemiol Community Health* 1992;**46**:1–8.

6 Elford J, Whincup P, Shaper AG. Early life experience and adult cardiovascular disease—longitudinal and case-control studies. *Int J Epidemiol* 1991;**20**:833–44.

7 Bock GR, Whelan J, eds. *The childhood environment and adult disease*. Ciba Foundation Symposium 156. Chichester: Wiley, 1991.

8 Williams H, McNichol KN. Prevalence, natural history, and relationship of wheezy bronchitis and asthma in children. An epidemiological study. *BMJ* 1969;**ii**:321–8.

9 Godfrey S. What is asthma? *Arch Dis Child* 1985;**60**:997–1000.

10 Burr ML, Butland BK, King S, Vaughan-Williams E. Changes in asthma prevalence: two surveys 15 years apart. *Arch Dis Child* 1989;**64**:1452–6.

11 Ninan TK, Russell G. Respiratory symptoms and atopy in Aberdeen schoolchildren: evidence from two surveys 25 years apart. *BMJ* 1992;**304**:873–5.

12 Urrusti J, Yoshida P, Velasco L, Frenk S, Rosado A, Sosa A *et al*. Human fetal growth retardation: clinical features of sample with intrauterine growth retardation. *Pediatrics* 1972;**50**:547–58.

13 Villar J, Belizan JM. The timing factor in the pathophysiology of the intrauterine growth retardation syndrome. *Obstet Gynecol Surv* 1982;**37**:499–506.

14 Chiswick ML. Intrauterine growth retardation. *BMJ* 1985;**291**;845–8.

15 Wigglesworth JS. Aetiology of fetal undergrowth. In: Sharp F, Fraser RB, Milner RDG, eds. *Fetal growth*. London: Springer-Verlag, 1989:185–95.

16 Kramer MS, Olivier M, McLean FH, Dougherty GE, Willis DM, Usher RH. Determinants of fetal growth retardation and body proportionality. *Pediatrics* 1990:**86**;707–13.

17 Bonds DR, Gabbe SG, Kumar S, Taylor T. Fetal weight/placental weight ratio and perinatal outcome. *Am J Obstet Gynecol* 1984;**149**:195–200.

18 Moxon ER. In discussion of Thornburg KL. Fetal response to intrauterine stress. In:

Bock GR, Whelan J, eds. *The childhood environment and adult disease*. Ciba Foundation Symposium 156. Chichester: Wiley, 1991:32.

19 Office of Population Censuses and Surveys. *Key population and vital statistics: local and health authority areas*. London: HMSO, 1990. (Series VS No 16, PP1 No 12.)

20 Lumey H. Obstetric performance of women after in utero exposure to the Dutch famine (1944–1945). New York: Columbia University, 1988. (PhD thesis.)

21 Court SDM. *Fit for the future: report of the committee on child health services*. London: HMSO, 1976.

22 Townsend P, Davidson N. *Inequalities in health: the Black report*. Harmondsworth: Penguin, 1982.

23 Delamothe T. Social inequalities in health. *BMJ* 1991;**303**:1046–50.

24 Popper KL. *Conjectures and refutations: the growth of scientific knowledge*. 5th ed. London: Routledge and Kegan Paul, 1974:66.

25 Burke TE. *The philosophy of Popper*. Manchester: Manchester University Press, 1983.

PART I
GEOGRAPHICAL STUDIES

1: Infant mortality, childhood nutrition, and ischaemic heart disease in England and Wales

D J P BARKER, C OSMOND

Although the rise in ischaemic heart disease in England and Wales has been associated with increasing prosperity, death rates are highest in the least affluent areas. On division of the country into 212 local authority areas a strong geographical relation was found between ischaemic heart disease mortality in 1968–78 and infant mortality in 1921–5. Of the 24 other common causes of death only bronchitis, stomach cancer, and rheumatic heart disease were similarly related to infant mortality. These diseases are associated with poor living conditions, and mortality from them is declining. Ischaemic heart disease is strongly correlated with both neonatal and postneonatal mortality. It is suggested that poor nutrition in early life increases susceptibility to the effects of an affluent diet.

Introduction

In England and Wales, death rates during the past hundred years have been consistently higher in the north and west of the country than in the south and east.[1] Formerly this reflected differences in the incidences of infective diseases that were attributable to inequalities of living standards. Today it reflects differences in mortality from chronic diseases, most importantly ischaemic heart disease. It is a paradox that although the steep increase in ischaemic heart disease during this century[2 3] has been associated with rising prosperity, the disease is now more common in poorer areas[4] and lower income groups.[5]

We have explored the association between poor living standards and ischaemic heart disease by a detailed geographical comparison of infant mortality in 1921–5 and death in adults from ischaemic heart disease and other leading causes in 1968–78.

Methods

The Office of Population Censuses and Surveys made available to us extracts from all death certificates in England and Wales during 1968–78. There were 25 causes of death, as coded under the eighth revision of the International Classification of Diseases (ICD), for which more than 10 000 deaths occurred in each sex, or in the sex usually affected. These were: cancers at 12 sites (oesophagus, stomach, colon, rectum, pancreas, lung, breast, cervix, uterus, ovary, prostate, and bladder); ischaemic heart disease; rheumatic heart disease; subarachnoid haemorrhage; stroke; diabetes; prostatic hyperplasia; traffic accidents; falls; aortic aneurysm; pulmonary embolism; pneumococcal pneumonia; bronchitis; and suicide.[6 7] Death rates for each sex for each local authority area were calculated from the 1971 census data, which we grouped according to pre-1974 local authority boundaries. Death rates were expressed as standardised mortality ratios.

We have compared adult mortality (1968–78) with infant mortality in the four main geographical groups used by the registrar general since 1911[1]—that is, county boroughs, London boroughs, urban areas, and rural areas within counties. Eighty three towns were recognised as county boroughs before the 1974 reorganisation. Three of these became county boroughs after 1960 and in the analysis are classed as metropolitan boroughs. The London Government Act of 1963 defined 33 London boroughs: 15 were aggregates of 32 former London boroughs; 18 were previously urban areas of four counties adjacent to London and are classed as such in our analysis. There are 58 counties but we included an additional county, Middlesex (metropolitan boroughs and urban districts only), which had been absorbed into London after the 1963 Act. In this chapter England and Wales is therefore divided into 212 local authority areas comprising 80 county boroughs, 15 London boroughs, 59 urban areas, and 58 rural areas.

We have divided the causes of infant deaths into five groups according to Woolf's[8] classification: congenital causes (registrar general, 1921, short list nos 27, 28); bronchitis and pneumonia (18–19); infectious diseases (2–9, 13); diarrhoea (1, 22); and other. Because specific causes of infant death are recorded only from 1921, our analysis is based on the five years 1921–5. We have examined the relation between different causes of adult and infant death by age, sex, and geographical area using correlation coefficients and scatter plots. The coefficients are influenced by the numbers of deaths as well as by the strength of the relation. During 1921–5 there were 291 082 infant deaths, 127 796 in the first month of life (neonatal) and 163 286 thereafter (postneonatal). Death was attributed to congenital causes in 118 514, bronchitis and pneumonia in 61 770, infectious diseases in 20 668, diarrhoea in 31 147, and other reasons in 58 983. Calculations of rates for ischaemic heart disease during 1968–78 for people aged 35 to 74 are based on 649 817 deaths in men and 273 017 in women: the average annual rates were 5722 deaths per million men and 2184 per million women. Deaths from other causes ranged from 48 636 for rheumatic heart disease up to 279 343 for lung cancer.

Results

The infant mortality rate during 1921–5 was 76 per 1000 births. It ranged from 44 per 1000 births in rural West Sussex to 114 in Burnley county borough. The overall rates were 88 for the county boroughs, 70 for the London boroughs, 73 for the urban areas, and 65 for the rural areas. Standardised mortality ratios for ischaemic heart disease ranged from 70 to 140 in men and from 46 to 148 in women. In men they were 107 for the county boroughs, 90 for the London boroughs, 101 for the urban areas, and 91 for the rural areas. The corresponding figures for women were 109, 83, 99, and 92.

The correlations between infant mortality and the standardised mortality ratios from the leading causes of death during 1968–78 are shown in table I. There was a high correlation for ischaemic heart disease (0·73); and, in descending order, chronic bronchitis and emphysema, cancer of the stomach, and chronic rheumatic heart disease, were similarly highly correlated. Below these were cervical cancer (0·60), stroke (0·54, defined as cerebrovascular disease other than subarachnoid haemorrhage), cancer of the rectum (0·51), accidental falls (0·49), and lung cancer (0·46). Stroke is included in subsequent analyses because of its association with hypertension, a risk factor for ischaemic heart disease; and lung cancer is included

TABLE I—*Correlation of cause of death (standardised mortality ratios) at ages 35–74, in both sexes, and infant mortality*

Cause of death	ICD No (8th revision)	Correlation coefficient
Ischaemic heart disease	410–414	0·73
Bronchitis	490–492	0·82
Stomach cancer	151	0·79
Rheumatic heart disease	393–398	0·72
Stroke	431–438	0·54
Lung cancer	162	0·46

TABLE II—*Correlation of causes of death (standardised mortality ratios) and infant mortality by sex and age*

Cause of death	Age group (years)				
	35–44	45–54	55–64	65–74	35–74
Men					
Ischaemic heart disease	0·57	0·68	0·69	0·57	0·69
Bronchitis	0·42	0·78	0·82	0·76	0·81
Stomach cancer	0·30	0·47	0·59	0·69	0·74
Rheumatic heart disease	0·44	0·51	0·50	0·25	0·60
Stroke	0·33	0·55	0·64	0·49	0·60
Lung cancer	0·47	0·64	0·55	0·37	0·52
Women					
Ischaemic heart disease	0·48	0·69	0·73	0·67	0·73
Bronchitis	0·42	0·68	0·72	0·72	0·77
Stomach cancer	0·14	0·39	0·53	0·70	0·73
Rheumatic heart disease	0·63	0·71	0·58	0·43	0·70
Stroke	0·26	0·37	0·41	0·34	0·40
Lung cancer	0·44	0·45	0·09	−0·20	0·09

because of its association with cigarette smoking. We also calculated correlations with infant mortality in each successive five-year period from 1911 to 1960. For the diseases in table I the coefficients for 1911–15 were close to those for 1921–5. After this the coefficients became lower: for ischaemic heart disease they had fallen to 0·56 by 1956–60.

Table II shows the correlations with infant mortality during 1921–25 by sex and age group. For ischaemic heart disease, bronchitis, stomach cancer, and rheumatic heart disease the coefficients were similar in the two sexes,

TABLE III—*Correlation of causes of death (standardised mortality ratios) and infant mortality in three geographical groups in men and women*

Cause of death	Geographical group			
	County and London boroughs	Urban areas	Rural areas	All areas
Men				
Ischaemic heart disease	0·65	0·70	0·75	0·69
Bronchitis	0·75	0·74	0·66	0·81
Stomach cancer	0·73	0·63	0·73	0·74
Rheumatic heart disease	0·51	0·51	0·56	0·60
Stroke	0·68	0·56	0·75	0·60
Lung cancer	0·41	0·20	−0·13	0·52
Women				
Ischaemic heart disease	0·73	0·68	0·72	0·73
Bronchitis	0·73	0·68	0·53	0·77
Stomach cancer	0·68	0·66	0·78	0·73
Rheumatic heart disease	0·64	0·60	0·49	0·70
Stroke	0·51	0·49	0·72	0·40
Lung cancer	−0·06	−0·32	−0·56	0·09

but those for stroke and lung cancer differed, being higher in men than in women. In each age group, death from ischaemic heart disease was highly correlated with infant mortality.

Table III shows the correlations according to the geographical groups— that is, county boroughs, London boroughs, urban areas, and rural areas. The coefficients for ischaemic heart disease, stomach cancer, and rheumatic heart disease varied little between the groups. In women from rural areas there was a lower correlation for bronchitis. The highest correlations for stroke were in the rural areas. Correlations for lung cancer were negative in men from rural areas and in women from each group.

The association between death from ischaemic heart disease in men and women and infant mortality is shown in figs 1 and 2. The statistical dependence is such that an increase in 10 infant deaths per 1000 births corresponds with increases in standardised mortality ratios of 6·0 in men and 9·0 in women. Standardised mortality ratios for ischaemic heart disease

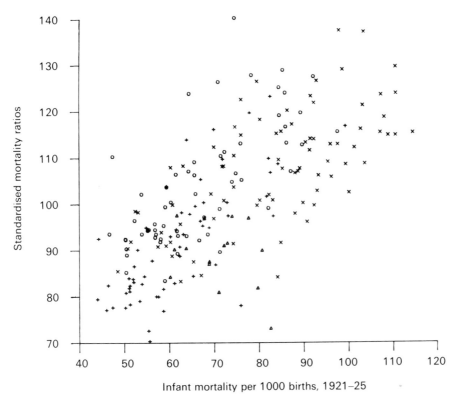

FIG 1—*Standardised mortality ratios for ischaemic heart disease in 1968–78 at ages 35– 74, men, and infant mortality per 1000 births in 1921–25 in the 212 areas of England and Wales. (X = County boroughs, △ = London boroughs, ○ = urban areas, + = rural areas).*

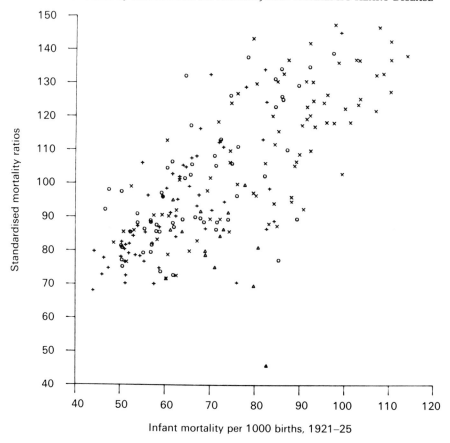

FIG 2—*Standardised mortality ratios for ischaemic heart disease, women, and infant mortality.* (X = *County boroughs,* △ = *London boroughs,* ○ = *urban areas,* + = *rural areas*).

were correlated with those for the other causes of death. The rank order of the coefficients, in both sexes combined, is stroke (0·70), stomach cancer (0·65), bronchitis (0·63), rheumatic heart disease (0·58), and lung cancer (0·26). These values may be compared with 0·73 for infant mortality (table I). Table IV shows the coefficients according to sex and geographical area. Among men the values for stroke were similar to those for infant mortality, whereas among women the overall coefficient was less because of a lower value in urban areas. Correlations with other causes of death were generally lower than those with infant mortality.

Table V shows the correlations between causes of death, neonatal and postneonatal mortality, and causes of infant mortality. There were similar correlations between ischaemic heart disease and neonatal and postneonatal

TABLE IV—*Correlation of death from ischaemic heart disease and from other causes of death (standardised mortality ratios) in three geographical groups in men and women*

Cause of death	Geographical group			
	County and London boroughs	Urban areas	Rural areas	All areas
Men				
Bronchitis	0·49	0·49	0·67	0·58
Stomach cancer	0·48	0·72	0·53	0·62
Rheumatic heart disease	0·27	0·48	0·58	0·45
Stroke	0·73	0·68	0·78	0·72
Lung cancer	0·18	−0·09	−0·03	0·30
Infant mortality 1921–25	0·65	0·70	0·75	0·69
Women				
Bronchitis	0·59	0·64	0·50	0·60
Stomach cancer	0·64	0·36	0·43	0·57
Rheumatic heart disease	0·50	0·46	0·52	0·55
Stroke	0·73	0·44	0·70	0·59
Lung cancer	−0·16	−0·09	−0·40	−0·03
Infant mortality 1921–25	0·73	0·68	0·72	0·73

TABLE V—*Correlation of causes of death (standardised mortality ratios) in both sexes, and specific infant mortality*

Cause of death	Period of infant death		Cause of infant death					
	Neonatal	Post-neonatal	Congenital	Bronchitis + pneumonia	Infectious diseases	Diarrhoea	Other	All
Ischaemic heart disease	0·69	0·68	0·61	0·68	0·48	0·48	0·62	0·73
Bronchitis	0·58	0·83	0·53	0·85	0·61	0·74	0·55	0·82
Stomach cancer	0·61	0·78	0·52	0·71	0·66	0·63	0·69	0·79
Rheumatic heart disease	0·55	0·72	0·45	0·73	0·52	0·65	0·54	0·72
Stroke	0·66	0·44	0·60	0·40	0·34	0·24	0·52	0·54
Lung cancer	0·13	0·55	0·16	0·56	0·50	0·62	0·14	0·46

mortality, 0·69 and 0·68, respectively (figs 3 and 4). By contrast bronchitis was more highly correlated with postneonatal mortality (figs 5 and 6) as were stomach cancer and rheumatic heart disease; whereas stroke correlated more closely with neonatal mortality.

In his detailed analysis of infant mortality in the county boroughs during 1928–38 Woolf found that more than 80% of neonatal deaths were certified as congenital whereas bronchitis and pneumonia was the most common cause of postneonatal death:[8] in keeping with this, the highest correlations with congenital death were for ischaemic heart disease and stroke (table V). Correlations with infant death due to bronchitis and pneumonia were highest for bronchitis. In the London boroughs neonatal death rates were

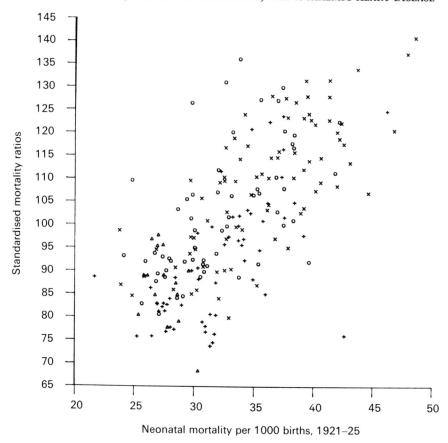

FIG 3—*Standardised mortality ratios for ischaemic heart disease, both sexes, and neonatal mortality. (X = County boroughs, △ = London boroughs, ○ = urban areas, + = rural areas).*

low whereas postneonatal rates were high (figs 3 to 6). Correspondingly, standardised mortality ratios for ischaemic heart disease were low whereas those for bronchitis were high.

Discussion

We have shown a close geographical relation between current mortality from ischaemic heart disease and past infant mortality. Our study was based on the whole of England and Wales, whereas previous reports on the distribution of ischaemic heart disease have been based on selected areas such as towns,[9] or on large geographical areas such as counties and regions.[10 11]

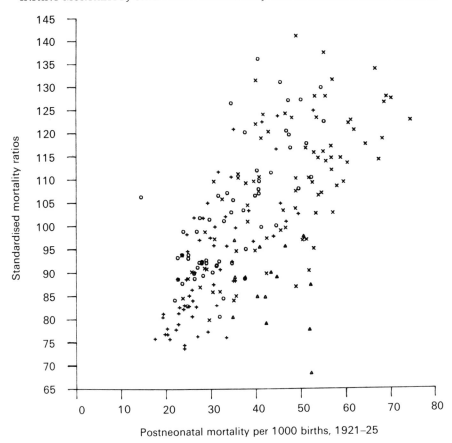

FIG 4—*Standardised mortality ratios for ischaemic heart disease, both sexes, and postneonatal mortality.* (X = *County boroughs,* △ = *London boroughs,* ○ = *urban areas,* + = *rural areas*).

The positive correlations we found between ischaemic heart disease mortality and infant mortality are remarkably consistent in both sexes, in all age groups, and in the different geographical areas. Among the other 24 common causes of death only bronchitis, stomach cancer and chronic rheumatic heart disease have a similarly close geographical relation to infant mortality: this is to be expected as the three diseases are associated with low socioeconomic groups and their rates, like those for infant mortality, are declining. In 1921 infant mortality increased from 38 per 1000 births in socioeconomic group I to 97 per 1000 in group V.[12] In 1971 standardised mortality ratios for bronchitis and emphysema among men aged 15 to 64 years rose from 36 in group I to 188 in group V. There were similar rises in standardised mortality ratios for stomach cancer (50 to 147)

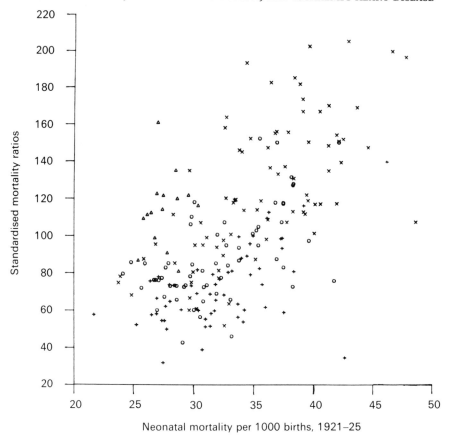

FIG 5—*Standardised mortality ratios for bronchitis, both sexes, and neonatal mortality.*
(X = County boroughs, △ = London boroughs, ○ = urban areas, + = rural areas).

and chronic rheumatic heart disease (77 to 124).[5] Infant mortality began to decline at the turn of the century and fell almost without interruption from 154 per 1000 births in 1900 to 22 per 1000 live births in 1960. Death rates from bronchitis, stomach cancer, and rheumatic fever have all declined this century, particularly since 1930.

The geographical relation between past infant mortality and current mortality from three diseases associated with poor living conditions emphasises the paradox of its close relation with ischaemic heart disease, whose rates have increased with greater prosperity. Analysis of the geographical correlations between death from ischaemic heart disease and from other diseases (table IV) gives no additional insight: there are consistent positive correlations with all three diseases and with stroke, as is to be expected from the similar distributions of cerebrovascular and

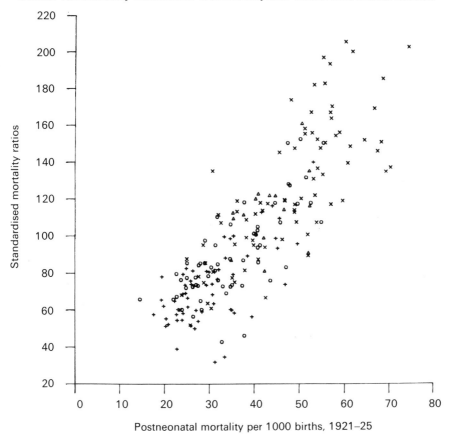

FIG 6—*Standardised mortality ratios for bronchitis, both sexes, and postneonatal mortality. (X = County boroughs, △ = London boroughs, ○ = urban areas, + = rural areas).*

cardiovascular disease in British towns.[13] Apart from stroke no common cause of adult death in 1968–78 correlates as consistently and highly with ischaemic heart disease as does infant mortality during 1921–5.

It is possible that this correlation depends on a factor that is independently related to ischaemic heart disease and infant mortality, although the nature of such an influence is not apparent. The findings for lung cancer show that the social conditions that give rise to infant death do not regularly lead to higher cigarette smoking and hence to raised heart disease rates. In the large county boroughs the hardness of drinking water is negatively correlated with both ischaemic heart disease and infant mortality.[13] However, if there is a causal relation between water hardness and cardiovascular mortality it seems to be weak.[14] Other environmental influences suspected as being causes of ischaemic diseases—for example, dietary fat intake or psychosocial stress—are not known to have the same geographical variations as past infant mortality.

The close geographical similarity between previous infant mortality and current ischaemic heart disease mortality is most readily reconciled with their opposing time trends by the hypothesis that adverse influences in childhood, associated with poor living standards, increase susceptibility to other influences, associated with affluence, encountered in later life.

Findings from other studies support the hypothesis that childhood influences increase the risk of adult heart disease. Rose reported that siblings of ischaemic heart disease patients had stillbirth and infant mortality rates twice those of controls.[15] The inverse relation, among London civil servants, between mortality and height suggests that factors operating in early life could influence adult death rates from ischaemic heart disease and other diseases, and hence contribute to mortality differences between socioeconomic groups.[16] Forsdahl reported a positive correlation between arteriosclerotic heart disease and past infant mortality rates in the 20 counties of Norway and suggested that a poor standard of living in childhood and adolescence was a risk factor in heart disease.[17] Among long term employees of the Bell System company in the USA, men whose parents had been in "white-collar" occupations had a lower incidence of ischaemic heart disease than those from "blue-collar" families: this was consistent in all job categories and areas of the country.[18]

Examination of the causes of infant death elucidates possible childhood influences on heart disease. Woolf reported that much of the variation in stillbirth and neonatal death rates depended on variations in poverty (measured by the percentages of unemployed and employed men in groups IV and V).[8] He attributed this to the adverse effects of poverty on maternal nutrition and lactation. By contrast, postneonatal mortality was influenced by overcrowding (persons per room, population density, and family size), the effect of which was attributed to greater exposure to respiratory infection. In our study adult mortality from bronchitis and chronic rheumatic heart disease are more closely correlated with the geographical variations in postneonatal than neonatal mortality and with infant deaths from bronchitis and pneumonia. Death rates for ischaemic heart disease and stroke, however, have a strong correlation with neonatal death, and hence deaths attributed to congenital causes. The low cardiovascular disease rates in the London boroughs emphasise the geographical correlation with neonatal death rates, which are low in London whereas postneonatal rates are high.

The association of ischaemic heart disease with neonatal mortality suggests that the childhood influences predisposing to it are related to nutrition during prenatal and early postnatal life. The association with postneonatal mortality suggests a continued relation with nutrition throughout infancy. Nutrition in the subsequent years of childhood may also play a part as infant mortality was closely correlated with mortality at ages 1 to 5 years.[19]

Early in this century many infants were poorly nourished. Maternal malnutrition and ill health and frequent infant intercurrent infection impaired nutrition. Bottle feeding was becoming more common although breast feeding remained usual.[20] The composition of artificial infant foods varied and some patent foods were mainly starches.[21] Artificial feeding practices were related to increased infant mortality.[22] The excess deaths were due to a range of illnesses, including both enteric and respiratory infections.[23 24]

The idea that the manner of infant feeding influences metabolism in later life was put forward by Chapin in 1909.[25] As animal fat is the main source of calories in human milk and is suspected as being a cause of ischaemic heart disease, fat metabolism could be one of the links between infant nutrition and the disease. In infants there is evidence of differences in serum cholesterol according to type of feeding.[26 27] In women who had been exclusively breast fed during the first five months of life mean serum cholesterol concentrations were significantly lower than in those who had not been breast fed; for men the difference was smaller and not significant.[28]

We suggest that the geographical distribution of ischaemic heart disease in England and Wales reflects variations in nutrition in early life, which are expressed pathologically on exposure to later dietary influences. One adult disease whose geographical distribution in England and Wales largely depends on the environment in early life is toxic nodular goitre. Its distribution is determined not by the small variations in the current high levels of dietary iodine intake but by the large variations in earlier low intakes,[29 30] and it is now common only where iodine deficiency was prevalent 60 years ago.

Our hypothesis could account for a number of hitherto unexplained aspects of the epidemiology of ischaemic heart disease. Fifty years ago death from ischaemic heart disease was more common in socioeconomic groups I and II than in IV and V. By 1961 the position was reversed, with a larger difference in the younger age groups.[31] In 1971 standardised mortality ratios for ischaemic heart disease increased from 88 in group I to 111 in group V. Such a change is explicable if historically the higher socioeconomic groups were the first to be exposed to "affluence", and as all groups became more prosperous the difference in ischaemic heart disease death rates became dependent on susceptibility. The higher past infant mortality in Scotland than in England and Wales matches the higher mortality from heart disease.[11] The high heart disease mortality among immigrants from the Indian subcontinent could also be due to poor childhood nutrition.[32]

We are exploring the cohort time trends of neonatal and postneonatal mortality, ischaemic heart disease, and stroke, in small areas within

England and Wales. This may give closer insight into whether a fall in mortality from these diseases will follow improvements in nutrition in early childhood.

1 Office of Population Censuses and Surveys. *Registrar general's statistical review of England and Wales. Part 1. Tables, medical.* London: HMSO, 1880 and following years.
2 Ryle JA, Russell WT. The natural history of coronary disease. A clinical and epidemiological study. *Br Heart J* 1949;**11**:370–89.
3 Morris JN. Recent history of coronary disease. *Lancet* 1951;**i**:1–7.
4 Gardner MJ, Crawford MD, Morris JN. Patterns of mortality in middle and early old age in the county boroughs of England and Wales. *Br J Prev Soc Med* 1969;**23**:133–40.
5 Registrar general's decennial supplement, occupational mortality, England and Wales 1970–72. London: HMSO, 1978.
6 Gardner MJ, Winter PD, Taylor CP, Acheson ED. Atlas of cancer mortality in England and Wales 1968–78. Chichester: Wiley, 1983.
7 Gardner MJ, Winter PD, Barker DJP. Atlas of mortality from selected diseases in England and Wales 1968–78. Chichester: Wiley, 1984.
8 Woolf B. Studies on infant mortality: part II, social aetiology of stillbirths and infant deaths in county boroughs of England and Wales. *Br J Social Med* 1947;**2**:73–125.
9 Pocock SJ, Shaper AG, Cook DG, *et al.* British regional heart study: geographic variations in cardiovascular mortality, and the role of water quality. *BMJ* 1980;**i**:1243–9.
10 Knox EG. Ischaemic heart disease mortality and dietary intake of calcium. *Lancet* 1973;**i**:1465–7.
11 Fulton M, Adams W, Lutz W, Oliver MF. Regional variations in mortality from ischaemic heart and cerebrovascular disease in Britain. *Br Heart J* 1978;**40**:563–8.
12 Registrar general's decennial supplement, England and Wales 1921. London: HMSO, 1927.
13 Morris JN, Crawford MD, Heady JA. Hardness of local water-supplies and mortality from cardiovascular disease in the county boroughs of England and Wales. *Lancet* 1961;**i**:860–2.
14 Shaper AG. Geographic variations in cardiovascular mortality in Great Britain. *Br Med Bull* 1984;**40**:366–73.
15 Rose G. Familial patterns in ischaemic heart disease. *Br J Prev Soc Med* 1964;**18**:75–80.
16 Marmot MG, Shipley MJ, Rose G. Inequalities in death-specific explanations of a general pattern? *Lancet* 1984;**i**:1003–6.
17 Forsdahl A. Are poor living conditions in childhood and adolescence an important risk factor for ateriosclerotic heart disease? *Br J Prev Soc Med* 1977;**31**:91–5.
18 Hinkle LE. Coronary heart disease and sudden death in actively employed American men. *Bull NY Acad Med* 1973;**49**:467–74.
19 Thirty-ninth annual report of the local government board 1909–10. Supplement on infant and child mortality. London: HMSO, 1910.
20 National health insurance medical research committee. The mortalities of birth, infancy and childhood. Special report series No 10. London: HMSO. 1917.
21 Coutts FJH. *On the use of proprietary foods for infant feeding.* London: HMSO, 1914. (Reports to the local government board on public health and medical subjects, No 80.)
22 Howarth WJ. The influence of feeding on the mortality of infants. *Lancet* 1905;**ii**:210–3.
23 Robinson M. Infant morbidity and mortality: a study of 3266 infants. *Lancet* 1951;**i**:788–94.
24 Douglas JWB. The extent of breast feeding in Great Britain in 1946, with special reference to the health and survival of children. *J Obstet Gynaecol Br Emp* 1950;**57**:335–61.

25 Chapin HD. Biology as the basic principle in infant feeding. *Postgraduate (NY)* 1909;**24**:272–80.
26 Foman SJ. A pediatrician looks at early nutrition. *Bull NY Acad Med* 1971;**47**:569–78.
27 Darmady JM, Fosbrooke AS, Lloyd JK. Prospective study of serum cholesterol levels during first year of life. *BMJ* 1972;**ii**:685–8.
28 Marmot MG, Page CM, Atkins E, Douglas JWB. Effect of breast-feeding on plasma cholesterol and weight in young adults. *J Epidemiol Community Health* 1980;**34**:164–7.
29 Barker DJP, Phillips DIW. Current incidence of thyrotoxicosis and past prevalence of goitre in 12 British towns. *Lancet* 1984;**ii**:567–70.
30 Phillips DIW, Barker DJP, Rees-Smith B, Didcote S, Morgan D. The geographical distribution of thyrotoxicosis in England according to the presence or absence of TSH-receptor antibodies. *Clin Endocrinol* 1985;**23**:283–7.
31 Marmot MG, Adelstein AM, Robinson N, Rose GA. Changing social-class distribution of heart disease. *BMJ* 1978;**ii**:1109–12.
32 McKeigue PM, Adelstein AM, Shipley MJ, *et al*. Diet and risk factors for coronary heart disease in Asians in northwest London. *Lancet* 1985;**ii**:1086–9.

2: Death rates from stroke in England and Wales predicted from past maternal mortality

D J P BARKER, C OSMOND

Geographical differences in maternal mortality in England and Wales during 1911–14 correlate closely with death rates from stroke in the generation born around that time. The geographical distribution of stroke is more closely related to past maternal mortality than to any leading cause of death, past or present, except ischaemic heart disease, for which correlation coefficients with stroke are similar.

This relation is new evidence that poor health and physique of mothers are important determinants of the risk of stroke among their offspring.

Introduction

There are large and unexplained differences in death rates from stroke in different parts of England and Wales.[1] We have noted previously a geographical relation between mortality from stroke and neonatal mortality 60 years ago (chapter 1). As neonatal mortality was previously linked to poor maternal health and physique[2 3] we made a detailed geographical comparison of maternal mortality in the early years of this century and the death rates from stroke in the generation born during the same period.

Methods

Maternal mortality in England and Wales during the early years of the century has been analysed in two government publications covering the years 1911–14 and 1919–22, respectively.[4 5] Maternal mortality was defined as death directly attributable to pregnancy or childbirth. During 1911–14 there were 14 045 maternal deaths. These were divided into two groups—namely, those due to puerperal fever (4951) and those due to "other complications of pregnancy and parturition" (9094). During 1919–22 there were 13 465 deaths, with 5137 and 8328, respectively, occurring in these two groups. From 1921 all deaths of women in different areas were divided into 32 groups according to cause of death.[1] We derived crude death rates for 1921–5 using data from the population at the 1921 census.

The numbers of neonatal deaths (deaths in the first month of life) in different areas were published from 1911 onward.[1] To match the data on maternal mortality, rates per 1000 births were calculated for 1911–14, when there were 137 960 neonatal deaths.

The Office of Population Censuses and Surveys made available extracts from all death certificates in England and Wales during 1968–78 (chapter 1), the period covered by the eighth revision of the International Classification of Diseases. Our analysis is based on mortality at ages 55–74, as these are deaths occurring in the generation born around 1911–14. Sex specific rates were based on data from the 1971 census and were expressed as standardised mortality ratios. Stroke was defined as ICD 431–438, which is cerebrovascular disease other than subarachnoid haemorrhage. The stroke rates were based on 142 975 deaths in men and 134 503 deaths in women. The average annual rates were 2876/million men and 2233/million women.

We analysed mortality in the 154 local authority areas used by the registrar general since 1911—that is, 80 county boroughs (larger towns), 15 London boroughs, and 59 administrative counties (aggregates of metropolitan boroughs, urban districts, and rural areas). The data for maternal mortality do not allow separate analysis of local authority groupings within administrative counties.

We used correlation coefficients and scatter plots to examine the relation among adult, maternal, and neonatal death rates. The values of the coefficients reflect not only the strength of a relation but also the numbers of deaths. The coefficient describing a relation will tend to have a larger absolute value with increasing numbers of deaths. To allow for differences in the size of the population among areas, the correlation coefficients with maternal and neonatal death rates were weighted according to the numbers of deaths from stroke at ages 55–74 expected in each area, as calculated from national rates.

Results

Maternal mortality in England and Wales during 1911–14 was 4·0/1000 births. The rates ranged from 1·9/1000 in Rutland to 8·7/1000 in Merioneth. During 1919–22 the rate was 4·1/1000 births, ranging from 1·5/1000 in Rutland to 7·9/1000 in Brecon. The geographical distribution was similar during the two periods and was described as follows: "Maternal mortality tends to be highest in rural, sparsely populated counties, and in industrial districts, notably those associated with the textile industries in Lancashire and Yorkshire, and with coal mining; and tends to be lowest in the South of England, in districts in and around London, and in certain large towns, such as Birmingham, Manchester and Liverpool."[5] During 1911–14 the rates of maternal death from causes other than puerperal fever were 2·6/1000 in the county boroughs, 1·6/1000 in the London boroughs, and 2·6/1000 in the administrative counties. For deaths from puerperal fever the corresponding figures were 1·5/1000, 1·5/1000, and 1·4/1000.

Table I shows the causes, other than puerperal fever, of maternal death that were published for the two years 1913 and 1922.[45] The three leading causes were toxaemia (puerperal albuminuria and convulsions), puerperal haemorrhage, and other accidents of childbirth. Together these accounted for 67% of all "other" maternal deaths.

The standardised mortality ratios for stroke during 1968–78 among men aged 55–74 ranged from 60 in Westminster to 158 in Dewsbury and among women from 25 in the City of London to 146 in Wakefield. Their geographical distribution has been described elsewhere.[6] Among men the standardised mortality ratio was 110 in the county boroughs, 75 in the London boroughs, and 98 in the administrative counties; the corresponding figures for women were 105, 74, and 100.

We examined the correlation coefficients between maternal mortality during 1911–14 and standardised mortality ratios from the 25 leading causes of death at ages 55–74 during 1968–78. Leading causes of death were those for which more than 10 000 deaths occurred in each sex, or in the sex usually affected, during 1968–78. For total maternal mortality the highest correlation was with stroke (0·55) and, in descending order, ischaemic heart disease (0·47), stomach cancer (0·37), subarachnoid haemorrhage (0·30),

TABLE I—*Numbers (percentages) of maternal deaths by cause in 1913 and 1922, excluding deaths from puerperal fever**

Cause of death	1913	1922
Toxaemia	755 (32)	556 (29)
Puerperal haemorrhage	507 (21)	390 (21)
Other accidents of childbirth	374 (16)	304 (16)
Abortion	120 (5)	92 (5)
Other accidents of pregnancy	257 (11)	218 (12)
Puerperal embolism and sudden death	332 (14)	296 (16)
Puerperal insanity	28 (1)	30 (2)
Puerperal diseases of the breast	11	6
Total	2384 (100)	1892 (100)

*There were 1108 deaths from puerperal fever in 1913 and 1079 in 1922.

TABLE II—*Correlations between causes of death (standardised mortality ratios ages 55–74, 1968–78, both sexes) and maternal mortality (1911–14) in 154 areas of England and Wales*

Cause of death	ICD No (8th revision)	Puerperal fever	"Other" causes	All maternal mortality
Stroke	431–438	0·21	0·65	0·55
Ischaemic heart disease	410–414	0·17	0·56	0·47
Stomach cancer	151	0·21	0·40	0·37
Lung cancer	162	−0·24	−0·47	−0·43

chronic rheumatic heart disease (0·25), and cervical cancer (0·25). The coefficient for chronic bronchitis and emphysema was 0·02. Table II and subsequent analyses include lung cancer (−0·43) because of its association with cigarette smoking, a risk factor for vascular disease.

The correlation between maternal mortality and stroke depends on causes other than puerperal fever (figure). The coefficient is 0·65 (table II), and the statistical dependence is such that an increase of one maternal death from "other" causes/1000 births corresponds to an increase of 12 in the standardised mortality ratio for stroke.

Table III shows the correlations between causes of death in each sex and maternal mortality from other causes within county and London boroughs, administrative counties, and all areas combined. The coefficients for stroke were consistently high. Those for ischaemic heart disease were comparable, but for stomach cancer they were lower. All coefficients for lung cancer were negative. When mortality from stroke was correlated with maternal mortality from other causes during the later period, 1919–22, the coefficients were lower. The consistent relation between maternal mortality and both stroke and ischaemic heart disease, however, remained, whereas the relation with stomach cancer was greatly reduced. The coefficients for lung cancer were negative.

The correlations between the leading causes of death and neonatal mortality during 1911–14 differed from those between leading causes of death and maternal mortality from other causes during the same period. Though coefficients for stroke (0·60) and ischaemic heart disease (0·65) were similarly high, those for some other causes increased. In descending order they were: cancer of the rectum (0·57), stomach cancer (0·55), chronic bronchitis and emphysema (0·50), and cervical cancer (0·46). The coefficient for lung cancer was −0·01. Within each sex and geographical group the correlation between stroke and neonatal mortality (table IV) was less than that between stroke and maternal mortality from other causes (table III).

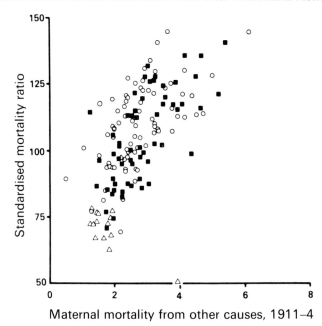

Standardised mortality ratios for stroke (1968–78) at ages 55–74, both sexes, and maternal mortality/1000 births (1911–14) from causes other than puerperal fever in 154 areas of England and Wales. ○ = County boroughs. △ = London boroughs. ■ = Administrative counties.

When standardised mortality ratios for stroke were correlated with those for other leading causes of death at ages 55–74 the rank order of the coefficients was ischaemic heart disease (0·72), stomach cancer (0·53), cervical cancer (0·49), cancer of the rectum (0·48), diabetes (0·42), and chronic bronchitis and emphysema (0·40). Within each sex and geographical group only coefficients for ischaemic heart disease were as high and consistent as those for maternal mortality from other causes during 1911–14 (table V).

Maternal mortality from other causes during 1911–14 was correlated with mortality from other causes of death among women during 1921–5. The highest coefficients were for acute and chronic nephritis (0·57), non-respiratory tuberculosis (0·35), and cerebral haemorrhage (0·34). These were high in both geographical groups. For nephritis the coefficient was 0·45 in the county and London boroughs and 0·72 in the counties. For non-respiratory tuberculosis the corresponding figures were 0·29 and 0·60. For cerebral haemorrhage they were 0·31 and 0·31, respectively.

The standardised mortality ratios for stroke were correlated with the crude death rates in both sexes for all 32 causes of death during 1921–5.

TABLE III—Correlations between causes of death (standardised mortality ratios ages 55–74, 1968–78) and maternal mortality (1911–14 and 1919–22) from causes other than puerperal fever in two geographical groups

| | 1911–14 | | | | | | 1919–22 | | | | | |
| | County and London boroughs | | Administrative counties | | All areas | | County and London boroughs | | Administrative counties | | All areas | |
Cause of death	Men	Women	Men	Women	Men	Women	Men	Women	Men	Women	Men	Women
Stroke	0·64	0·53	0·66	0·71	0·61	0·63	0·52	0·48	0·45	0·55	0·38	0·36
Ischaemic heart disease	0·76	0·72	0·72	0·47	0·60	0·46	0·62	0·59	0·49	0·45	0·40	0·35
Stomach cancer	0·43	0·47	0·60	0·62	0·38	0·36	0·23	0·33	0·41	0·51	0·04	0·11
Lung cancer	−0·22	−0·48	−0·49	−0·66	−0·39	−0·59	−0·37	−0·51	−0·52	−0·51	−0·39	−0·36

TABLE IV—*Correlations between causes of death (standardised mortality ratios ages 55–74, 1968–78) and neonatal mortality (1911–4) in two geographical groups*

| | Geographical group | | | | | |
| | County and London boroughs | | Administrative counties | | All areas | |
Cause of death	Men	Women	Men	Women	Men	Women
Stroke	0·56	0·46	0·52	0·55	0·61	0·54
Ischaemic heart disease	0·57	0·57	0·53	0·67	0·63	0·65
Stomach cancer	0·50	0·54	0·48	0·50	0·47	0·54
Lung cancer	0·04	−0·51	−0·18	−0·54	0·09	−0·38

TABLE V—*Correlations between causes of death from stroke and other causes (standardised mortality ratios ages 55–74, 1968–78) in two geographical groups*

| | Geographical group | | | | | |
| | County and London boroughs | | Administrative counties | | All areas | |
Cause of death	Men	Women	Men	Women	Men	Women
Ischaemic heart disease	0·72	0·73	0·77	0·59	0·73	0·64
Stomach cancer	0·48	0·50	0·68	0·64	0·53	0·47
Lung cancer	0·03	−0·56	−0·18	−0·70	0·01	−0·60
"Other" maternal mortality 1911–14	0·64	0·53	0·66	0·71	0·61	0·63

After maternal deaths from other causes (0·66) and a group of causes of infant death (0·54, shortlist No 28) the highest coefficients were for non-respiratory tuberculosis (0·46), rheumatic fever (0·42), influenza (0·40), and cerebral haemorrhage (0·37).

Discussion

We have shown that current death rates from stroke in different areas of England and Wales can be closely predicted from maternal mortality, from causes other than puerperal fever, 75 years ago (figure). This geographical relation is consistently close in both sexes, in towns, and in counties (table III). Its specificity is remarkable. Among other current causes of death only ischaemic heart disease correlates as closely with both current mortality from stroke and past maternal mortality (tables II, III, and V). The relation between stroke and maternal mortality is so strong that the correlations exceed those between either cause of death and past mortality from any cause.

The relation is closer for maternal mortality around the years of birth of the people who died from stroke than for later years (table III). It is restricted to maternal death from causes other than puerperal fever. The geographical distribution of deaths from puerperal fever differed from that of maternal deaths from other causes and was thought to be determined largely by midwifery practices.[5] Most "other" deaths, which made up 65% of all maternal deaths, were certified as being due to toxaemia, puerperal haemorrhage, or other accidents of childbirth (table I). Their geographical distribution was similar to that of mortality from two chronic diseases: nephritis and non-respiratory tuberculosis.

Campbell et al's analyses of the causes of maternal mortality in Britain clearly implicated the poor physique and health of mothers.[5 7] This was a result of poor nutrition and ill health among young girls and of rickets and the industrial employment of children. Stroke is more closely and specifically related to maternal mortality than to neonatal mortality (table IV) despite the small number of maternal deaths—10% of the total of neonatal deaths—which would tend to diminish correlations. This emphasises an association with maternal influences rather than the neonatal environment. The strong negative correlations with lung cancer (tables II, III, and V) show that the relation between stroke and maternal mortality is not determined by a confounding relation with cigarette smoking.

Hypertension is one of the possible links between maternal health and stroke. A parental history of hypertension increases the risk of hypertension in the offspring,[8 9] and hypertension is a risk factor for stroke.[10] There is increasing evidence that hypertension originates in childhood.[11] The persistence of rank order of blood pressure between patients examined at intervals—so called "tracking"—has been repeatedly observed in longitudinal studies of children as well as of adults,[12–15] though the tracking coefficients in children are lower than those in adults.[11] Three studies of infants have shown small correlations between maternal blood pressure and systolic or diastolic pressure in the neonatal period.[16–18] In one of the studies the correlations with both systolic and diastolic pressure were shown to persist at 12 months.[17]

A link between the intrauterine environment and hypertension is suggested by the negative relation between birth weight and blood pressure. In a national sample of 3240 children born in Britain and followed up to the age of 36 there was an inverse relation between birth weight and systolic pressure in both men and women.[19] Two studies have shown a similar inverse relation in children aged 7 and 10 years.[20 21] As an alternative to a direct intrauterine influence on blood pressure Ounsted has suggested that the accelerated growth of healthy babies of low birth weight during the first six months may be accompanied by an accelerated increase in blood pressure.[22] The resulting above average values may persist.

Studies of the relation between body weight and stroke point to the importance of growth during adolescence. Evidence whether obesity is a risk factor for stroke is conflicting,[10] but three studies have shown that obesity at around 20 years of age is associated with an increased risk.[23-25] In one of these studies short stature was also a risk factor.[23]

Baird has related the large geographical differences in perinatal mortality in Britain during this century to differences in the physique and health of women.[2] Poor living standards, which accompanied industrialisation or economic depression in certain areas, adversely affected the development of young girls and impaired their subsequent reproductive efficiency. We suggest that the close geographical relation between past maternal mortality and current mortality from stroke indicates that this impaired reproductive efficiency is also expressed as an increased risk of stroke in the surviving offspring.

This interpretation may explain the paradox that while the time trends of stroke and ischaemic heart disease in Britain are in opposite directions the geography of the two diseases is similar, both being more common in poorer areas and lower income groups.[26] The increased incidence in ischaemic heart disease during this century is attributed to affluence, in particular diet, during adult life. We have previously suggested that, in contrast, the geography of the disease reflects differences in susceptibility related to adverse maternal and early postnatal influences (chapter 1). We suggest here that both the decrease in mortality from stroke during the past 40 years and its geographical distribution reflect a dominant effect of maternal physique and health.

1 Office of Population Censuses and Surveys. *Registrar general's statistical reviews of England and Wales 1911 and following years.* Part 1. Tables, medical. London: HMSO, 1911 and following years.

2 Baird D. Environment and reproduction. *Br J Obstet Gynaecol* 1980;**87**:1057–67.

3 Baird D. Social factors in obstetrics. *Lancet* 1949;**i**:1079–83.

4 Local Government Board. *Forty-fourth annual report 1914–15.* Supplement *Maternal mortality in connection with childbearing.* London: HMSO, 1916.

5 Campbell JM. *Maternal mortality.* London: HMSO, 1924. (Ministry of Health Reports on Public Health and Medical Subjects, No 25.)

6 Gardner MJ, Winter PD, Barker DJP. *Atlas of mortality from selected diseases in England and Wales 1968–78.* Chichester: Wiley, 1984.

7 Campbell JM, Cameron D, Jones DM. *High maternal mortality in certain areas.* London: HMSO, 1932. (Ministry of Health Reports on Public Health and Medical Subjects, No 68.)

8 Hamilton M, Pickering GW, Roberts JAF. The aetiology of essential hypertension. 4. The role of inheritance. *Clin Sci* 1954;**13**:273–304.

9 Stamler R, Stamler J, Reidlinger WF, Algera G, Roberts RH. Family (parental) history and prevalence of hypertension. Results of a nationwide screening programme. *JAMA* 1979;**241**:43–6.

10 Evans JG. The epidemiology of stroke. *Age Ageing* 1979;**8**:(suppl):50–6.

11 Hofman A. Blood pressure in childhood: an epidemiological approach to the aetiology of hypertension. *Journal of Hypertension* 1984;**2**:232–8.

12 de Sweit M, Fayers P, Shinebourne EA. Blood pressure survey in a population of newborn infants. *BMJ* 1976;**ii**:9–11.

13 Beaglehole R, Salmond CE, Eyles EF. A longitudinal study of blood pressure in Polynesian children. *Am J Epidemiol* 1977;**105**:87–9.

14 Clarke WR, Schrott H, Leaverton PE, Connor WE, Laver RM. Tracking of blood lipids and blood pressure in school age children: the Muscatine study. *Circulation* 1978;**58**:626–34.

15 Voors W, Webber LS, Berenson GS. Time course studies of blood pressure in children: the Bogalusa heart study. *Am J Epidemiol* 1979;**109**:320–34.

16 Lee YH, Rosner B, Gould JB, Lowe EW, Kass EH. Familial aggregation of blood pressure of newborn infants and their mothers. *Pediatrics* 1976;**58**:722–9.

17 Zinner SH, Rosner B, Oh W, Kass EH. Significance of blood pressure in infancy: familial aggregation and predictive effect on later blood pressure. *Hypertension* 1985;**7**:411–6.

18 Ibsen KK, Gronback M. Familial aggregation of blood pressure in newly born infants and their mothers. *Acta Paediatr Scand* 1980;**69**:109–11.

19 Wadsworth MEJ, Cripps HA, Midwinter RE, Colley JRT. Blood pressure in a national birth cohort at the age of 36 related to social and familial factors, smoking, and body mass. *BMJ* 1985;**291**:1534–8.

20 Simpson A, Mortimer JG, Silva PA, Spears G, Williams S. In: Onesi G, Kim KE, eds. *Hypertension in the young and old.* New York: Grune and Stratton, 1981:153–63.

21 Cater J, Gill N. The follow-up study: medical aspects. In: Illsey R, Mitchell RG, eds. *Low birthweight, a medical, psychological and social study.* Chichester: Wiley, 1984:191–205.

22 Ounsted MK, Cockburn JM, Moar VA, Redman CWG. Factors associated with the blood pressures of children born to women who were hypertensive during pregnancy. *Arch Dis Child* 1985;**60**:631–5.

23 Paffenberger RS, Wing AL. Characteristics in youth predisposing to fatal stroke in later years. *Lancet* 1967;**i**:753–4.

24 Heyden S, Hames CG, Bartel A, Cassel JC, Tyroler HA, Cornoni JC. Weight and weight history in relation to cerebrovascular and ischaemic heart disease. *Arch Intern Med* 1971;**128**:956–60.

25 Evans JG, Prudham D, Wandless I. Risk factors for stroke in the elderly. In: Sangiorgi GB, Exton-Smith AN, eds. *The ageing brain, neurological and mental disturbances.* New York: Plenum, 1980;113–26.

26 Acheson RM, Williams DRR. Epidemiology of cerebrovascular disease: some unanswered questions. In: Rose FC, ed. *Clinical neuroepidemiology.* London: Pitman Medical, 1980:88–104.

3: Childhood respiratory infection and adult chronic bronchitis in England and Wales

D J P BARKER, C OSMOND

The high mortality from chronic bronchitis in England and Wales and the excess of urban over rural mortality are unexplained. On dividing England and Wales into 212 local authority areas a strong geographical relation was found between death rates from chronic bronchitis and emphysema in 1959–78 and infant mortality from bronchitis and pneumonia during 1921–5. It was concluded that this relation provided strong evidence of a direct causal link between acute lower respiratory infection in early childhood and chronic bronchitis in adult life. Regression analysis suggested that infection in early childhood had a greater influence than cigarette smoking in determining the geographical distribution of chronic bronchitis. National time trends reflected the influence of both factors.

Chronic air pollution in adult life may be less important a cause of chronic bronchitis than previously supposed.

Introduction

Britain has a higher mortality from chronic bronchitis than any other country in western Europe.[1] This cannot be explained by international differences in environmental influences, such as cigarette smoking and atmospheric pollution, nor by differences in death certification practices.[2] The excess of urban over rural mortality and morbidity from bronchitis, which is characteristic of Britain, is also unexplained.[3]

Reid and others conjectured that respiratory disease in childhood was a cause of chronic bronchitis in later life.[4-6] Recent findings have shown that bronchiolitis, bronchitis, and pneumonia in infancy lead to persisting damage to the airways during childhood, with cough, wheeze, bronchial reactivity, and impaired ventilatory function.[7-10] In the long term follow up of a national sample of British children born in 1946, young adults who had had one or more lower respiratory infections before 2 years of age had a higher prevalence of chronic cough.[11 12] There is, however, no direct evidence to link respiratory infection during childhood with clinically established chronic bronchitis in adult life.

We have examined the geographical relation between past infant death rates from lower respiratory tract infection and current adult mortality from chronic bronchitis in England and Wales. We have also analysed the time trends in mortality from chronic bronchitis over the past 40 years.

Methods

The Office of Population Censuses and Surveys made available extracts from all death certificates in England and Wales during 1959–78. Our previous analysis of these data in relation to past infant mortality was based on the 11 years 1968–78 (chapter 1), the period covered by the eighth revision of the International Classification of Diseases (ICD). For this analysis we added data on four selected causes of death during 1959–67. Death rates at ages 35–74 years were calculated for each sex and each local authority area grouped according to boundaries before 1974. For 1968–78 rates were based on data from the 1971 census, whereas for 1959–67 data from the 1961 census were used. Rates were expressed as standardised mortality ratios. We used published mortality rates[13] for 1941–80 to analyse the time trends of chronic bronchitis and emphysema (ICD codes 106 b,c, 113 (5th revision); 501–502, 527 (6th revision); 501–502, 527.1 (7th revision); 490–492 (8th and 9th revisions)).

In England and Wales numbers of infant deaths by specific cause were published only from 1921, and this analysis is based on the years 1921–5. We divided causes of infant deaths into five groups using Woolf's classification[14]—congenital, bronchitis and pneumonia, infectious diseases, diarrhoea, and others.

We compared adult mortality (1959–78) with infant mortality (1921–5) in the same 212 local authority areas used in the analysis in chapter 1.

We used correlation coefficients, regression analysis, and scatter plots to examine the relation between different causes of adult and infant deaths. The coefficients are influenced by the numbers of deaths as well as by the strength of the relation. During 1921–5 there were 291 082 infant deaths, 127 796 in the first month of life (neonatal) and 163 286 thereafter (postneonatal). Death was attributed to bronchitis and pneumonia in 61 770.

Calculations of mortalities from bronchitis during 1959–78 for ages 35–74 years are based on 256 470 deaths in men and 121 157 deaths in women.

We have summarised trends in age specific mortality for bronchitis and lung cancer by a set of birth cohort (generation) values and period of death values. This method has been described.[15] Cohort values summarise the mortality experience of a generation, while period values summarise the experience of all age groups at one point in time. Each age specific rate contributes to both a cohort and a period value by reference to all other rates at that age. Cohort and period values are adjusted to give an average of unity and are similar to relative risks in having no units.

Results

Infant mortality in England and Wales during 1921–5 was 76/1000 births. Of these deaths, 16/1000 births were attributed to bronchitis and pneumonia, with rates among boys of 19/1000 and among girls of 14/1000. Mortalities from bronchitis and pneumonia in the 212 local authority areas varied from two to 33/1000 births. They were highest in the county boroughs at 20/1000 and fell to 16 in the London boroughs, 15 in the urban areas, and 11 in the rural areas. Standardised mortality ratios for bronchitis among men aged 35–74 during 1968–78 ranged from 26 to 205 and among women from 27 to 292. Again standardised mortality ratios were highest in the county boroughs at 121 for men and 126 for women and fell to 113 for each sex in the London boroughs, 97 and 94 respectively in the urban areas, and 74 and 73 respectively in the rural areas.

During 1968–78 there were 25 causes of death for which more than 10 000 deaths occurred in each sex or in the sex usually affected.[16 17] Table I shows the coefficients of correlation between infant mortality caused by bronchitis and pneumonia in the 212 local authority areas and the leading causes of death in both sexes at ages 35–74. In descending order the coefficients were 0·85 for bronchitis, 0·73 for chronic rheumatic heart disease, 0·71 for cancer of the stomach, 0·68 for ischaemic heart disease, and 0·56 for lung cancer. Table I also shows that infant deaths from bronchitis and pneumonia correlated more highly with adult bronchitis than did infant deaths in any of the other four cause groups. Among the infectious diseases only measles had a high correlation ($r = 0·77$), the next highest ($r = 0·29$) being for whooping cough.

When infant respiratory mortality during 1921–5 was correlated with the other causes of infant death the coefficients were lower than that with adult bronchitis during 1968–78 (table I). Similarly, when standardised mortality ratios for bronchitis during 1968–78 were correlated with those for the other causes of adult death the coefficients were lower than that with infant respiratory mortality during 1921–5 (table I). The strength of the relation was further emphasised by the low correlation ($r = 0·20$) between infant

TABLE I—*Correlation of causes of infant death (rates) during 1921–5 and of adult deaths (standardised mortality ratios) during 1968–78 in 212 geographical areas of England and Wales*

	Infant mortality from bronchitis and pneumonia 1921–5	Adult mortality from bronchitis 1968–78
Infant mortality 1921–5		
Bronchitis and pneumonia	1·00	0·85
Congenital	0·60	0·53
Diarrhoea	0·78	0·74
Infectious diseases	0·65	0·61
Other	0·65	0·55
Adult mortality 1968–78		
Bronchitis	0·85	1·00
Rheumatic heart disease	0·73	0·78
Stomach cancer	0·71	0·71
Ischaemic heart disease	0·68	0·63
Lung cancer	0·56	0·62
Pneumococcal pneumonia	0·38	0·34

respiratory mortality in 1921–5 and mortality from bronchitis at all other ages during those same years.

Figures 1 and 2 show the close geographical relation between infant deaths from bronchitis and pneumonia and subsequent adult deaths from bronchitis in each sex. The statistical dependence is such that an increase among areas of 10 infant deaths per 1000 births corresponds with increases in standardised mortality ratios for bronchitis of 45 in men and 53 in women.

Table II shows correlations by sex and age group within the 212 areas. Rheumatic heart disease is included because it is known to be caused by respiratory borne infection in childhood, pneumococcal pneumonia because it is caused by adult respiratory infection. Lung cancer is associated with cigarette smoking, a known risk factor for bronchitis. The coefficients for bronchitis were consistently high in both sexes and each age group above 45. The lower values in the youngest age group may reflect the smaller number of deaths. Most coefficients for rheumatic heart disease, pneumococcal pneumonia, and lung cancer were lower than those for bronchitis.

The coefficients for bronchitis and rheumatic heart disease varied little among the three geographical groups—county boroughs and London boroughs, urban areas, and rural areas (table III). Those for pneumococcal pneumonia, however, were negative among women in urban and rural areas. For lung cancer they were low among men in rural areas and zero or negative among women.

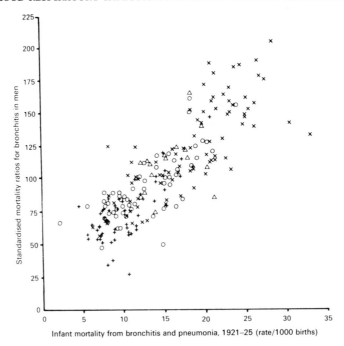

FIG 1—*Standardised mortality ratios for chronic bronchitis in men aged 35–74 during 1968–78 and infant mortality from bronchitis and pneumonia per 1000 births in 1921–5 in 212 areas of England and Wales.* × = County boroughs. △ = London boroughs. ○ = Urban areas. + = Rural areas.

TABLE II—*Correlation of causes of death (standardised mortality ratio) in 1968–78 and infant death rates from bronchitis and pneumonia in 1912–5 by age and sex in 212 geographical areas of England and Wales*

Cause of death	Age group (years)				
	35–44	45–54	55–64	65–74	35–74
Men					
Bronchitis	0·43	0·79	0·84	0·79	0·84
Rheumatic heart disease	0·50	0·54	0·49	0·25	0·61
Pneumococcal pneumonia	0·27	0·37	0·40	0·36	0·41
Lung cancer	0·46	0·68	0·62	0·48	0·61
Women					
Bronchitis	0·44	0·70	0·73	0·74	0·80
Rheumatic heart disease	0·65	0·71	0·57	0·46	0·71
Pneumococcal pneumonia	0·19	0·30	0·21	0·18	0·26
Lung cancer	0·46	0·49	0·19	−0·09	0·20

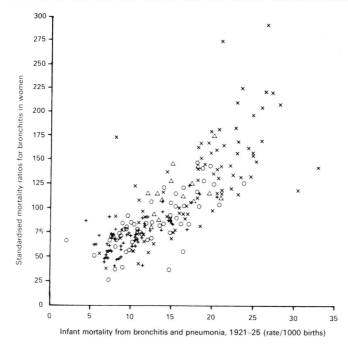

FIG 2—*Standardised mortality ratios for chronic bronchitis in women aged 35–74 during 1968–78 and infant mortality from bronchitis and pneumonia per 1000 births in 1921–5 in 212 areas of England and Wales.* × = *County boroughs.* △ = *London boroughs.* ○ = *Urban areas.* + = *Rural areas.*

TABLE III—*Correlation of causes of death (standardised mortality ratios) in 1968–78 and infant death rates from bronchitis and pneumonia in 1921–5 in three geographical groups in men and women*

Cause of death	Geographical group			
	County and London boroughs	Urban areas	Rural areas	All areas
Men				
Bronchitis	0·75	0·77	0·75	0·84
Rheumatic heart disease	0·48	0·63	0·53	0·61
Pneumococcal pneumonia	0·26	0·42	0·36	0·41
Lung cancer	0·46	0·23	0·04	0·61
Women				
Bronchitis	0·70	0·74	0·68	0·80
Rheumatic heart disease	0·61	0·56	0·59	0·71
Pneumococcal pneumonia	0·23	− 0·05	− 0·10	0·26
Lung cancer	0·00	− 0·23	− 0·39	0·20

For deaths during the period 1959–67 the coefficients for chronic bronchitis and rheumatic heart disease were again consistently high in the three geographical groups in either sex (table IV). Those for pneumococcal pneumonia were negative in rural areas, whereas those for lung cancer were positive only among men in county boroughs.

Table V shows the correlations between standardised mortality ratios for bronchitis during 1968–78 and those for rheumatic heart disease, pneumococcal pneumonia, and lung cancer. For rheumatic heart disease correlations were consistently high in each geographical group and in either sex. They were, however, lower than those with infant respiratory mortality.

The statistical dependence of the geographical distribution of chronic bronchitis on geographical variations in past infant deaths from bronchitis and pneumonia and variations in smoking, as indicated by current deaths from lung cancer, is described by the regression equations: standardised mortality ratio for bronchitis in men = 0·60 infant death rate + 0·41 standardised mortality ratio for lung cancer in men; standardised mortality ratio for bronchitis in women = 0·79 infant death rate + 0·22 standardised mortality ratio for lung cancer in women. In these equations the mean infant death rate was standardised to a value of 100 and adult death rates during 1968–78 were used.

Figures 3 and 4 show the age specific mortality trends for bronchitis and lung cancer during 1941–80 summarised by birth cohort and period values. The cohort values relate to successive generations born from 1856 to 1951. Among men they rose to a peak for both diseases in generations born around 1900–5; among women they rose to a later peak in generations born around 1925, again for both diseases. Period values for lung cancer were

TABLE IV—*Correlation of causes of death (standardised mortality ratios) in 1959–67 and infant death rates from bronchitis and pneumonia in 1921–5 in three geographical groups in men and women*

	Geographical group			
Cause of death	County and London boroughs	Urban areas	Rural areas	All areas
Men				
Bronchitis	0·69	0·73	0·67	0·80
Rheumatic heart disease	0·40	0·51	0·46	0·54
Pneumococal pneumonia	0·27	0·36	−0·05	0·43
Lung cancer	0·23	−0·05	−0·24	0·43
Women				
Bronchitis	0·70	0·58	0·54	0·77
Rheumatic heart disease	0·56	0·60	0·52	0·68
Pneumococcal pneumonia	0·29	0·21	−0·03	0·31
Lung cancer	−0·03	−0·25	−0·51	0·11

TABLE V—*Correlation of mortality from chronic bronchitis with other causes of death (standardised mortality ratios) during 1968–78 in three geographical groups in men and women*

Cause of death	Geographical group			
	County and London boroughs	Urban areas	Rural areas	All areas
Men				
Rheumatic heart disease	0·48	0·57	0·60	0·61
Pneumococcal pneumonia	0·20	0·27	0·24	0·35
Lung cancer	0·47	0·30	0·40	0·66
Infant bronchitis and pneumonia, 1921–5	0·75	0·77	0·75	0·84
Women				
Rheumatic heart disease	0·63	0·48	0·64	0·70
Pneumococcal pneumonia	0·16	− 0·12	0·17	0·25
Lung cancer	0·12	− 0·06	0·02	0·33
Infant bronchitis and pneumonia, 1921–5	0·70	0·74	0·68	0·80

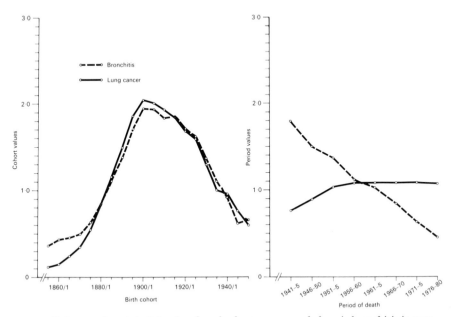

FIG 3—*Cohort and period of death values for lung cancer and chronic bronchitis in men aged over 25 in England and Wales during 1941–80.*

55

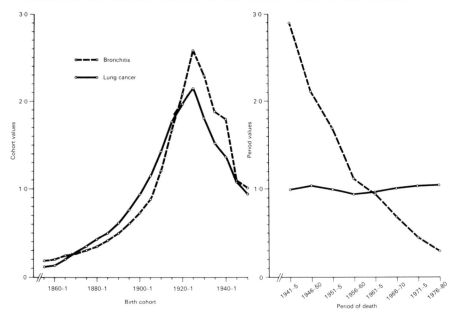

FIG 4—*Cohort and period of death values for lung cancer and chronic bronchitis in women aged over 25 in England and Wales during 1941–80.*

close to unity for both sexes throughout 1941–80, but for bronchitis they declined steadily, falling fourfold in men and ninefold in women during the 40 years.

Discussion

There was a close geographical relation between adult mortality from bronchitis and emphysema and past infant mortality from bronchitis and pneumonia (figs 1 and 2). Our analyses were based on adult mortality over 20 years and on the whole of England and Wales divided into the 212 areas used by the registrar general. The correlations between mortality from bronchitis during 1959–78 and infant respiratory mortality during 1921–5 were consistent in both sexes and at all ages in the different geographical groups and throughout the 20 years (tables II–IV). They were remarkably high, particularly in view of known inaccuracies in death certification.

From detailed studies of death certification and results of prevalence surveys in Britain it is reasonable to conclude that geographical differences in mortality certified as due to chronic bronchitis and emphysema reflect differences in the prevalence of these diseases.[2]

Past infant respiratory mortality correlated more closely with current adult mortality from bronchitis than it did with any other common cause of death, or with any other cause of past infant death, or with past mortality from bronchitis at all other ages (table I). No other cause of infant death correlated more closely with bronchitis, though the correlation with measles was similarly high. Adult bronchitis correlated more closely with rheumatic heart disease than with any other leading cause of adult death, but the coefficients were below those with past infant respiratory mortality (table V).

A pointer to the possible role of childhood respiratory infection in the causation of adult chronic bronchitis comes from the broad similarity in the international geography and time trends of respiratory disease at different ages.[5] Migrant studies also suggest that determinants of chronic bronchitis act in early life. For example, among British born men who migrated to the United States the prevalence of chronic bronchitis, after allowing for smoking habits, was higher than among migrants from Norway. It was higher among those born in urban areas of Britain and was unrelated to age at migration.[2]

Follow up studies of infants and young children who have had bronchiolitis have shown persisting abnormalities of pulmonary function.[7-9] For example, among 130 children in Tyneside reviewed 10 years after admission to hospital in infancy with respiratory syncytial virus infection (the most common cause of bronchiolitis) there was a threefold increase in bronchial lability compared with controls.[9] A study of 7 year old children suggested that bronchial reactivity and persisting abnormalities of ventilatory function may result after acute lower respiratory tract infection in infancy at any site—that is, bronchitis, bronchiolitis, or pneumonia.[10] The simplest interpretation of these observations is that infection of the lung during the period of rapid growth in infancy has deleterious effects on lung function which persist into childhood. An alternative explanation is that influences such as atopy render some infants more susceptible to symptomatic lower respiratory tract infection and independently determine respiratory abnormalities in later childhood. While this cannot be discounted, recent studies have not shown a relation between atopy and lower respiratory infection in children.[18 19]

In a national sample of 3899 children born in 1946 and followed up to the age of 20, those with a history of one or more lower respiratory tract infections before 2 years of age had a higher reported prevalence of cough during the day or at night in the winter.[11] This association strengthened after follow up to 25 years.[12] There is, however, no direct evidence linking respiratory infection in early childhood with chronic bronchitis in adults.

Arguably the geographical relation between infant mortality from respiratory infection and adult mortality from bronchitis depends on persistence over the years of geographical differences in the environment related to respiratory disease at all ages. Air temperature is a possible example.[20]

Several determinants of bronchitis, however, act only at certain ages.[21] The risk of infant respiratory infection may be reduced by breast feeding[19 22] and is increased by overcrowding, the number and age of other siblings, their presence in the same room at night, respiratory infection among them, and parental smoking.[23-25] Domestic air pollution may also have an effect on infant respiratory infection, though the balance of evidence suggests that this is small.[25]

Among adults cigarette smoking is the main known risk factor.[3] Mortality from lung cancer, however, did not correlate consistently with infant respiratory mortality (tables II–IV). This suggests that the geography of smoking differs from that of the determinants of respiratory disease in early childhood. Despite the influence of smoking on adult bronchitis, the urban to rural and social class gradients of infant and adult mortality were strikingly similar. When standardised to a value of 100 for England and Wales infant respiratory mortality during 1921–5 declined from 125 in the county boroughs to 98 in the London boroughs, 93 in urban areas, and 70 in rural areas. The corresponding figures for adult mortality during 1968–78 were 122, 113, 96, and 74. Similarly the standardised mortality ratios for infants in 1921 rose progressively from 21 in social class I to 131 in social class V, and standardised mortality ratios for adults in 1970–2 rose from 36 to 188.[26]

The close geographical relation between bronchitis and chronic rheumatic heart disease, in contrast with the low correlations with pneumococcal pneumonia (tables II–IV), is further evidence for a strong link between bronchitis and past respiratory infection. Most deaths from bronchitis during 1968–78 at ages 35–74 occurred among people born before 1921–5, the earliest years for which cause specific infant mortality data were published. Total postneonatal death rates, however, are available from 1911[13] and may be used as a proxy for respiratory deaths in infants. Respiratory infection is the main cause of postneonatal mortality and was closely correlated with it geographically during 1921–5 ($r = 0.94$). The correlation coefficients between postneonatal mortality and adult mortality from bronchitis during 1968–78 in both sexes were the same ($r = 0.83$) for postneonatal rates throughout 1911–20 as for 1921–5. This is consistent with a relation between adult bronchitis and respiratory infection in early childhood. Follow up studies of children suggest that this relation is determined mainly in infancy.

We conclude that the close geographical relation between infant mortality from respiratory infection and adult mortality from bronchitis provides strong evidence of a direct causal link between lower respiratory infection in early childhood and chronic bronchitis. The regression equations of adult mortality from bronchitis in relation to deaths in infants and from lung cancer may be interpreted as showing the relative importance of early childhood infection and cigarette smoking in determining the prevalence of the disease. They suggest that in both men and women smoking is subordinate.

Figures 3 and 4 show that the bronchitis time trends may be partitioned into two components. The cohort component corresponds remarkably closely to that found for lung cancer and may be attributed to the different smoking habits of successive generations of men and women. The other component, described by the steeply declining period values, indicates that the age specific rates had fallen progressively since 1941. This pattern is quite different from that found for lung cancer, for which the period values were almost constant, and suggests another cause. The decline in infant bronchitis and pneumonia in the early decades of this century[21] may have determined the subsequent fall in age specific mortality from bronchitis in adults. The steeper fall among women than men is consistent with the lesser contribution of smoking to their mortality. Improved treatment after the advent of antibiotics may have contributed to the decline in both sexes.

The Clean Air Act 1956 was not followed by a change in the rate of decline. This is evidence that chronic air pollution in adult life, as opposed to short episodes of high pollution, may be a less important cause of mortality from bronchitis than previously supposed. A survey of respiratory symptoms in a sample of British adults showed that in the absence of cigarette smoking the influence of air pollution was small.[3] There is suggestive evidence that children exposed to high levels of air pollution may have an increased risk of serious respiratory disease, but this is not conclusive. One inconsistency is the high rates for respiratory disease recorded in south Wales at a time when air pollution was relatively low.[27 28]

We interpret our findings as strong support for the hypothesis that pulmonary infection during infancy may have persisting effects and cause chronic bronchitis in adult life. Our results throw no light on the nature or site of pulmonary infection except in so far as adult mortality from bronchitis is related to infant bronchitis and pneumonia, to measles, but not to whooping cough. Recent findings have shown that apart from bronchiectasis, which is no longer common, whooping cough is not followed by persisting abnormalities of lung function in childhood.[29 30]

We have previously suggested that the geographical distribution of ischaemic heart disease in England and Wales reflects social conditions in the early years of the century that adversely affected childhood nutrition (chapter 1). We now conclude that the high mortality from chronic bronchitis in England and Wales, especially in the towns, is another legacy of poor social conditions which led to high rates of respiratory infection in young children. Particular adverse influences which have been implicated include abandonment of breast feeding, inadequate housing, large family size, and overcrowding in the home.

1 Holland WW, Gilderdale S. Epidemiology of chronic bronchitis. In: Scadding JG, Cumming G, Thurlbeck WM, eds. *Scientific foundations of respiratory medicine.* London: Heinemann. 1981:18–29.
2 Reid DD, Fletcher CM. International studies in chronic respiratory disease. *Br Med Bull* 1971;**27**:59–64.
3 Lambert PM, Reid DD. Smoking, air pollution, and bronchitis in Britain. *Lancet* 1970;i:853–7.
4 Orie NGM, Sluiter HJ, eds. *Bronchitis—an international symposium.* Groningen, the Netherlands: Assen Royal Vengorium, 1961.
5 Reid DD. The beginnings of bronchitis. *Proceedings of the Royal Society of Medicine* 1969;**62**:311–6.
6 Holland WW, Halil T, Bennett AE, Elliott A. Factors influencing the onset of chronic respiratory disease. *BMJ* 1969;ii:205–8.
7 Kattan M, Keens TG, Lapierre JG, Levison H, Bryan AC, Reilly BJ. Pulmonary function abnormalities in symptom-free children after bronchiolitis. *Pediatrics* 1977;**59**:683–8.
8 Gurwitz D, Mindorff C, Levison H. Increased incidence of bronchial reactivity in children with a history of bronchiolitis. *Pediatrics* 1981;**98**:551–5.
9 Pullan CR, Hey EN. Wheezing, asthma, and pulmonary dysfunction 10 years after infection with respiratory syncytial virus in infancy. *BMJ* 1982;**284**:1665–9.
10 Mok JYQ, Simpson H. Outcome for acute bronchitis, bronchiolitis, and pneumonia in infancy. *Arch Dis Child* 1984;**59**:306–9.
11 Colley JRT, Douglas JWB, Reid DD. Respiratory disease in young adults: influence of early childhood lower respiratory tract illness, social class, air pollution, and smoking. *BMJ* 1973;iii:195–8.
12 Kiernan KE, Colley JRT, Douglas JWB, Reid DD. Chronic cough in young adults in relation to smoking habits, childhood environment and chest illness. *Respiration* 1976;**33**:236–44.
13 Office of Population Censuses and Surveys. *Registrar general's statistical review of England and Wales. Part I. Tables, medical.* London: HMSO, 1911 and following years.
14 Woolf B. Studies on infant mortality: part II. Social aetiology of stillbirths and infant deaths in county boroughs of England and Wales. *British Journal of Social Medicine* 1947;**2**:73–125.
15 Osmond C, Gardner MJ. Age, period and cohort models applied to cancer mortality rates. *Statistics in Medicine* 1982;**1**:245–59.
16 Gardner MJ, Winter PD, Taylor CP, Acheson ED. *Atlas of cancer mortality in England and Wales 1968–78.* Chichester: Wiley, 1983.
17 Gardner MJ, Winter PD, Barker DJP. *Atlas of mortality from selected diseases in England and Wales 1968–78.* Chichester: Wiley, 1984.
18 Mok JYQ, Simpson H. Symptoms, atopy, and bronchial reactivity after lower respiratory infection in infancy. *Arch Dis Child* 1984;**59**:299–305.
19 Sims DG, Gardner PS, Weightman D, Turner MW, Soothill JF. Atopy does not predispose to RSV bronchiolitis or postbronchiolitic wheezing. *BMJ* 1981;**282**:2086–8.
20 Boyd JT. Climate, air pollution and mortality. *British Journal of Preventive and Social Medicine* 1960;**14**:123–35.
21 Colley JRT. Respiratory disease in childhood. *Br Med Bull* 1971;**27**:9–14.
22 Downham MAPS, Scott R, Sims DG, Webb JKG, Gardner PS. Breast feeding protects against respiratory syncytial virus infections. *BMJ* 1976;ii:274–6.
23 Leeder SR, Corkhill R, Irwig LM, Holland WW, Colley JRT. Influence of family factors on the incidence of lower respiratory illness during the first year of life. *British Journal of Preventive and Social Medicine* 1976;**30**:203–12.
24 Pullan CR, Toms GL, Martin AJ, Gardner PS, Webb JKG, Appleton DR. Breast feeding and respiratory syncytial virus infection. *BMJ* 1980;**281**:1034–8.
25 Ogston SA, Florey C du V, Walker CHM. The Tayside infant morbidity and mortality study: effect on health of using gas for cooking. *BMJ* 1985;**290**:957–60.

26 Registrar general. *Decennial supplement, occupational mortality, England and Wales 1921, 1970–2*. London: HMSO, 1927, 1978.

27 Colley JRT, Reid DD. Urban and social origins of childhood bronchitis in England and Wales. *BMJ* 1970;ii:213–7.

28 Royal College of Physicians of London. *Air pollution and health*. London: Pitman 1970.

29 Johnston IDA, Anderson HR, Lambert HP, Patel S. Respiratory morbidity and lung function after whooping cough. *Lancet* 1983;ii:1104–8.

30 Swansea Research Unit of the Royal College of General Practitioners. Respiratory sequelae of whooping cough. *BMJ* 1985;**290**:1937–40.

4: Intrauterine and early postnatal origins of cardiovascular disease and chronic bronchitis

D J P BARKER, C OSMOND, C M LAW

Geographical differences in mortality from cardiovascular disease and chronic bronchitis within England and Wales are closely related to past differences in infant mortality (chapters 1–3). This chapter examines the separate relations of mortality during 1968–78 with neonatal and postneonatal mortality during 1911–25. These divisions of infant mortality are indicators of the intrauterine and early postnatal environments respectively. Stroke is related to neonatal mortality and therefore to the intrauterine environment. Prenatal determinants of blood pressure levels may be one mechanism underlying this. Bronchitis is related to postneonatal mortality and therefore to the postnatal environment. This may reflect the long term effects of lower respiratory tract infection in early childhood. Ischaemic heart disease is related to both neonatal and postneonatal mortality and therefore to the intrauterine and postnatal environments. The links may include blood pressure and as yet unknown processes established in early postnatal life.

Introduction

Within England and Wales there is a close relation between geographical differences in mortality from cardiovascular disease and differences in infant mortality 70 and more years ago (chapters 1 and 2). A similar relation between current cardiovascular mortality and past infant mortality has been shown within three other countries: in the 20 counties of Norway,[1] in east and west Finland,[2] and in 17 registration states within the United States of America.[3]

The data from England and Wales are based on the largest numbers of deaths. They allow detailed examination based on the 212 local authority areas into which the country was formerly divided, and they allow analyses for ischaemic heart disease and stroke separately. The completeness and detail of infant mortality records from 1911 onwards enable examination of the relations with infant mortality at different ages and from different causes. In particular they distinguish neonatal mortality (deaths before 1 month of age) from postneonatal mortality (deaths from 1 month to 1 year).

Findings in Norway and Finland were interpreted as evidence that adverse living conditions during childhood, for example housing and recurrent infection, increased the risk of ischaemic heart disease.[1 2] The study in the USA found a closer relation with infant mortality from diarrhoeal disease than from other causes.[3] In our first analysis we found that, whereas the geographical correlations of cardiovascular disease with previous neonatal and postneonatal death rates were similar when expressed as correlation coefficients, the position of the 15 London boroughs on the scattergram suggested a more consistent relation with neonatal mortality (chapter 1). London has low cardiovascular mortality and had low neonatal mortality but high postneonatal mortality in the past.

Seventy years ago most neonatal deaths occurred within a week of birth and depended mainly on prenatal rather than postnatal influences.[4] This pointer to a relation with the intrauterine environment is reinforced by the relation between cardiovascular disease and past maternal mortality, a relation which is especially strong for stroke (chapter 2).

We present here an analysis which discriminates more closely between the geographical relations of cardiovascular disease with past neonatal and postneonatal mortality. The findings are contrasted with those for chronic bronchitis, where the geographical distribution is closely related to past variations in postneonatal mortality from respiratory infection and is therefore determined by the postnatal environment (chapter 3). Lower respiratory tract infections in infancy and early childhood are a known risk factor for chronic bronchitis.

Methods

Numbers of neonatal deaths and of postneonatal deaths in different areas of England and Wales were published from 1911 onwards.[5] We calculated rates per 1000 births for 1911–25. During this time there were 436 087 neonatal deaths and 668 115 postneonatal deaths.

We analysed the mortality data that are described in chapter 1, that is death rates from stroke, ischaemic heart disease, and chronic bronchitis at ages 35–74 during 1968–78 in the 212 local authority areas of England and Wales. We ordered the areas according to neonatal mortality during 1911–25 and derived five groups of 42 or 43 areas with increasing mortality. We similarly derived five groups with increasing postneonatal mortality. In this way mortality at ages 35–74 was examined within a grid of 25 cells.

Results

Table I shows the numbers of areas of England and Wales within each neonatal and postneonatal mortality group. Neonatal mortality rose from 30 per 1000 births in group 1 to 44 in group 5. Postneonatal mortality rose from 32 per 1000 in group 1 to 73 in group 5. Most areas were on the diagonal of the grid. Areas with low neonatal but high postneonatal mortality were mostly in London but included the county boroughs of Chester and Great Yarmouth. Areas with high neonatal but low postneonatal rates were scattered through the north and west and included the rural areas of Anglesey, Northumberland, and Staffordshire.

Table II shows mortality from stroke, ischaemic heart disease, and chronic bronchitis within the grid defined in table I. Within any of the five bands of postneonatal mortality, standardised mortality ratios for stroke increased sharply with increasing neonatal mortality. There was no independent trend in stroke mortality with postneonatal mortality. Mortality from ischaemic heart disease had similar but separate trends with neonatal and postneonatal mortality. Mortality from chronic bronchitis showed a steep increase with increasing postneonatal mortality, but no independent trend with neonatal mortality.

Discussion

This analysis shows that mortality from cardiovascular disease and

TABLE I—*Division of the 212 areas of England and Wales according to neonatal and postneonatal mortality during 1911–25.*

	Postneonatal mortality					Neonatal deaths/1000 births
	lowest			highest		
	1	2	3	4	5	
Neonatal mortality						
1 lowest	21	11	5	4	1	30
2	11	16	9	5	2	33
3	8	11	14	5	4	36
4	0	5	11	18	9	39
5 highest	2	0	3	11	26	44
Postneonatal deaths/1000 births	32	40	50	61	73	

TABLE II—*Death rates from stroke, ischaemic heart disease, and chronic bronchitis (standardised mortality ratios, ages 35–74, both sexes, 1968–78) in the 212 areas of England and Wales grouped by neonatal and postneonatal mortality (1911–25).*

Neonatal mortality	Postneonatal mortality						
	lowest	1	2	3	4	5	highest
Stroke							
1 lowest		85	81	79	78	79	
2		86	90	98	74	76	
3		102	100	104	104	104	
4		—	108	110	115	117	
5 highest		124	—	121	123	117	
Ischaemic heart disease							
1 lowest		84	89	91	88	98	
2		85	93	95	88	91	
3		86	94	99	106	113	
4		—	98	109	111	115	
5 highest		83	—	114	119	116	
Chronic bronchitis							
1 lowest		67	78	106	115	161	
2		64	84	85	104	126	
3		69	65	89	88	151	
4		—	91	99	120	142	
5 highest		41	—	108	123	144	

chronic bronchitis has different geographical relations with past differences in the intrauterine and early postnatal environments, as indicated by the distribution of neonatal and postneonatal mortality in England and Wales during 1911–25. Stroke is related to the intrauterine environment; chronic bronchitis is related to the postnatal environment; and ischaemic heart disease is related to both.

The median year of birth of people dying before 75 years of age during 1968–78, the years included in our analysis, is around 1905. The data on infant mortality are for 1911–25 and do not exactly correspond with this. Data published before 1911, however, do now allow such a detailed geographical analysis. The distributions of neonatal and postneonatal mortality changed little throughout 1911–25, despite a fall in the rates, and there is no reason to think that they differed much from those in the previous decade.

We have suggested that blood pressure is one link between an adverse intrauterine environment and the risk of cardiovascular disease (chapter 2). In a large national sample of adults aged 36 in Britain, blood pressure was inversely related to birth weight.[6] In the past most neonatal deaths in Britain occurred during the first week after birth and were attributed to prematurity or low birth weight.[4] The geographical distribution of maternal mortality, from causes other than puerperal fever, was closely similar to neonatal mortality. Poor physique of the mothers was clearly implicated as a cause of high maternal mortality, and was itself a result of poor nutrition and impaired growth of young girls.[7] The aggregation of high perinatal mortality, low birth weight, and poor maternal physique in certain areas of the country was first shown in national surveys during 1910–30, and has been repeatedly confirmed in perinatal surveys since the second world war.[8] The magnitude of past differences in birth weight is illustrated by the birth weight distribution of babies born in maternity hospitals in Preston and London around 1930. In Preston, which had high neonatal and maternal mortality, mean birth weight was 289 g below that in London, which had low mortality (unpublished data).

Several mechanisms could link an adverse intrauterine environment, reduced fetal growth, and higher blood pressure. Pressure in the fetal circulation could be raised as a method of maintaining placental perfusion, and the raised pressures may persist after birth.[9] Retardation of intrauterine growth may lead to accelerated postnatal growth accompanied by an accelerated increase in blood pressure.[10]

There is considerable evidence linking serious or recurrent lower respiratory tract infection before the age of 2 years with increased risk of chronic bronchitis in adult life, though the mechanism underlying this association is not understood.[11 12] Part of this evidence comes from the remarkably close and specific geographical relation between past infant mortality from bronchitis or pneumonia and current mortality from chronic bronchitis in England and Wales (chapter 3).

Failure of long term "programming" of lipid metabolism during infancy, as a result of infant feeding, is a possible link between infancy and ischaemic heart disease for which there is increasing evidence in experimental animals.[13]

Mortality from stroke has fallen in Britain over the past 40 years.[5] This is consistent with past improvements in the intrauterine environment, as a result of improved maternal physique. Bronchitis mortality has also fallen, in keeping with past improvements in housing and reduction of overcrowding. Ischaemic heart disease mortality, however, has risen steeply. It may therefore have two groups of causes, one acting through the mother and in infancy, and associated with poor living standards, the other acting in later life, and associated with affluence.

1 Forsdahl A. Are poor living conditions in childhood and adolescence an important risk factor for arteriosclerotic heart disease? *Br J Prev Soc Med* 1977;**31**:91–5.
2 Notkola V. *Living conditions in childhood and coronary heart disease in adulthood.* Helsinki: Finnish Society of Science and Letters, 1985.
3 Buck C, Simpson H. Infant diarrhoea and subsequent mortality from heart disease and cancer. *J Epidemiol Community Health* 1982;**36**:27–30.
4 Local Government Board. *Thirty-ninth annual report 1909–10. Supplement on infant and child mortality.* London: HMSO, 1910.
5 Office of Population Censuses and Surveys. *Registrar general's statistical reviews of England and Wales 1911.* Part 1. Tables, medical. London: HMSO, 1911 and following years.

6 Wadsworth MEJ, Cripps HA, Midwinter RE, Colley JRT. Blood pressure in a national birth cohort at the age of 36 related to social and familial factors, smoking, and body mass. *BMJ* 1985;**291**:1534–8.

7 Campbell JM, Cameron D, Jones DM. *High maternal mortality in certain areas.* London: HMSO, 1932. (Ministry of Health Reports on Public Health and Medical Subjects, No. 68).

8 Butler N, Alberman ED. *Second report on the 1958 British perinatal mortality survey.* Edinburgh and London: Livingstone, 1969.

9 Gennser G, Rymark P, Isberg PE. Low birth weight and risk of high blood pressure in adulthood. *BMJ* 1988;**296**:1498–9.

10 Ounsted MK, Cockburn JM, Moar VA, Redman CWG. Factors associated with the blood pressures of children born to women who were hypertensive during pregnancy. *Arch Dis Child* 1985;**60**:631–5.

11 Colley JRT, Douglas JWB, Reid DD. Respiratory disease in young adults: influence of early childhood lower respiratory tract illness, social class, air pollution, and smoking. *BMJ* 1973;**iii**:195–8.

12 Holland W, Halil T, Bennett AE, Elliot A. Factors influencing the onset of chronic respiratory disease. *BMJ* 1969;**ii**:205–8.

13 Mott GE. Deferred effects of breastfeeding versus formula feeding on serum lipoprotein concentrations and cholesterol metabolism in baboons. In: Filer LJ Jr, Fomon SJ, eds. *The breastfed infant: a model for performance.* Report of the 91st Ross conference on pediatric research. Columbus, Ohio: Ross Laboratories, 1986: 144–9.

5: Inequalities in health in Britain: specific explanations in three Lancashire towns

D J P BARKER, C OSMOND

The reasons that mortality is higher in the poorer areas of Britain are largely unknown. Thus how to reduce inequalities in health is a matter of conjecture. In three neighbouring towns in northern England the rates of death from all causes differ greatly. Socioeconomic conditions in the towns are similar though below average for England and Wales. The pattern of disease specific rates was analysed and related to past differences in infant mortality.

It is suggested that past differences in maternal health and physique and in the postnatal environment, particularly infant feeding, housing, and overcrowding, may be determinants of current differences in adult mortality.

Introduction

The geographical and social class differences in mortality in Britain reflect differences in death rates from several chronic diseases. They correlate with variations in a range of socioeconomic indexes, with rates being higher in poorer places and groups.[1][2] How specific socioeconomic influences determine variations in mortality from chronic diseases is, however, largely unknown, and therefore how inequalities in mortality can be reduced is a matter of conjecture.[3]

During 1968–78 variations in ischaemic heart disease, chronic bronchitis, and stroke accounted for 93% of the total variance in mortality from all causes between the 212 local authority groupings in England and Wales—that is, the county boroughs (large towns), London boroughs, urban areas within counties, and rural areas. We have shown that these three diseases have a close geographical relation with certain causes of infant mortality during the early years of the century (chapters 1–3). We interpret this as evidence that events in prenatal life and early childhood are important in the aetiology of these diseases. Specifically, the physique and health of the mother and the prenatal and postnatal growth and development of the infant may be determinants of ischaemic heart disease and stroke, and respiratory infection in early childhood may be a determinant of chronic bronchitis.

It follows that differences in maternal characteristics and in the postnatal environment may be determinants of the current differences in adult mortality. Census data from the past give some insight into the childhood environment. Indexes of crowded housing and of family income were geographically correlated with infant mortality.[4] The value of such indexes, however, is limited because they do not, for example, describe nutrition.

In 1914, after a national survey,[5] the Local Government Board published a report on infant mortality in Lancashire.[6] The report focused on the three neighbouring towns of Burnley, Colne, and Nelson, situated side by side on the western slopes of the Pennine Hills (figure). Each had developed as a

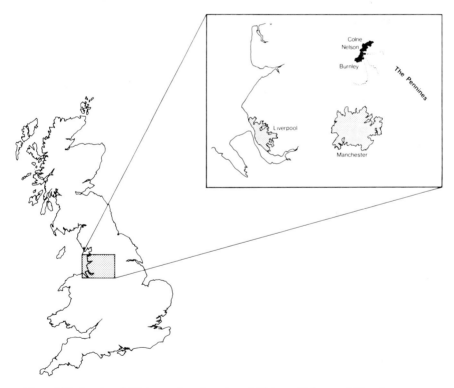

Map of England and Wales to show location of Nelson, Colne, and Burnley

cotton weaving town, and for the six miles from the centre of Burnley through Nelson to Colne there was hardly a break in the line of houses. Yet the infant mortality rates differed greatly. In 1911–13 there were 177 deaths per 1000 births in Burnley, 130 in Colne, and 87 in Nelson.

The current mortality in the towns differs also. During 1968–78 mortality at all ages and from all causes was 21% above the national average in Burnley, 10% above in Colne, and 4% above in Nelson.[7] The detailed description of the towns in the 1914 report gives an insight into the way in which past environmental differences that affected the health and development of infants might have determined the current differences in mortality among adults.

Methods

Data on past conditions in the three towns were taken from the 1911 census[8] and from two Local Government Board reports, the first (1913) covering all 241 urban areas of England and Wales[9] and the second (1914) covering Lancashire.[6] Published data from the 1971 census allowed current occupation, housing, and other socioeconomic indexes to be compared.[10] Additional data on infant mortality in 1921–5 came from the registrar general's statistical reviews.[11]

The Office of Population Censuses and Surveys made available to us extracts from all death certificates in England and Wales during 1968–78, the period covered by the eighth revision of the International Classification of Diseases. Death rates for each sex for each local authority area were calculated from 1971 census data, grouped according to local authority boundaries before 1974.[7 12] Death rates were expressed as standardised mortality ratios.

Results

INFANT MORTALITY RATES

Table I shows infant mortality rates in the towns for four periods from 1896 to 1925.[6 9] Throughout this time there was a gradient in the rates from Nelson to Colne to Burnley. Rates in Burnley were much above the average for England and Wales, being consistently among the highest of any town. National rates fell from 155 per 1000 in 1896–8 to 76 in 1921–5.

Data for 1911–13 show that there were gradients from Nelson to Colne to Burnley for both neonatal and postneonatal deaths (table I) and for deaths from the three main groups of causes—that is, the so called "group of five" diseases (premature birth, congenital defects, birth injury, want of breast milk, and atrophy, debility, and marasmus), bronchitis and pneumonia, and diarrhoea. Most deaths in this first group were recorded as being due to

TABLE I—*Nelson, Colne, and Burnley: infant mortality rates per 1000 births from 1896 to 1925 and infant mortality by period and cause, child mortality, and birth rate 1911 to 1913*

	Nelson	Colne	Burnley	England and Wales
Infant mortality/1000 births, 1896–1925:				
1896–8	154	170	197	155
1907–10	107	130	171	113
1911–13	87	130	177	111
1921–5	79	109	114	76
Rates from 1911 to 1913:				
Infant mortality/1000 births				
Neonatal	38	37	49	
Postneonatal	49	93	128	
Cause:				
Group of five diseases*	35	33	53	
Bronchitis and pneumonia	17	25	26	
Diarrhoea	16	30	48	
Mortality at age 1–5 years/1000				
survivors at age 1	58	85	96	
Birth rate/1000 population	18	21	23	

*Premature birth, congenital defects, birth injury, want of breast milk, and atrophy, debility, and marasmus.

premature birth or congenital defects. The gradient in neonatal deaths, however, and in the group of five diseases which is their main cause, was less steep than for postneonatal deaths. Differences in mortality between the towns persisted through early childhood to 5 years.

Data from the 1913 report allow rates for the earlier period 1907–10 to be compared with those in all 241 urban areas in England and Wales. Neonatal death rates and those for the "group of five" diseases in Burnley during 1907–10 were 13% and 18% above the urban average; rates for bronchitis and pneumonia were 73% above and for diarrhoea 105% above. Rates in Nelson were mostly below the average, those for diarrhoea being 55% below.

There was a gradient in birth rates from 18 per 1000 population in Nelson up to 23 in Burnley (table I).

CONDITIONS IN THE TOWNS[6]

Most of Burnley is in the valley where the rivers Brun and Calder meet. Nelson and Colne lie above it on the western slopes of the Pennines. The climate is cold and damp, and rainfall is above average, particularly in Nelson. Low lying areas of Burnley were persistently damp, especially those below the high embankment that carries the Leeds–Liverpool canal through the town. During the early 1800s there was extensive house building on land near Burnley town centre that was so marshy that it was unfit for farming.

In all three towns the level of employment was high, and wages were relatively good. The staple industry was cotton weaving (table II). The textile industry employed roughly 40% of all the women aged 10 years and over. In Burnley a small percentage (8·7%) of the men worked in coal and shale mines. Otherwise the distribution of occupations among men and women in the three towns was similar.

Many of the women who worked in the weaving mills of Burnley and Colne were from the second or third generation of Lancashire industrial workers. Nelson, however, had developed more recently and had an eightfold increase in population between 1871 and 1911. Most of the people were immigrants from adjacent areas, especially from parts of Yorkshire. "This fact has an important bearing on the question of infantile mortality, owing to the general good health and the habits of cleanliness and thrift characteristic of these immigrants from rural districts." The women were described as "sturdier and healthier" than those in Burnley.

There were no crêches at the mills. Usually the return of the mothers to work was soon followed by complete weaning and the infant, together with other children in the family below school age, was placed in the care of an untrained "minder" who was paid by the mother. "In view of the fact that so many mothers are anxious, for the sake of the wages, to get back to employment in the mills as soon as possible after childbirth, a large proportion of children born in Burnley are deprived of the advantages of breast feeding after the first few weeks of life. . . . In Colne and still more in Nelson breast feeding is usually continued longer than in Burnley." An inquiry in Burnley showed that at the end of six months 36% of infants

TABLE II—*Distribution (%) of men and women aged 10 years and over by occupation and percentage of married women employed, 1911*

Occupation	Nelson	Colne	Burnley
Men:			
Textiles	59·4	47·0	36·0
Coal and shale mine workers	0·7	0·5	8·7
Building and construction	4·9	6·2	5·2
General engineering	1·9	6·0	5·7
All other occupations	24·0	30·7	33·7
Retired or unoccupied	9·1	9·6	10·7
Women:			
Textiles	45·0	39·0	43·6
All other occupations	9·7	11·5	12·7
Retired or unoccupied	45·3	49·5	43·7
Percentage of married women employed	37·1	32·2	41·4

were breast fed, 34% had mixed breast and artificial feeding, and 27% had artificial feeding alone.

Most houses in the towns were similarly built of stone. In Nelson, however, houses were newer and tended to be more spacious (table III). Mean family size in the towns was similar. The worst houses were the back to back houses in the oldest parts of Burnley and Colne. These were small, had no means of ventilation to the outside air, and lacked facilities for the storage of food and milk. Infant mortality was much higher in such houses—248 per 1000 in the back to back houses of Colne, for example, during 1912 compared with 80 in the so called "through" houses. Much of the excess mortality was due to diarrhoea. Resettlement of families from back to back houses to "through" houses was accompanied by a fall in infant mortality to around the average for "through" houses, showing that high mortality was a consequence of the structure of back to back houses rather than of the habits of those who occupied them. There were 2371 of these houses in Burnley and 1000 in Colne but only 52 in Nelson (table III).

Sanitary conditions in Nelson were better than those in the other two towns. In Nelson the women kept the streets outside their houses clean, "more water being said to be used for this purpose in Nelson than in any other town in Lancashire." In Nelson communal pits, used for disposal of household refuse, were small and covered and were "in striking contrast" to the large open pits in Burnley and Colne, which favoured the breeding of flies. Refuse collected from the pits and bins in Nelson and Colne was destroyed, whereas in Burnley around half was put on to "tips," which were sites for breeding flies. In Nelson, and to a lesser extent Colne, the manure pits around stables and cowsheds were disinfected in summer to prevent flies breeding. Sanitary regulations that were related to the production and sale of milk were more strictly enforced in Nelson.

TABLE III—*Housing conditions, mean family size, and total population, 1911*

	Nelson	Colne	Burnley	England and Wales
Percentage of population in dwellings of less than four rooms	5·6	15·1	13·6	19·4
Percentage of population living more than two persons to a room	3·7	6·6	9·5	9·1
Percentage (number) of dwellings back to back or single room	0·6 (52)	17·0 (1000)	9·9 (2371)	—
Mean family size	4·3	4·3	4·4	4·4
Total population	39 479	25 689	106 322	

CURRENT MORTALITY

Table IV shows standardised mortality ratios for 1968–78 at ages 55–74. Most people who died at these ages belong to the generation to whose childhood environment the 1914 report relates.[6] Analysis of all deaths in the towns during 1969–72 shows that 85% of people aged 55–74 who died in Burnley were born in Lancashire. The corresponding figures for Nelson and Colne are 80% and 79%. More details are available for Burnley, where 65% of the people were born in the town itself. Analysis of a sample of 471 death certificates for people aged 55–74 years who died in the towns in 1973 showed that 79% who died in Burnley were born within a 12 mile radius of the Nelson town centre. Corresponding figures for Nelson and Colne are 75% and 73%. The percentages of people who were born and died in the same town are 68 in Burnley, 36 in Nelson, and 50 in Colne.

The gradient in standardised mortality ratios from all causes from Nelson to Colne to Burnley was shown by both sexes. Ratios for men were 99 in Nelson, 110 in Colne, and 120 in Burnley; the corresponding ratios for women were 105, 112, and 125. For both sexes combined mortality in Nelson (standardised mortality ratio 100) was exactly the national average. The gradient in standardised mortality ratios for all causes is reflected in gradients for ischaemic heart disease, bronchitis, pneumonia, and stroke.

Standardised mortality ratios for lung cancer were low, although there was a trend between the towns. Ratios for all cancers other than stomach or lung were also around 100, with no trend.

Of the 971 deaths in Burnley that were in excess of those expected from national rates, 63% were caused by ischaemic heart disease (280 deaths), bronchitis (235), or stroke (97). A further 17% were certified as due to bronchopneumonia (167 deaths).

TABLE IV—*Standardised mortality ratios for causes of death at ages 55–74 years in 1968–78, both sexes (figures in parentheses are numbers of deaths)*

Cause of death	ICD No (8th revision)	Nelson	Colne	Burnley
All causes	001–999	100 (2258)	109 (1468)	121 (5646)
Ischaemic heart disease	410–414	106 (707)	119 (473)	120 (1662)
Bronchitis	490–492	134 (175)	132 (102)	188 (503)
Pneumonia	480–486	108 (120)	125 (82)	174 (392)
Stroke	431–438	101 (242)	121 (171)	120 (582)
Lung cancer	162	81 (160)	83 (99)	100 (415)
Stomach cancer	151	106 (66)	127 (47)	132 (170)
Other cancers	140–209 less 151, 162	87 (310)	102 (219)	96 (720)
Other causes	Codes 001–009 not used above	97 (478)	93 (275)	117 (1202)

CURRENT SOCIOECONOMIC CONDITIONS

Data from the 1971 census (table V) show that compared with England and Wales the three towns have a higher percentage of men in social classes III manual, IV, and V. This excess is greatest in Nelson. For housing, overcrowding, car ownership, and other socioeconomic indexes the towns are also worse than the average for England and Wales, with the exception of domestic overcrowding in Colne. Only in the percentage of households owning a car, which is an indicator of income, is there a worsening gradient from Nelson to Colne to Burnley. The outstanding feature of the industry in the towns has been the decline in cotton weaving, less than 20% of the workforce in any of the towns being employed in the cotton industry in 1971. New industries include light engineering and the manufacture of aerospace equipment. The pattern of employment in the towns is similar.

Discussion

In three industrial towns in nothern England that are situated side by side there are large differences in current death rates. In Burnley (famous through its association with Sir James MacKenzie, who practised medicine there from 1879 to 1907) adult mortality at ages 55–74 is one of the highest in any of the large towns in England and Wales. In Colne mortality is only 9% above average, whereas in Nelson, which is situated between the others, mortality is average (table IV). Eighty per cent of the excess mortality in Burnley is certified as due to ischaemic heart disease, chronic bronchitis, stroke, or bronchopneumonia. The last of these is given as the underlying cause of death from several types of chronic disease. Excluding cancer of the stomach, cancer mortality is around the national average.

TABLE V—*Socioeconomic indexes in 1971 and infant mortality 1968–72*

	Nelson	Colne	Burnley	England and Wales
Employed men in social classes (%):				
I	2	3	3	5
II	13	14	13	18
IIIN	8	10	10	12
IIIM	48	47	45	38
IV	18	16	20	18
V	11	11	10	9
Households with exclusive use all amenities (%)*	67	72	63	82
People living more than one person per room (%)	14	10	14	12
Households in dwellings of less than five rooms (%)	55	44	51	36
Households owning a car (%)	40	36	34	52
Infant mortality 1968–72	20	19	22	18
Total population	31 249	18 940	76 513	

*Hot water, fixed bath, inside lavatory.

Mortality from lung cancer, which is an index of cigarette smoking, is average or below average.

The close proximity of the towns precludes explaining the large differences in mortality in terms of environmental variables such as rainfall. Nor is it likely that there are important differences in medical care. The hospital services for the towns are centred on Burnley. Rather the effect of socioeconomic factors is suggested. Recent census data show all three towns to be among the poorer towns in England and Wales as indicated by the high percentage of manual workers, by type of housing, and by income. Differences between Nelson and Burnley, however, are small and less than the differences from the national average. Interestingly, Nelson has the greatest excess of manual workers but nevertheless has a mortality rate from all causes that is equal to the national average.

The present similarity of the towns belies the large differences that formerly existed and led to large differences in mortality among infants and young children. These differences included the health and physique of mothers, infant feeding practices, housing, and sanitation but not income or occupation.

Nelson is newer than the other two towns. The people were recent migrants from nearby rural areas rather than second or third generation industrial workers. More of the women—described as "sturdier and healthier" than those in Burnley—breast fed their infants and did so for longer. The birth rate in Nelson was the lowest of the three towns. The housing was more spacious, and domestic overcrowding, measured by the percentage of the population living more than two persons to a room, was less. There were fewer back to back houses and single room dwellings than in the other towns. The effects of poor housing in Burnley may have been compounded by unusually damp soil. Nelson had better sanitation than the other two towns as a result of better refuse disposal and street cleaning and more vigorous action against fly breeding.

We have shown that within the 212 local authority groupings in England and Wales there is a close geographical relation between neonatal mortality during 1921–5 and ischaemic heart disease and stroke mortality in 1968–78 (chapter 4). We interpret this as evidence that poor maternal health and physique and impaired prenatal and postnatal growth and development of the infant are major risk factors for the two diseases. In addition, ischaemic heart disease is related to postneonatal mortality. Thus giving artificial feeds to infants, early weaning, and frequent respiratory or enteric infection in infancy may also be risk factors for the disease. We suggest that past variations in prenatal and early postnatal influences determined the current geographical distribution of ischaemic heart disease and stroke in England and Wales. The gradient in neonatal mortality and the "group of five" diseases during 1911–13 from Nelson up to Burnley, the description of better maternal physique and health in Nelson, and the lower birth rate accord with the current lower rates of ischaemic heart disease and stroke in the town.

We have also shown a close geographical relation between past infant mortality from bronchitis and pneumonia and current mortality from chronic bronchitis and emphysema in England and Wales (chapter 3). We interpret this as strong support for the hypothesis that pulmonary infection during infancy may have persisting effects and lead to chronic bronchitis in adult life. The gradient in postneonatal mortality, specifically mortality from bronchitis and pneumonia, from Nelson up to Burnley accords with the current lower rates of chronic bronchitis in Nelson. Aspects that are likely to have determined the lower infant mortality from respiratory disease in Nelson include better housing, lower level of domestic over-crowding, and more infants being breast fed.

The findings presented in this chapter allow interpretations of differences in adult mortality other than as a major effect of the prenatal and early postnatal environment. Although mortality from cancer, apart from lung and stomach cancer, is little different in Nelson and Burnley and below the national average in both, mortality from all causes other than ischaemic heart disease, stroke, bronchitis, pneumonia, and cancer is highest in Burnley. Diseases contributing to this excess include those with origins in early life—for example, chronic rheumatic heart disease—and others with more immediate origins, such as accidents, poisonings, and violence.

Our evidence for the importance of the prenatal and early postnatal environment rests on close geographical correlations that are remarkably consistent in both sexes, all age groups, and the different geographical areas throughout England and Wales (chapters 1–4). The findings in Burnley, Colne, and Nelson add little to the evidence. They do, however, give a detailed insight into differences in maternal characteristics and the postnatal environment which might have determined current differences in adult mortality.

The inability to find specific explanations for the geographical differences in mortality in Britain has led to a variety of hypotheses. The Black report concluded that "much, we feel, can only be understood in terms of the more diffuse consequences of the class structure."[1] We suggest that specific explanations may be found in the environmental influences that determined past differences in child development. These explanations may allow a national strategy for reducing inequalities in health to be developed.

We thank Dr Peter Grime, district medical officer for Burnley, and Pendle and Rossendale Health Authority for help in obtaining information about the three towns.

1 Townsend P, Davidson N. *Inequalities of health: the Black report*. Harmondsworth: Penguin, 1982.
2 Barker DJP. Geographical variations in disease in Britain. *BMJ* 1981;**283**:398–400.
3 Smith R. Whatever happened to the Black report? *BMJ* 1986;**293**:91–2.
4 Woolf B. Studies on infant mortality: part II, social aetiology of stillbirths and infant deaths in county boroughs of England and Wales. *British Journal of Social Medicine* 1947;**2**:73–125.
5 Local Government Board. *Thirty ninth annual report, 1909–10. Supplement to the report of the board's medical officer*. London: HMSO, 1910.
6 Local Government Board. *Forty third annual report, 1913–14. Supplement in continuation of the report of the medical officer of the board for 1913–14*. London: HMSO, 1914.
7 Gardner MJ, Winter PD, Barker DJP. *Atlas of mortality from selected diseases in England and Wales 1968–1978*. Chichester: Wiley, 1984.
8 Census Office. *Census of England and Wales 1911*. London: HMSO, 1917.
9 Local Government Board. *Forty second annual report, 1912–13. Supplement in continuation of the report of the medical officer of the board for 1912–13*. London: HMSO, 1913.
10 Office of Population Censuses and Surveys. *Census of England and Wales 1971*. London: HMSO, 1975.
11 Office of Population Censuses and Surveys. *Registrar general's statistical review of England and Wales*. Part 1. Tables, medical. London: HMSO, 1921 and following years.
12 Gardner MJ, Winter PD, Taylor CP, Acheson ED. *Atlas of cancer mortality in England and Wales 1968–1978*. Chichester: Wiley, 1983.

6: Risk of death from cardiovascular disease and chronic bronchitis determined by place of birth in England and Wales

C OSMOND, D J P BARKER, J M SLATTERY

The death certificates of nearly 2 million people who died in England and Wales from April 1969 to December 1972 were used to examine the relation between place of birth and cause of death.

Persons born in northern counties and industrial towns, and in Wales, had increased risk of ischaemic heart disease and stroke, which persisted whether or not they had moved to other parts of the country. A low risk of cardiovascular disease among people born in and around London went with them when they moved. People born in cities and large towns had an increased and persisting risk of chronic bronchitis.

These findings are evidence that past geographical differences in fetal and infant growth, and in exposure to respiratory infection in early childhood, partly determine today's differences in adult death rates.

Introduction

The environment in intrauterine life and early childhood may influence adult health more than has previously been supposed (chapters 1 to 5). Evidence for this comes mainly from epidemiological studies, and the underlying processes are not well understood.

In the early years of this century, when people now dying in middle and late life were born, there were large differences in the early environment between one part of Britain and another. These were determined by differences in the health and physique of mothers, infant rearing practices, overcrowding in the home, and population density.[12] The effects on child growth and health were reflected in large differences in child mortality. In 1911–15, for example, infant mortality ranged from 68 per 1000 births in rural Sussex to 171 in Burnley.

If the environment in early life has an important effect, a person's risk of disease will be predicted by place of birth. This can be explored by examining disease rates in people who migrate from their place of birth, as the effects of the environment in early life can be distinguished from that encountered later on. Disease in migrants can be analysed using data from death certificates because place of birth is recorded. We have analysed cause of death in 2 million people born in England and Wales, half of whom migrated to another part of the country during their lives.

We present findings for ischaemic heart disease, stroke, and chronic bronchitis. Death rates from each of these serve as a useful indicator of incidence, and the numbers of deaths are sufficient to allow detailed geographical analysis. Death rates from ischaemic heart disease and stroke are higher in the north and west of the country, whereas for chronic bronchitis they are higher in the towns. There is epidemiological evidence that the early life environment is important in all three diseases (chapters 1 to 4). In bronchitis the evidence is supported by studies of migrants from one country to another.[3] Among British born men who migrated to the United States the prevalence of chronic bronchitis, after allowing for smoking habits, was higher than among migrants from Norway. It was higher among those born in urban areas of Britain and was unrelated to age at migration.

Methods

Place of birth within England and Wales is recorded on death certificates, but not routinely coded. For a trial period from April 1969 to December 1972, however, the Office of Population Censuses and Surveys (OPCS) did code the place of birth. These data, which have not been analysed before, were made available to us. There were 1 907 999 deaths in England and Wales among people who were also born there. For each death we had seven items of information; place of birth, place of usual residence at time of death, sex, age at death in years, year of death, underlying cause of death coded to the eighth revision of the International Classification of Diseases (ICD), and occupation (for 1970–2 only, used to estimate social class).

Place of birth and death were coded to the 80 county boroughs, that is large towns, 15 London boroughs, and 57 administrative counties, which together comprise England and Wales. The OPCS coded Montgomeryshire and Radnorshire administrative counties identically; and births in Rutlandshire administrative county were coded as occurring in Leicestershire administrative county. Some places of birth were given as "London" without specifying the borough, and were analysed separately. The analyses were therefore based on 153 areas.

We grouped ages at death into 10 year bands, from 0 to 9 up to 90 and over. We ignored year of death because the data spanned less than four years. We analysed death from ischaemic heart disease (ICD 410–414), stroke (ICD 431–438), and chronic bronchitis (ICD 490–492).

The place where each individual lived was known only at birth and death. There was no denominator to calculate death rates for those who were born in one area and died in another, and we therefore used the proportion of all deaths that were due to each cause. To explore how these proportions varied according to birthplace and place of death we used a log linear regression.[4] For each disease and place this gave two numbers which were based on proportions of deaths in each age, sex, and social class stratum. These represented the effect on the disease of either birth or death in that place. We refer to the numbers as the "place of birth" and the "place of death" effects. Their average value is 1·00.

Results for men and women were similar. We used deaths from stomach cancer, which show a steep social class gradient,[5] to explore the effect of social class on place of birth effects. Values after adjustment for social class were similar to those unadjusted, the largest differences being 0·01. We therefore present unadjusted values for men and women combined.

The size of the place of birth effects does not necessarily represent the strength of their effect on disease risk. They are based on proportions of deaths from one cause in relation to all other causes. A high value may reflect deficits of deaths from other causes rather than a high risk associated with the place of birth. This is the fundamental disadvantage of proportional data analysis. The range of values taken by the place of birth effects is not immediately comparable across diseases which occur with different frequency, diseases which cause fewer deaths tending to have a greater range.

Results

From April 1969 to December 1972 there were 475 547 deaths from ischaemic heart disease, 251 565 from stroke, and 94 707 from chronic bronchitis among men and women who were born in England and Wales. For each disease there was a considerable spread in the place of birth effects. As predicted from the numbers of deaths from each cause, the range of place of birth effects was smallest for ischaemic heart disease and highest for chronic bronchitis. The range for ischaemic heart disease was from 0·89 to 1·12, for stroke from 0·86 to 1·19, and for chronic bronchitis from 0·83 to 1·24.

We calculated χ^2 statistics for the variation in place of birth effects both independently of and in relation to place of death effects (table I). The "joint" χ^2 statistic was derived from the model. For the "conditional" statistic all possible variation was conceded to the place of death effect. Each disease had joint and conditional place of birth effects, which were strongly significant.

Tables II and III list places where the place of birth effects were in the bottom and top tenth of the distributions and were significantly different from unity using a test at the 5% level. For ischaemic heart disease there were high place of birth effects in a number of industrial towns and counties in the north and west. The striking feature for stroke was the low place of birth effects in a group of London boroughs. For chronic bronchitis there were high place of birth effects in a group of towns and London boroughs and in two industrialised counties in South Wales.

We examined the relation between place of birth effects and standardised mortality ratios. To obtain stable estimates we calculated standardised mortality ratios for the 11 years 1968–78, which is the period covered by the eighth revision of the ICD. For each cause of death the geographical distribution of place of birth effects correlated positively with the distribution of standardised mortality ratios. The correlation coefficients were 0·63 for ischaemic heart disease, 0·56 for stroke, and 0·38 for chronic bronchitis. These correlations would have been influenced by use of an analysis based upon proportional mortality. For example, Burnley county borough had a low place of birth effect for stroke (table II), but a standardised mortality ratio of 120. Because mortality ratios from other leading causes were even higher, the proportion of deaths due to stroke was below average, and the low place of birth effect is likely to reflect this.

Discussion

This analysis of 2 million men and women, half of whom migrated from one part of England and Wales to another, shows that a person's risk of dying from ischaemic heart disease, stroke, and chronic bronchitis is predicted by place of birth, independently of place of death. Part of the increased risk of ischaemic heart disease and stroke among people born in many northern counties and industrial towns, and in Wales, persists whether or not they move to other areas of the country. The low risk of cardiovascular disease, especially stroke, among people born in and around London goes with them when they move. People born in cities and large towns have an increased and persisting risk of chronic bronchitis.

Our analysis had to be based on the proportion of all deaths due to one

TABLE I—χ^2 *statistics with 152 degrees of freedom, for strength of place of birth effects: values exceeding 189 are significant at the 5% level*

	Ischaemic heart disease	Stroke	Chronic bronchitis
Independent	1547	2077	2242
Joint	587	567	522
Conditional	320	372	327

TABLE II—*Areas with place of birth effects for ischaemic heart disease, stroke, and chronic bronchitis in the bottom tenth of the distribution and significantly different from unity*

Ischaemic heart disease	Stroke	Chronic bronchitis
Bournemouth CB	Birkenhead CB	Bradford CB
Great Yarmouth CB	Bootle CB	Halifax CB
Nottingham CB	Burnley CB	Norwich CB
Anglesey AC	Dudley CB	Essex AC
Caernarvonshire AC	Grimsby CB	Lincolnshire (Kesteven) AC
Somerset AC	Camden LB	Norfolk AC
Sussex, East AC	Hackney LB	Yorkshire East Riding AC
Sussex, West AC	Hammersmith LB	
Wight, Isle of AC	Lewisham LB	
	Newham LB	
	Southwark LB	
	Tower Hamlets LB	
	Westminster LB	

CB = county borough; AC = administrative county; LB = London borough

TABLE III—*Areas with place of birth effects for ischaemic heart disease, stroke, and chronic bronchitis in the top tenth of the distribution and significantly different from unity*

Ischaemic heart disease	Stroke	Chronic bronchitis
Bradford CB	Blackburn CB	Birkenhead CB
Dewsbury CB	Preston CB	Cardiff CB
Halifax CB	Southport CB	Grimsby CB
Huddersfield CB	Wigan CB	Hastings CB
Preston CB	Anglesey AC	St Helens CB
Cardiganshire AC	Cambridgeshire AC	Stockport CB
Carmarthenshire AC	Denbighshire AC	Warley CB
Cumberland AC	Lincolnshire (Kesteven) AC	Wigan CB
Northumberland AC	Northamptonshire AC	Westminster LB
Westmorland AC	Yorkshire North Riding AC	Glamorganshire AC
Yorkshire West Riding AC		Monmouthshire AC

CB = county borough; AC = administrative county; LB = London borough

83

cause, rather than on death rates. For the reasons given, the values of place of birth effects for each disease do not necessarily represent the strength of their effect on disease risk. The finding of a strong effect of birthplace on risk of chronic bronchitis is, however, consistent with a similar effect found in migrants from Britain to the United States.[3] Additional analyses, published elsewhere, also show a strong effect of birthplace on risk of stomach cancer, another disease for which studies of international migrants show a large effect.[6]

Our results conflict with the conclusions of a recent analysis based on 43 episodes of ischaemic heart disease in 1177 middle aged men who migrated from one of three regions of England and Wales, or from Scotland, to another region.[7] The absence of an important effect of place of birth in that analysis contrasts with the large effect we have observed for men and women, at all ages and in 153 areas. We have assigned our 153 areas to the three regions of England and Wales and find in our data that the independent, joint, and conditional χ^2 statistics (table I) all give values that are higher for place of birth than for place of death. In each region the proportion of deaths due to ischaemic heart disease is greatest among those born in the northern region.

Studies of migrants need careful interpretation as their risk of disease is unlikely to be representative of the populations they leave. Furthermore, in our study the place where each individual lived was known only at birth and death and we cannot determine the age at which the place of birth acts in the genesis of each disease. A place of birth effect could reflect predisposition to disease related to social customs that are acquired in childhood, but which migrants take with them and which act in later life, dietary customs for example. Place of birth effects could also reflect genetic variations in susceptibility, although the large changes in incidence of each of the diseases during this century point to the dominance of the environment in determining their distribution.

Other evidence suggests that, though influences on the adult environment such as cigarette smoking are important, the environment in early life also has a major effect on the risk of cardiovascular disease and chronic bronchitis. The geographical distribution of cardiovascular mortality throughout England and Wales is closely related to maternal and neonatal mortality 70 and more years ago (chapter 4). The effect of place of birth may therefore depend on past differences in maternal health and fetal and infant growth. Blood pressure levels in adult life are inversely related to fetal growth and are one possible link between birthplace and cardiovascular risk.

The effect of birthplace on the risk of chronic bronchitis may be determined by past differences in the incidence of lower respiratory tract infection in early life (chapter 3). These in turn depended on differences in housing, family size, crowding in the home, and infant feeding. Evidence that childhood respiratory function is causally linked to chronic bronchitis comes from prospective studies showing that lower respiratory infection before the age of 2 may be followed by respiratory symptoms and abnormalities of pulmonary function in later childhood and early adult life.[8-11]

This analysis of one million people who moved from one part of England and Wales to another is further evidence that the environment in intrauterine life and early childhood has a larger effect on adult cardiovascular disease than has previously been supposed, and partly determines today's geographical inequalities in health. Measurements of this effect must, however, await the results of prospective studies which are now in progress.

1 Local Government Board. *42nd annual report, 1912–13. Supplement in continuation of the report of the medical officer of the board for 1912–13*. London: HMSO, 1913.
2 Campbell JM. *Maternal morality*. London: HMSO, 1924. (Ministry of Health Reports on Public Health and Medical subjects. No. 25).
3 Reid DD, Fletcher CM. International studies in chronic respiratory disease. *Br Med Bull* 1971;**27**:59–64.
4 Osmond C, Slattery JM, Barker DJP. Mortality by place of birth. In: *Mortality and geography*. London: HMSO, 1990. (Office of Population Censuses and Surveys Decennial Supplement No. 9).
5 Coggon D, Acheson ED. The geography of cancer of the stomach. *Br Med Bull* 1984;**40**:335–41.
6 Coggon D, Osmond C, Barker DJP. Stomach cancer and migration within England and Wales. *Br J Cancer* 1990;**61**:573–4.
7 Elford J, Phillips AN, Thomson AG, Shaper AG. Migration and geographic variations in ischaemic heart disease in Great Britain. *Lancet* 1989;i:343–6.
8 Gurwitz D, Mindorff C, Levison H. Increased incidence of bronchial reactivity in children with a history of bronchiolitis. *Pediatrics* 1981;**98**:551–5.
9 Pullan CR, Hey EN. Wheezing, asthma, and pulmonary dysfunction 10 years after infection with respiratory syncytial virus in infancy. *BMJ* 1982;**284**:1665–9.
10 Mok JYQ, Simpson H. Outcome of acute bronchitis, bronchiolitis, and pneumonia in infancy. *Arch Dis Child* 1984;**59**:306–9.
11 Kierman KE, Colley JRT, Douglas JWB, Reid DD. Chronic cough in young adults in relation to smoking habits, childhood environment and chest illness. *Respiration* 1976;**33**:236–44.

7: Height and mortality in the counties of England and Wales

D J P BARKER, C OSMOND, J GOLDING

Average heights of adults and children in the counties of England and Wales were examined using national samples of people born between 1920 and 1970. Although height increased over this 50 year period, the differences between counties persisted. Average height in a county is closely related to its pattern of death rates, which were derived from all deaths during 1968–78. Counties with taller populations have lower mortality from chronic bronchitis, rheumatic heart disease, ischaemic heart disease, and stroke, and higher mortality from three hormone related cancers, of the breast, prostate and ovary. The inverse relation of height with bronchitis and cardiovascular disease is further evidence of risk factors acting in early childhood. The positive relation between height and cancers of the breast, ovary, and prostate could suggest that promotion of child growth has disadvantages as well as benefits.

Introduction

Promotion of the growth of children by better nutrition, hygiene, housing, and child care has been a major public health objective in Britain since the turn of the century. In the early years importance was attached to improving the physique of young men whose poor state, especially in some northern areas, was revealed during recruitment for the South African war.[1] The relation between poor physique in women and maternal mortality was recognised later.[2] From the beginning better child growth was assumed to reflect better child health and to lead to improved health in adult life. Adult height increased progressively,[3] but large differences between geographical areas and social groups persisted, at least up to the second world war.[4]

Recent epidemiological findings, described in previous chapters of this book, suggest that the risks of several important causes of adult death, including ischaemic heart disease, stroke, and bronchitis, are partly determined by influences which act during early childhood. Height is largely determined by growth in childhood,[5] and relations between adult diseases and childhood influences can therefore be explored through associations between the diseases and height.

We have used data on height in three national surveys of children and their parents to examine the trends and differences between the counties in England and Wales, over the past 60 years. We have related average heights in the counties to the pattern of adult mortality.

Methods

HEIGHTS

1946 Cohort: The 1946 cohort was taken from 82% of all infants born alive in Britain during one week in March 1946.[6] Twins and illegitimate children were not followed up. Of the remainder, all who were the children of non-manual and agricultural workers were followed up together with one in four children of manual workers. Our analysis is based on 3503 children born in England and Wales, whose heights were measured at age 11 years, and on the self reported heights of their parents.

1958 Cohort: 98·5% of all births in Britain during one week in March 1958 were included in the British perinatal mortality survey.[7] Mother's height was measured antenatally and social class of the head of the household was recorded. The surviving children were followed up at 11 years, when their heights were measured and those of their fathers were reported. Our analysis is based on the 10 445 children born in England and Wales and their parents.

1970 Cohort: 97·5% of all births in Britain during one week in April 1970 were included in the British births survey.[8][9] Social class of the head of the household was recorded. The surviving children were followed up at 10 years when their heights were measured and parents' heights were reported. Our analysis is based on the 10 602 children born in England and Wales and their parents.

MORTALITY

The Office of Population Censuses and Surveys made available extracts from all death certificates in England and Wales during 1968–78, the period covered by the 8th revision of the International Classification of Diseases.[10] Our analysis is based on mortality at ages 35–74 in both sexes combined or in the sex usually affected. Rates for each of the 60 counties were based on population data from the 1971 census and were expressed as standardised mortality ratios.

Results

We ordered the 60 counties according to the average heights of parents and children in the three cohorts. We divided the counties into five groups such that the numbers of people in each group were as similar as possible. Table I lists the counties in each group. The counties with the shortest people were in the north or west of the country. Most of those with the tallest people were in the south and east, around London.

Table II shows the mean heights of men, women, boys, and girls in the five groups of counties. We used age at the time of birth of their children to estimate average year of birth of the adults. Within each group of counties average height of men increased from the oldest, born around 1920, to the youngest, born around 1945. There was no similar increase in average height of women. Heights of children were not comparable because they were measured at different ages. There was a consistent increase in height from group 1, the shortest group, up to group 5, the tallest, in each generation and in both sexes. The difference between groups 1 and 5 ranged from 1·5 to 2·6 cms. Standard errors in this table range from 0·06 to 0·17. Standardisation for each person's social class made little difference. Table II gives social class standardised heights in the shortest and tallest groups. They are similar to the unstandardised heights.

Table III shows standardised mortality ratios from leading causes of adult death in the five groups of counties during 1968–78. All standardised mortality ratios are based on a minimum of 3500 deaths. In men and

TABLE I—*The counties of England and Wales grouped according to average height*

Group	Counties
1 (shortest)	Durham, Hereford, Lancashire, Northumberland, Caernarvon, Cardigan, Carmarthen, Glamorgan, Merioneth, Monmouth, Radnor
2	Cumberland, Gloucestershire, Lincolnshire (Holland), Lincolnshire (Lindsey), Staffordshire, Yorkshire (East, North and West Riding), Anglesey, Brecknock, Denbigh, and Montgomery
3	Cornwall, London, Nottinghamshire, Shropshire, Warwick, Worcestershire, Flint, Pembroke
4	Bedfordshire, Berkshire, Cambridgeshire, Cheshire, Derbyshire, Essex, Huntingdonshire, Leicestershire, Middlesex, Norfolk, Oxfordshire, Suffolk (East), Wiltshire
5 (tallest)	Buckinghamshire, Devon, Dorset, Hampshire, Hertfordshire, Kent, Lincolnshire (Kesteven), Northamptonshire, Rutland, Somerset, Suffolk (West), Surrey, Sussex (East and West), Westmorland, Isle of Wight

TABLE II—*Mean heights in centimetres of men, women, boys and girls in three national surveys in the counties of England and Wales grouped by average height*

Survey	Year of birth	Group of counties					Social class standardised heights	
		1 Short	2	3	4	5 Tall	Group 1	Group 5
Men								
1946 cohort	ca 1920	172·4	172·9	173·9	173·3	174·4	172·5	174·4
1958 cohort	ca 1930	173·7	174·4	174·5	175·5	175·5	173·8	175·2
1970 cohort	ca 1945	174·3	175·1	175·4	175·6	176·4	174·6	176·2
Women								
1946 cohort	ca 1920	160·0	160·9	161·7	161·6	162·1	160·1	162·1
1958 cohort	ca 1930	160·3	161·1	161·1	161·7	162·1	160·4	162·0
1970 cohort	ca 1945	160·4	161·2	161·4	161·7	162·7	160·5	162·6
Boys								
1946 cohort (age 11)	1946	140·2	140·2	141·0	141·7	141·8	140·3	141·8
1958 cohort (age 11)	1958	142·9	143·7	144·4	145·0	145·0	143·1	144·9
1970 cohort (age 10)	1970	138·0	138·4	138·9	138·9	139·5	138·2	139·4
Girls								
1946 cohort (age 11)	1946	139·5	139·9	142·3	141·6	142·1	139·6	142·0
1958 cohort (age 11)	1958	143·5	144·4	145·9	145·5	146·1	143·6	146·0
1970 cohort (age 10)	1970	137·7	137·8	138·9	138·8	139·3	137·8	139·2

women standardised mortality ratios for bronchitis, rheumatic heart disease, ischaemic heart disease, and stroke fell progressively from the shortest to the tallest group of counties. Prostatic, breast, and ovarian cancer showed an opposite trend. There was no clear trend for lung cancer.

Discussion

There is a remarkably close relation between average height in the counties of England and Wales and patterns of mortality. In the three national cohorts the heights of parents were self reported, except for those of mothers in the 1958 cohort whose heights were measured. Those of men show, however, the progressive increase in successive generations which would be expected from other data.[3] The heights of children were measured. Despite changes in average height, differences between the counties of England and Wales have remained stable (table II). They are still evident in 10 year old children born in 1970. The differences do not

TABLE III—*Standarised mortality ratios at ages 35–74, 1968–78, in the counties of England and Wales grouped by average height*

Cause of death	Group of counties				
	1 Short	2	3	4	5 Tall
Men					
All causes	114	105	102	92	89
Bronchitis	131	113	108	84	73
Rheumatic heart disease	118	109	106	90	79
Ischaemic heart disease	115	107	95	93	90
Stroke	121	113	96	89	84
Prostatic cancer	92	96	101	101	107
Lung cancer	109	101	108	95	90
Women					
All causes	113	105	99	94	90
Bronchitis	138	113	107	82	68
Rheumatic heart disease	125	112	107	88	72
Ischaemic heart disease	124	113	91	90	83
Stroke	117	110	93	93	88
Breast cancer	93	96	102	103	105
Ovarian cancer	88	103	98	102	106
Lung cancer	99	90	111	98	102

depend on the varying social class composition of the populations of the counties, as adjustment of mean height for social class has little effect (table II). The stability of the differences could result from either prenatal or postnatal influences on child growth. The large movements of population within England and Wales during the industrial revolution make it unlikely that genetic influences determine them.[11] Stability of influences in the prenatal environment through successive generations is suggested by the positive correlation between the birth weights of mothers and their babies.[12] The postnatal influences on growth which persist in a place could include infant feeding practices, housing, and population density.[13]

Counties with taller populations have lower mortality from chronic bronchitis, chronic rheumatic heart disease, ischaemic heart disease, and stroke, and higher mortality from three hormone related cancers, in the breast, ovary, and prostate.

The inverse geographical relation of height with chronic bronchitis and cardiovascular disease is consistent with other evidence of risk factors for these diseases acting in childhood. Acute lower respiratory tract infections in early childhood are thought to be a major determinant of risk of chronic bronchitis in adult life (chapter 3). Evidence for this comes from several sources including the close geographical relation between infant mortality from lower respiratory tract infections in England and Wales during the early years of this century and current mortality from chronic bronchitis. Respiratory borne infection in childhood is also known to be the cause of chronic rheumatic heart disease. The link between chronic bronchitis, rheumatic heart disease, and shorter stature may be through a direct effect of recurrent respiratory infection in childhood on growth rates.[14] The lack of a consistent trend in lung cancer mortality with height (table III) suggests that the link is not through an association between cigarette smoking and height.

Evidence that an adverse environment during early childhood has an important effect on the later risk of cardiovascular disease rests on the close geographical relation between maternal and neonatal mortality in England and Wales 70 and more years ago and current cardiovascular mortality (chapters 1 and 2). This is interpreted as evidence that maternal health and fetal and infant growth partly determine later risk of cardiovascular disease. Blood pressure levels in adult life are inversely related to fetal growth and are one possible link between early growth and cardiovascular risk (chapter 15). An inverse relation between height and cardiovascular disease has been found in prospective studies of three populations: 1·8 million people in Norway who attended for mass radiography,[16] 17 000 male civil servants in London,[17] and 1700 men in Finland.[18]

Early menarche is one of the four major risk factors for breast cancer[19 20] and the positive relation between height and breast cancer mortality in the counties is consistent with an association between improvement in growth in populations and earlier age at menarche.[3] To our knowledge there is no known link between childhood growth and cancers in the ovary and prostate. However, the positive geographical association between these three cancers and height within England and Wales is reflected in their international distribution and time trends. All three are more common in wealthier countries. In England and Wales as height has increased rates of the cancers have risen. Breast cancer mortality in England and Wales has increased continuously over 30 years; ovarian cancer mortality has risen in women aged over 55; prostatic cancer mortality has increased for the past 15 years.[21] One interpretation of these associations between greater height and hormone related cancers is that promotion of child growth has disadvantages as well as benefits.

We thank Peter Thomas and Richard Belli, who helped with the computing.

1 Smyth AM. *Physical deterioration, its causes and the cure*. London: John Murray, 1904.
2 Campbell JM. *Maternal mortality*. London: HMSO, 1924. (Ministry of Health Reports on Public Health and Medical Subjects, No 25).
3 Wieringen J Van. Secular growth changes. In: Falkner F, Tanner J, eds. *Human growth*. 2nd ed, Vol 3. New York: Plenum, 1986.
4 Orr JB. *Food, health and income*. London: MacMillan, 1936.
5 Tanner J, Healy M, Lockhart R, MacKenzie J, Whitehouse R. Aberdeen growth study. 1. The prediction of adult body measurements from measurements taken each year from birth to 5 years. *Arch Dis Child* 1956;**31**:372.
6 Wadsworth M. Follow-up of the first national birth cohort: findings from the Medical Research Council National Survey of Health and Development. *Paediatr Perinat Epidemiol* 1987;**1**:95–116.

7 Davie R, Butler NR, Goldstein H. *From birth to seven: a report of the National Child Development Study.* London: Longman, 1972.
8 Butler NR, Golding J, Haslum M, Stewart-Brown S. Recent findings of the 1970 child health and education study: preliminary communication. *J R Soc Med* 1982;75:781–4.
9 Butler NR, Golding J. *From birth to five: a study of the health and behaviour of Britain's five year olds.* Oxford: Pergamon, 1986.
10 Gardner MJ, Winter PD, Barker DJP. *Atlas of mortality from selected diseases in England and Wales 1968–78.* Chichester: Wiley, 1984.
11 Office of Population Censuses and Surveys. *Census of England and Wales 1911. Volume IX. Birthplaces.* London: HMSO, 1913.
12 Little RE. Mother's and father's birthweight as predictors of infant birthweight. *Paediatr Perinat Epidemiol* 1987;1:19–31.
13 Falkner F, Tanner JM. Methodology, ecological, genetic and nutritional effects on growth. In: *Human growth, a comprehensive treatise.* 2nd ed, Vol 3. New York and London: Plenum, 1986.
14 Rona RJ, Florey C du V. National study of health and growth: respiratory symptoms and height in primary schoolchildren. *Int J Epidemiol* 1980;9:35–43.
15 Wadsworth MEJ, Cripps HA, Midwinter RE, Colley JRT. Blood pressure in a national birth cohort at the age of 36 related to social and familial factors, smoking, and body mass. *BMJ* 1985;291:1534–8.
16 Waaler HT. Height, weight and mortality. The Norwegian experience. *Acta Med Scand [Suppl]* 1984;679:1–56.
17 Marmot MG, Shipley MJ, Rose G. Inequalities in death—specific explanations of a general pattern? *Lancet* 1984;i:1003–6.
18 Notkola V. *Living conditions in childhood and coronary heart disease in adulthood.* Helsinki: Finnish Society of Sciences and Letters, 1985.
19 Armstrong B, Doll R. Environmental factors and cancer incidence and mortality in different countries, with special reference to dietary practices. *Int J Cancer* 1975;15:617–31.
20 Pike MC, Ross RK. Breast cancer. *Br Med Bull* 1984;40:351–4.
21 Office of Population Censuses and Surveys. *Registrar general's statistical review of England and Wales.* Part 1. Tables, medical. London: HMSO, 1911 and following years.

8: Diet and inequalities in health in three English towns

J E CADE, D J P BARKER, B M MARGETTS,
J A MORRIS

The diets of 2340 middle aged men and women living in three English towns were recorded. Consumption of fat and the other main nutrients was lowest in the northern industrial town, which had the highest death rates from ischaemic heart disease and from all causes combined.

The findings suggest that differences in diet in middle age are not a major cause of differences in adult mortality between one part of Britain and another.

Introduction

Differences in the diets of middle aged men and women are thought to contribute to the large geographical and social class differences in mortality and morbidity in Britain. Evidence, however, is lacking. The National Food Survey, which each year records food purchases within a sample of around 7500 households, is the only large source of data on the national diet, but it does not record consumption separately for men and women or at different ages.[1]

We describe the first large study comparing the diets of middle aged men and women in different areas of England with differing mortality and morbidity from diseases thought to have dietary causes.

Population and methods

The three towns studied, Ipswich, Stoke-on-Trent, and Wakefield, were included among nine towns in England and Wales previously selected for a series of morbidity surveys.[2] The towns were defined by the local authority boundaries used before the changes in 1974. Socioeconomic indices were abstracted from published data from the 1981 census.[3] The Office of

Population Censuses and Surveys made available to us extracts from all death certificates in England and Wales during 1968–78, the period covered by the eighth revision of the International Classification of Diseases (ICD). Death rates for each sex for each town were calculated from 1971 census data.[4] Death rates were expressed as standardised mortality ratios.

In each town a sample of men and women aged 35–54 was taken from the lists of general practitioners. To obtain a social class distribution representative of the town the practices were in different electoral wards. In Ipswich there were 14 practices from 10 of the 16 wards, in Stoke 16 practices from 16 of the 20 wards, and in Wakefield five practices from three of the four wards. People were selected by stratified random sampling to give equal numbers in each five year age group in each sex.

We recorded diet by using a 24 hour diary. In comparing the diets of populations it is statistically efficient to have only one day of recordings on each subject and to maximise the number of subjects rather than have two or more days of observations on fewer subjects.[5] Using data from previous dietary studies in Britain[6–8] we estimated that completion of a 24 hour dietary record by samples of 400 men and 400 women in each town would give a 90% chance of detecting differences between any two towns of 10% or more (at the 5% level of significance) in mean daily intakes of energy, total fat, carbohydrate, protein, and total dietary fibre. To achieve this sample size 1150 people were selected initially after a pilot study in Stoke had suggested that 30% of those approached would be unavailable for the survey — usually because they had moved from the address on the general practitioner's list. In each town the survey was carried out during 16 weeks evenly spread through the year May 1984 to April 1985.

An introductory letter signed by the general practitioner was sent to each subject. He or she was asked to complete a 24 hour dietary diary on a specified day during the following week. Days for diary keeping were allocated to give equal numbers for each day of the week. Subjects recorded quantities of food in terms of household measures. A pilot study of 33 people showed that, except for total dietary fibre and vitamin A, estimates of intake of the main nutrients based on household measures were within 10% of those based on weighed food records.

Before the survey a local interviewer was appointed in each town and trained. As soon as possible after the diary day, usually the next day, the local interviewer or one of us (JC) visited the subject at home. The diaries were checked, sizes of portions clarified by using standard models, and the volumes of household utensils measured. If the subject had not kept the diary either another day was allocated or a 24 hour recall for the previous day was taken at interview. Data on fatty foods and vitamins A and C were extended by means of a food frequency questionnaire.

The subjects were also asked about smoking, alcohol consumption, occupation, and residential history. Questions on alcohol were based on those used in the British regional heart study.[9] At interview subjects were weighed on a portable Seca scale and height measured by a stadiometer.

Nutrient intakes were derived from food consumption by using computerised food composition tables.[10-12] When intakes were not normally distributed by reference to the Kolmogorov-Smirnov goodness of fit test they were transformed by using a square root or natural logarithm value. Generalised linear interactive modelling was used for regression analyses.[13]

Results

Table I shows socioeconomic indices in the towns. The indices describe social class distribution, housing, and income, the last as indicated by the proportion of households owning their house or a car. In Ipswich, a southern market town with agricultural industries, the indices were generally around or better than the average for England and Wales. In Stoke, a Midlands town and centre for the pottery industry, and in Wakefield, a northern wool and coal mining town, socioeconomic conditions were generally below average. Stoke has a high proportion of people in manual occupations.

Table II shows the death rates and morbidity. All cause standardised mortality ratios at ages 35–74 were lowest in Ipswich (92 in men, 90 in women). Among men they were similarly high in Stoke and Wakefield (120, 118), whereas among women those in Wakefield were higher (131) than in Stoke (117). The pattern of ischaemic heart disease was similar,

TABLE I—*Socioeconomic indices in the three towns in 1981*

	Ipswich	Stoke	Wakefield	England and Wales
% Of people in social classes*:				
I	4·0	2·1	5·6	5·5
II	19·1	13·2	23·7	24·7
III Non-manual	13·5	8·8	9·6	11·3
III Manual	38·4	50·5	37·7	34·4
IV	15·2	16·0	15·7	16·0
V	6·9	7·3	6·1	6·0
% Of households with more than one person per room	2·0	3·9	3·5	3·4
% Of households in dwellings of fewer than five rooms	24·6	41·5	40·9	35·2
% Of households in owner occupied dwellings	58·1	56·4	41·5	58·1
% Of households owning a car	60·2	52·6	49·3	61·5
Total population	119 500	249 838	59 622	

* Figures for England and Wales are for male population aged 16 and over.

TABLE II—*Standardised mortality ratios and morbidity among men and women*

	Ipswich		Stoke		Wakefield	
	Men	Women	Men	Women	Men	Women
Standardised mortality ratios, 1968–78 (ages 35–74) from:						
All causes	92	90	120	117	118	131
Ischaemic heart disease	89	79	115	128	117	137
Breast cancer	—	103	—	93	—	98
Age standardised yearly incidence of colonic cancer/100 000, 1979–80 (ages <75)	25	18	19	20	12	15
Age standardised percentage prevalence of gall stones, 1977–8 (ages ⩾18)	14·4	29·0	13·5	17·1	6·1	13·4

rising in both sexes combined from 86 in Ipswich to 119 in Stoke and 123 in Wakefield. Trends in mortality from breast cancer, incidence of colonic cancer,[14] and prevalence of gall stones at necropsy[2] were in the opposite direction to those for ischaemic heart disease, rates in Ipswich being higher than in Wakefield.

Food records were obtained from 2340 subjects (1115 men, 1225 women), representing response rates of 86% in Ipswich, 85% in Stoke, and 84% in Wakefield among those who could be contacted. The social class distribution of respondents was closely similar to that of the towns except in Wakefield, where there was overrepresentation of class III non-manual and underrepresentation of class III manual.

TABLE III—*Mean daily intakes of nutrients among men in the three towns.*

	No of men	Energy (MJ) Mean	Energy (MJ) 95% Confidence interval	Fat (g) Mean	Fat (g) 95% Confidence interval	Polyunsaturated fatty acids (g) Mean	Polyunsaturated fatty acids (g) 95% Confidence interval	Saturated fatty acids (g) Mean
Ipswich								
JC	119	10·8	10·1 to 11·4	107·9	100 to 116	14·9	13 to 16	43·3
Local	244	10·5	10·0 to 10·9	105·0	100 to 111	14·8	14 to 16	42·3
Stoke								
JC	128	11·6	11·0 to 12·3	107·9	100 to 116	13·7	12 to 15	44·2
Local	249	11·4	10·9 to 11·9	112·0	106 to 118	14·5	14 to 16	45·1
Wakefield								
JC	110	10·1	9·5 to 10·7	96·5	89 to 104	13·2	12 to 15	38·6
Local	265	9·8	9·4 to 10·2	93·2	88 to 98	12·5	12 to 13	36·8

Though we sought to standardise the way in which dietary information was obtained, there were differences among the towns. More people in Stoke (25%) than in Ipswich (19%) and Wakefield (20%) had dietary records based on recall rather than diaries. More of the records in Wakefield (29%) than in Ipswich (13%) and Stoke (12%) were completed in the summer. One of us (JC) interviewed roughly one third of the respondents in Ipswich (33%), Stoke (35%), and Wakefield (29%). The mean nutrient intakes from her records tended to be higher than those recorded by the local interviewers. The mean daily nutrient intakes in the towns (tables III and IV) were therefore adjusted to take account of the use of diary or recall and the season. Results are shown separately for records completed by JC and the local interviewer.

Among men (table III) intakes of energy, fat, carbohydrate, protein, and total fibre were lowest in Wakefield. Differences in intakes of polyunsaturated and saturated fatty acids were such that in records completed by JC the polyunsaturated to saturated fatty acid ratios were 0·32 in Wakefield, 0·35 in Stoke, and 0·36 in Ipswich, whereas in those completed by local interviewers they were 0·29, 0·31, and 0·36.

Whereas total carbohydrate intake was highest in Stoke, intake of sugar (defined as naturally occurring and added monosaccharides and disaccharides) was highest in Ipswich. Protein intake was highest in Stoke but the proportions of protein derived from animal sources were similar in each town—around 60%. About 45% of the intake of fibre in each town came from cereal products and 16% from potatoes.

As would be expected, energy intakes were lower in women (table IV) and differences in nutrient intake among the towns were smaller. Similarly to men, however, intakes of energy, fat, carbohydrate, sugar, protein, and

Results shown separately for records completed by JC and local interviewer

Saturated fatty acids (g) 95% Confidence interval	Carbohydrate (g) Mean	95% Confidence interval	Sugars (g) Mean	95% Confidence interval	Protein (g) Mean	95% Confidence interval	Total fibre (g) Mean	95% Confidence interval
40 to 47	308·7	289 to 328	120·3	110 to 131	85·4	80 to 91	20·7	19 to 22
40 to 45	291·0	278 to 304	122·1	114 to 130	82·6	79 to 86	19·0	18 to 20
41 to 48	315·1	296 to 334	117·0	107 to 128	94·5	89 to 100	20·2	19 to 22
43 to 48	311·4	298 to 325	110·7	104 to 118	94·2	90 to 98	19·8	19 to 21
35 to 42	271·2	252 to 291	106·0	96 to 117	84·1	79 to 90	17·9	16 to 20
35 to 39	254·1	242 to 267	100·6	94 to 107	82·2	79 to 86	17·3	16 to 18

TABLE IV—*Mean daily intakes of nutrients among women in the three towns.*

	No of women	Energy (MJ) Mean	95% Confidence interval	Fat (g) Mean	95% Confidence interval	Polyunsaturated fatty acids (g) Mean	95% Confidence interval	Saturated fatty acids (g) Mean
Ipswich								
JC	129	7·1	6·7 to 7·5	73·0	67 to 79	10·1	9 to 11	29·7
Local	263	6·7	6·4 to 7·0	68·9	65 to 73	9·8	9 to 11	27·7
Stoke								
JC	150	7·3	6·9 to 7·7	72·4	67 to 78	8·5	8 to 9	31·2
Local	266	7·2	6·9 to 7·5	74·0	70 to 78	9·5	9 to 10	30·6
Wakefield								
JC	120	7·0	6·5 to 7·4	71·9	66 to 78	8·6	8 to 10	30·5
Local	297	6·4	6·2 to 6·7	65·1	61 to 69	8·7	8 to 9	26·1

total fibre were lowest in Wakefield. Carbohydrate and protein intakes were highest in Stoke. The polyunsaturated to saturated fatty acid ratios varied from 0·29 in Wakefield to 0·31 in Stoke and 0·36 in Ipswich for records completed by JC, and from 0·33 to 0·36 and 0·37 respectively for those completed by local interviewers. Higher consumption of vegetables other than potatoes among women in Ipswich resulted in only 37% of fibre coming from cereal products compared with 45% in the other towns.

Table V gives the mean intakes of fat, carbohydrate, and protein expressed as the percentage of total energy derived from them. Only results from interviews conducted by JC are shown. There were no large differences among the towns.

Social classes were combined to give three groups of similar size—I, II, and III non-manual; III manual; and IV and V. The lower energy intakes in Wakefield were seen in all social class groups. Table VI shows that the lower fat intakes in Wakefield were also not confined to any social class group. Intakes of the nutrients listed in tables III and IV did not show consistent trends with social class. Within each town and in both sexes, however, there was a decrease in intake of vitamin C from the highest to the lowest social class group.

Body mass index (weight (kg)/height (m)^2) was highest in Stoke. Among men mean values were 25·6 in Ipswich, 25·8 in Stoke, and 25·6 in Wakefield; among women they were 25·1, 25·4, and 24·6 respectively.

Table VII shows that Ipswich had the lowest proportion of heavy drinkers, defined as people having six or more drinks on one or two days a month or three or more drinks at weekends or on most days of the week. Among men the proportion of current cigarette smokers was highest in Stoke (43%); among women the proportion was highest in Wakefield (39%).

Results shown separately for records completed by JC and local interviewer

Saturated fatty acids (g) 95% Confidence interval	Carbohydrate (g) Mean	Carbohydrate (g) 95% Confidence interval	Sugars (g) Mean	Sugars (g) 95% Confidence interval	Protein (g) Mean	Protein (g) 95% Confidence interval	Total fibre (g) Mean	Total fibre (g) 95% Confidence interval
27 to 32	192·2	179 to 206	76·5	69 to 84	64·3	61 to 68	15·1	14 to 16
26 to 29	183·6	175 to 192	73·4	68 to 79	60·6	58 to 63	14·0	13 to 15
29 to 34	205·0	192 to 218	78·2	71 to 86	66·2	63 to 70	15·8	15 to 17
29 to 32	192·8	184 to 202	68·4	63 to 74	66·4	64 to 69	14·9	14 to 16
28 to 33	189·4	176 to 203	73·0	66 to 81	63·1	59 to 67	14·0	13 to 15
24 to 28	172·4	164 to 181	67·2	62 to 72	60·8	58 to 63	13·4	13 to 14

Discussion

This is the first large scale survey of nutrient intakes of people of middle age living in different areas of Britain. The samples were selected to be representative of the population of each town in the age range 35–54 years and were large enough to detect differences among the towns likely to be of biological importance. The response rate was 85%.

By comparison with international differences in dietary intakes the differences found among the towns in this study were small. This is in

TABLE V—*Mean daily intakes of fat, carbohydrate, and protein expressed as percentage of energy intake. Results for records completed by JC only*

	No of people	Fat Mean	Fat 95% Confidence interval	Carbohydrate Mean	Carbohydrate 95% Confidence interval	Protein Mean	Protein 95% Confidence interval
			Men				
Ipswich	119	37·8	36 to 39	48·5	47 to 50	13·5	13 to 14
Stoke	128	34·8	33 to 36	46·5	45 to 48	14·2	14 to 15
Wakefield	110	36·5	35 to 38	45·4	44 to 47	14·4	14 to 15
			Women				
Ipswich	129	38·8	37 to 40	46·1	45 to 48	15·8	15 to 17
Stoke	150	37·1	36 to 38	46·3	45 to 48	15·8	15 to 17
Wakefield	120	39·5	38 to 41	47·1	46 to 48	15·8	15 to 17

TABLE VI—*Mean daily intake of fat (g) stratified by social class. Results shown separately for records completed by JC and local interviewer*

	Social class								
	I–III Non-manual			III Manual			IV, V		
	No of people	Mean	95% Confidence interval	No of people	Mean	95% Confidence interval	No of people	Mean	95% Confidence interval
Men									
Ipswich									
JC	37	102·7	89 to 117	44	116·9	104 to 131	38	106·2	93 to 121
Local	86	103·1	94 to 112	87	110·2	101 to 120	67	102·1	92 to 113
Stoke									
JC	20	98·3	81 to 118	81	110·9	101 to 121	26	107·2	91 to 125
Local	56	103·0	92 to 115	128	113·8	106 to 122	63	118·4	107 to 130
Wakefield									
JC	55	105·6	94 to 118	28	79·6	66 to 94	26	87·9	73 to 104
Local	118	93·1	86 to 101	94	93·1	85 to 102	50	91·3	80 to 103
Women									
Ipswich									
JC	55	70·5	62 to 79	41	75·1	65 to 86	28	78·3	66 to 92
Local	98	75·6	69 to 82	93	63·0	57 to 69	62	67·2	60 to 75
Stoke									
JC	41	75·8	66 to 87	65	70·3	63 to 78	37	72·3	62 to 83
Local	75	70·9	64 to 78	125	74·8	69 to 81	53	76·6	68 to 86
Wakefield									
JC	52	71·5	63 to 81	31	74·5	63 to 87	33	70·1	60 to 82
Local	130	66·1	61 to 72	80	67·3	61 to 74	77	59·7	53 to 66

TABLE VII—*Percentage distribution of men and women in each town stratified by alcohol intake and cigarette smoking*

	Alcohol intake*				Cigarette smoking†			
	No of people	None	Light	Moderate/ heavy	No of people	Non- smoker	Ex- smoker	Current smoker
Men								
Ipswich	364	8	49	43	363	29	25	40
Stoke	378	6	27	67	378	23	26	43
Wakefield	375	5	35	60	373	28	25	36
Women								
Ipswich	392	17	72	11	388	52	16	32
Stoke	417	14	61	25	415	47	18	35
Wakefield	419	11	68	21	416	43	18	39

* See text for definition of levels.
† Six per cent of men in Ipswich, 8% in Stoke, and 11% in Wakefield were either past or current smokers of other tobacco products.

keeping with the small dietary differences among the regions of Britain estimated by the National Food Survey from household food purchases.[1]

The mean daily intakes of energy, fat, and all main nutrients were lower in the northern industrial town (Wakefield) than in the southern market town (Ipswich) among both men and women (tables III and IV). Though the social class distribution of these two towns was similar, socioeconomic conditions were worse in Wakefield, both in relation to quality of housing and in relation to income, as indicated by the proportion of households owning their own house or a car. The lower fat consumption in Wakefield was contrary to what might be expected from the high mortality from ischaemic heart disease. It was associated with a lower polyunsaturated to saturated fatty acid ratio and was largely due to lower consumption of milk, cheese, and fats in cakes and puddings. There were only small differences between any of the towns in the amounts of fat derived from meat, fried potatoes, butter, or margarine. When expressed as a proportion of total energy the consumption of fat in the three towns was similar (table V). There was not a consistent trend in fat consumption by social class within the towns (table VI). The survey was able to show social class differences in vitamin C intake similar to those reported by the National Food Survey.

The lower mean intakes of total fibre in Wakefield reflected lower consumption of vegetables other than potatoes. Consumption of cereal fibre, however, was lowest in Ipswich, with a mean of 7·4 g per person daily compared with 7·5 g in Wakefield and 8·4 g in Stoke. These findings are in keeping with the general trend of lower consumption of non-potato vegetables and higher consumption of cereals in less affluent communities within the British Isles.[15]

The mean daily intakes of energy and carbohydrate were highest in Stoke (tables III and IV). This town has the highest proportion of manual workers (table I). The higher intakes were seen, however, in all social classes and in both men and women. Mean body mass index was also highest in Stoke.

Our findings suggest that the geographical inequalities in mortality in Britain, in particular mortality from ischaemic heart disease, cannot be attributed to differences in consumption of energy or fat during middle life. There is evidence that cigarette smoking may contribute to the inequalities among men, as the regional heart study of 24 towns showed a correlation between smoking and the prevalence of ischaemic heart disease.[16] Information about women is lacking, except that throughout England and Wales mortality from ischaemic heart disease correlates negatively with mortality from lung cancer, an indicator of cigarette smoking (chapter 1). In the three towns in our study the small differences in cigarette smoking among men did not correspond with the differences in ischaemic heart disease, but the highest proportion of smokers among women was in Wakefield. The regional heart study has not found alcohol consumption to be an important determinant of variations in cardiovascular mortality.[9] In the three towns the proportion of heavy drinkers was, however, lowest in Ipswich.

Socioeconomic conditions are better in Ipswich than in the other two towns (table I). It might be expected that a more affluent town would tend to have higher rather than lower intakes of fat and other components of a Western diet. It is also consistent that it had higher rates of breast cancer, colonic cancer, and gall stones (table II), all of which are more common in affluent countries. The low mortality from ischaemic heart disease is paradoxical. The results of this study are in keeping with the findings described in previous chapters, which suggest that the explanation may lie more in the better development and health of infants in Ipswich in the past than in a more healthy diet among adults at present.

We are grateful to the subjects in the three towns who took part in this study and to their general practitioners. We also thank Dr Michael Nelson, who advised on dietary methods.

1 Ministry of Agriculture, Fisheries and Food. *Household food consumption and expenditure survey, 1985*. London: HMSO, 1987.
2 Barker DJP, Gardner MJ, Power C, Hutt MSR. Prevalence of gall stones at necropsy in nine British towns: a collaborative study. *BMJ* 1979;ii:1389–92.
3 Office of Population Censuses and Surveys. *Small area statistics, Census 1981*. London: HMSO, 1982.
4 Office of Population Censuses and Surveys. *Area mortality decennial supplement 1969–73, England and Wales*. London: HMSO, 1981. (Series DS, No 4.)
5 Cole T, Black A. Statistical aspects in the design of dietary surveys. In: *Dietary assessment of populations*. Southampton: Medical Research Council Environmental Epidemiology Unit, 1984. (Scientific report No 4.)
6 Bingham S, McNeil NI, Cummings JH. The diet of individuals: a study of a randomly-chosen cross section of British adults in a Cambridgeshire village. *Br J Nutr* 1981;45:23–35.
7 Thomson M, Logan RL, Sharman M, Lockerbie L, Riemersma RA, Oliver MF. Dietary survey in 40-year old Edinburgh men. *Hum Nutr Appl Nutr* 1982;36A:272–80.
8 Yarnell JWG, Fehily AM, Milbank JE, Sweetnam PM, Walker CL. A short dietary questionnaire for use in an epidemiological survey: comparison with weighed dietary records. *Hum Nutr Appl Nutr* 1983;37A:103–12.
9 Shaper AG, Phillips AN, Pocock SJ, Walker M. Alcohol and ischaemic heart disease in middle-aged British men. *BMJ* 1987;294:733–7.
10 Paul AA, Southgate DAT. *McCance and Widdowson's the composition of foods*. 4th ed. London: HMSO, 1978.
11 Paul AA, Southgate DAT, Russel J. *First supplement to McCance and Widdowson's the composition of foods*. London: HMSO, 1980.
12 Wiles SJ, Nettleton PA, Black AE, Paul AA. The nutrient composition of some cooked dishes eaten in Britain: a supplementary food composition table. *Journal of Human Nutrition* 1980;34:189–223.
13 Baker RJ, Nelder JA. *GLIM (generalised linear interactive modelling), release 3*, Oxford: Numerical Algorithms Group, 1978.
14 Barker DJP, Godfrey KM. Geographical variations in the incidence of colorectal cancer in Britain. *Br J Cancer* 1984;50:693–8.
15 Morris J, Barker DJP, Nelson M. Diet, infection and acute appendicitis in Britain and Ireland. *J Epidemiol Community Health* 1987;41:44–9.
16 Shaper AG. Geographic variations in cardiovascular mortality in Great Britain. *Br Med Bull* 1984;40:366–73.

9: Review: childhood causes of adult diseases

D J P BARKER

This review summarises the findings described in chapters 1–8. It points to the need for studies of individuals.

The search for influences in the adult environment which determine the risk of the major non-malignant diseases—cardiovascular disease and chronic bronchitis—has met with limited success. Cigarette smoking has been implicated; evidence on dietary fat has accumulated to the point where a public health policy of reduced intake is considered prudent, even if the case is not proved. Much, however, remains unexplained.

A puzzling aspect of the epidemiology of ischaemic heart disease, stroke, and chronic bronchitis in Britain is that they are more common in poorer areas and in lower income groups. Differences are large, greater than twofold. For ischaemic heart disease they are also paradoxical in that its steep rise in Britain and elsewhere has been associated with rising prosperity. Why should its rates be lowest in the most prosperous places, such as London and the home counties? Variations in cigarette smoking and adult diet do not explain these differences (chapter 8).

There is increasing evidence that they result from geographical and social class differences in child development and health 60 and more years ago. Past differences in child health were reflected in the wide range of infant mortality. For example in 1921–5 infant mortality ranged from 44 per 1000 births in rural West Sussex to 114 in Burnley. The highest rates were generally in northern counties where large manufacturing towns had grown up around the coal seams. Rates were also high in poor rural areas such as north Wales. They were lowest in counties in the south and east, which have the best agricultural land and are historically the wealthiest. A series of government inquiries on child and maternal mortality from 1910 onwards, prompted by revelations of the poor physique of military recruits, showed how these differences in infant mortality were related to differences in maternal physique and health, infant feeding, housing, and overcrowding.[1-3]

Mortality statistics for England and Wales can be used to compare the present distribution of adult death rates from specific causes with the past geographical distribution of causes of infant mortality. The comparisons can be made with the country divided into large towns and groupings of small towns and rural areas within counties, totalling 212 areas—a division of the country used in routine statistics since the turn of the century.

Mortality from chronic bronchitis and emphysema is concentrated in the large towns. Its geographical distribution correlates remarkably closely with infant mortality from bronchitis and pneumonia in the early years of the century (chapter 3). The coefficient of correlation is 0·85. A similarly high coefficient is seen for each sex separately and if comparisons are made between large towns only, or small towns or rural areas.

Suspicion that respiratory infection in early childhood might be a major cause of chronic bronchitis in adult life has been reinforced by follow up studies which show that, after bronchiolitis, bronchitis, or pneumonia, abnormalities of pulmonary function may persist through childhood.[4-7] In the national sample of children born in Britain during 1946 there was a strong association between the occurrence of one or more lower respiratory infections before 2 years of age and the prevalence of cough during the day, or at night in the winter, at the age of 25.[8]

The close geographical relation between infant mortality from respiratory infection and adult mortality from bronchitis may be interpreted as strong evidence for a direct causal link between respiratory infection in early childhood and chronic bronchitis. Regression analysis of bronchitis and lung cancer mortality suggests that childhood infection is more important than cigarette smoking in determining the prevalence of bronchitis. The high rates of chronic bronchitis in Britain, and its distribution within the country, are therefore a legacy of poor social conditions in the past. Particular adverse influences which are implicated include inadequate housing, large family size, overcrowding in the home, and the abandonment of breast feeding. This interpretation is consistent with the progressive decline in mortality from chronic bronchitis over the past 50 years.

Another close geographical relation in England and Wales is that between current mortality from stroke and maternal mortality from causes other than puerperal fever in the early years of the century (chapter 2). Toxaemia was the commonest cause of these maternal deaths. Hypertension may be the mechanism linking maternal health and risk of stroke in the offspring. Maternal hypertension increases the risk of hypertension in the children,[9] and hypertension is a risk factor for stroke. There is increasing evidence that hypertension originates in childhood.[10] "Tracking" of blood pressure has been repeatedly observed in longitudinal studies of children and adults.[11-14] A link between the intrauterine environment and hypertension is suggested by the negative relation between birth weight and blood pressure at age 36 in the 1946 cohort.[15] The distribution of stroke in Britain may therefore reflect the past distribution of poor living standards which accompanied industrialisation or economic depression in certain areas. These adversely affected the development of girls and increased the risk of stroke in their offspring, possibly through mechanisms associated with blood pressure and rates of growth in early life.

The geographical distribution of ischaemic heart disease in Britain is similar to that of stroke. A study in 24 British towns has shown that the mean blood pressure of adult men in a town correlates with the prevalence of ischaemic heart disease.[16] Childhood influences associated with blood pressure could determine the distribution of both diseases. Their time-trends, however, are opposite. Mortality from stroke has fallen in Britain over the past 40 years, which is consistent with past improvements in maternal health and physique. Ischaemic heart disease mortality, however, has risen steeply. This is attributed to increasing affluence, in particular diet, during adult life. Ischaemic heart disease may therefore have two groups of causes: one acting through the mother or in infancy, which is associated with poor living standards; the other acting in adult life, which is associated with affluence. Further evidence for the existence of the former comes from the inverse relation between ischaemic heart disease and height, which is largely determined by growth in childhood (chapter 7). Long term "programming" of lipid metabolism during infancy, as a result of infant feeding, is a mechanism for which there is increasing evidence in experimental animals, and which may be a link between childhood and the risk of ischaemic heart disease.[17]

A prediction from this is that the improvements in maternal and child health in generations born before the second world war will now be reflected in a fall in ischaemic heart disease. Rates are beginning to fall in many parts of Britain and there have already been substantial falls in the United States, Canada, Australia, and New Zealand.

Epidemiological investigation of the effect of childhood influences on the risk of cardiovascular disease and chronic bronchitis is being pursued in a variety of ways—through prospective and retrospective studies of individuals and by detailed analyses of time trends. If they show major effects we will need a new national strategy for reducing inequalities of health in Britain. The current strategy is focused on adult lifestyles. The new one will need to address differences in the development and health of children.

1 Local Government Board. *Forty-second annual report, 1912–13. Supplement in continuation of the report of the medical officer of the board for 1912–13.* London: HMSO, 1913.

2 Local Government Board. *Forty-fourth annual report, 1914–15. Supplement: maternal mortality in connection with childbearing.* London: HMSO, 1916.

3 Campbell JM, Cameron D, Jones DM. *High maternal mortality in certain areas.* London: HMSO, 1932. (Ministry of Health Reports on Public Health and Medical Subjects. No. 68.)

4 Kattan M, Keens TG, Lapierre JG, Levison H, Bryan AC, Reilly BJ. Pulmonary function abnormalities in symptom-free children after bronchitis. *Pediatrics* 1977;**59**:683–8.

5 Gurwitz D, Mindorff C, Levison H. Increased incidence of bronchial reactivity in children with a history of bronchiolitis. *Pediatrics* 1981;**98**:551–5.

6 Pullan CR, Hey EN. Wheezing, asthma, and pulmonary dysfunction 10 years after infection with respiratory syncytial virus in infancy. *BMJ* 1982;**284**:1665–9.

7 Mok JYQ, Simpson H. Outcome for acute bronchitis, bronchiolitis, and pneumonia in infancy. *Arch Dis Child* 1984;**59**:306–9.

8 Kiernan KE, Colley JRT, Douglas JWB, Reid DD. Chronic cough in young adults in relation to smoking habits, childhood environment and chest illness. *Respiration* 1976;**33**:236–44.

9 Stamler R, Stamler J, Riedlinger WF, Algera G, Roberts RH. Family (parental) history and prevalence of hypertension. Results of a nationwide screening programme. *JAMA* 1979;**241**:43–6.

10 Hofman A. Blood pressure in childhood: an epidemiological approach to the aetiology of hypertension. *J Hypertens* 1984;**2**:323–8.

11 de Swiet M, Fayers P, Shinebourne EA. Blood pressure survey in a population of newborn infants. *BMJ* 1976;**ii**:9–11.

12 Beaglehole R, Salmond CE, Eyles EF. A longitudinal study of blood pressure in Polynesian children. *Am J Epidemiol* 1977;**105**:87–9.

13 Clarke WR, Schrott H, Leaverton PE, Connor WE, Laver RM. Tracking of blood lipids and blood pressure in school age children: the Muscatine study. *Circulation* 1978;**58**:626–34.

14 Voors W, Webber LS, Berenson GS. Time course studies of blood pressure in children: the Bogalusa heart study. *Am J Epidemiol* 1979;**109**:320–34.

15 Wadsworth MEJ, Cripps HA, Midwinter RE, Colley JRT. Blood pressure in a national birth cohort at the age of 36 related to social and familial factors, smoking, and body mass. *BMJ* 1985;**291**:1534–8.

16 Shaper AG, Pocock SJ, Walker M, Cohen NM, Wale CJ, Thomson AG. British Regional Heart Study: cardiovascular risk factors in middle-aged men in 24 towns. *BMJ* 1981;**283**:179–86.

17 Mott GE. Deferred effects of breastfeeding versus formula feeding on serum lipoprotein concentrations and cholesterol metabolism in baboons. In: Filer LJ Jr, Fomon SJ, eds. *The breastfed infant: a model for performance. Report of the 91st Ross conference on paediatric research.* Columbus, Ohio: Ross Laboratories, 1986:144–9.

PART II
CHANGES IN DISEASE RATES
OVER TIME

10: Diet and coronary heart disease in England and Wales during and after the second world war

D J P BARKER, C OSMOND

During the second world war there were large changes in consumption of fats, fibre, and sugar in Britain. These changes matched recent recommendations made by the Committee on Medical Aspects of Food Policy with the object of reducing the incidence of coronary heart disease. It is widely believed that coronary heart disease mortality fell during the war. This paper re-examines coronary heart disease mortality among middle aged people in England and Wales from 1931 to 1967. After allowance for changes in the rules for coding cause of death, and for the sharp increase in all-causes mortality in 1940, there is little to suggest that time trends in coronary heart disease were much influenced by the war. Because of confounding variables, this does not argue against the Committee on Medical Aspects of Food Policy report. However, it gives no support to the view that compliance with the recommendations on fat, fibre, and sugar will lead, by itself, to an appreciable fall in coronary heart disease mortality in middle aged people.

Introduction

The recent report from the Committee on Medical Aspects of Food Policy recommends dietary changes in the United Kingdom with the object of reducing the incidence of coronary heart disease.[1] The recommendations include reduction in total fat intake, no further increase in intake of simple sugars, but an increase in consumption of fibre rich carbohydrates such as bread, cereals, fruit, and vegetables.

During the second world war government food policy effected major and widespread changes in the British diet. Fat and sugar consumption fell sharply[2] and fibre consumption rose.[3] It is therefore relevant to examine changes in mortality from coronary heart disease during and after the war. Previous analyses have concluded either that coronary heart disease mortality fell[4] or that its prewar increase was slowed.[5] In 1949 the registrar general wrote that whatever causes were responsible for the rapid increase in degenerative heart conditions during 1921–39 "must have been largely removed during the war". Such conclusions have been widely quoted.

Method

Interpretation of wartime rates in young adults is complicated by the large numbers of men who were in the armed forces overseas. In older age groups diagnosis of cause of death is often less accurate. This chapter therefore presents death rates for the civilian population aged 45–64.

In the registrar general's annual reviews[6] deaths in England and Wales were coded under the fourth revision of the International Classificaton of Disease (ICD) during 1931–9 and the fifth revision during 1940–9. The change in classification in 1940 was accompanied by a change in coding procedure whereby, when more than one cause of death was mentioned on the certificate, rules of allocation of the underlying cause were abandoned in favour of the certifying doctors' stated preference. To allow comparison between the old and new classifications and coding procedures the registrar general coded all 1939 deaths to the fourth and fifth revisions. In both classifications ICD 93 was "diseases of the myocardium" and ICD 94 was "diseases of the coronary arteries, angina pectoris". It was agreed that allocation to one or other of these codes was often arbitrary.[5 7] The table shows the number of 1939 deaths, at ages 45–64, coded to these causes under the rules of the fourth and fifth revisions. Under the fifth revision 2455 fewer deaths are coded to ICD 93 and 488 fewer to ICD 94. Most of these deaths were coded to bronchitis (ICD 106) for there were 2855 certificates on which bronchitis was given as the cause of death with myocardial disease as a contributory or secondary cause. The table shows that under the fifth revision 4076 more deaths were coded to bronchitis than under the fourth revision. These changes reflect the withdrawal of rules of allocation administered under the fourth revision, specifically "diseases of the heart (Nos 90–95) or kidney (Nos 130–133) to be preferred to any disease of the respiratory system (Nos 104–114)".[8]

During 1950–7 deaths in England and Wales were coded to the sixth ICD revision. As in 1939, the registrar general coded all 1949 deaths under both the existing classifications and the new one. Under the fifth revision 22 799 deaths were coded to ICD 93–94. Under the sixth revision 22 854 deaths were coded to ICD 420–422, "arteriosclerotic and degenerative

Number of deaths in 1939 in England and Wales coded to myocardial disease, coronary artery disease, and bronchitis under the fourth and fifth ICD revisions, men and women aged 45–64

		Men		Women	
Code	Description	ICD 4	ICD 5	ICD 4	ICD 5
93	Diseases of the myocardium	8960	7147	6844	6202
94	Diseases of the coronary arteries, angina pectoris	5498	5155	1705	1560
106	Bronchitis	2432	5189	918	2237

heart disease". The trends in ICD 93–94 from 1949 can therefore be extended into trends in ICD 420–422 from 1950 to 1957. The trends from 1957 can be extended into the period 1958–67 when deaths were coded to the seventh ICD revision but with minimal changes in classification or coding procedure for coronary heart disease.[9]

Results

Figure 1 shows data as published by the registrar general, that is, deaths coded to ICD 93 and 94 under the fourth revision during 1931–9 and under the fifth revision during 1940–9. In both men and women, mortality from

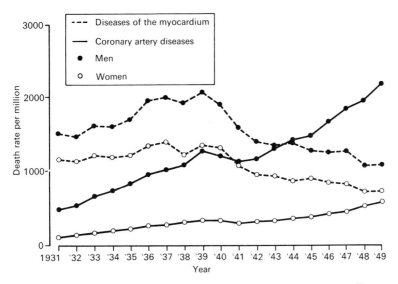

FIG 1—*Annual mortality from myocardial disease and coronary artery disease (ICD 93 and 94, fourth and fifth revisions) in England and Wales, men and women aged 45–64, 1931–49.*

diseases of the myocardium (ICD 93) rose to a peak in the late 1930s and thereafter declined, the steepest decline occurring in the war years. In contrast, mortality from coronary artery disease (ICD 94) rose progressively throughout the period except for a small decline in the early war years. As would be expected, rates were lower among women than men.

Figure 2 shows combined rates for myocardial and coronary artery disease during 1931–49 with rates for arteriosclerotic and degenerative heart disease (ICD 420–422) during 1950–67. Interrupted lines represent the 1931–9 rates as published by the registrar general, that is, coded to the fourth ICD revision. The dual coding of the 1939 data allows calculation of the proportion of these deaths, in each five year age and sex group, which would have been coded to other causes (mostly bronchitis) under the multiple cause coding rules which applied under the fifth revision from 1940 onwards. These proportions have been applied to the age and sex specific rates to give estimates for each year from 1931 to 1939. Continuous lines therefore represent the data for the entire 1931–49 period adjusted to the fifth ICD revision. A similar method, based on the dual coding of the 1949 and 1957 data, was used to adjust the 1950–67 data to the fifth ICD revision. An interrupted line shows the data as published, which are closely similar.

For men, the 1931–67 data as published showed a steep rise to a peak in 1939, followed by an abrupt reversal and fall. After 1942 there was again a rise, but the rates did not reach those of 1939 until the 1950s. Adjusted to

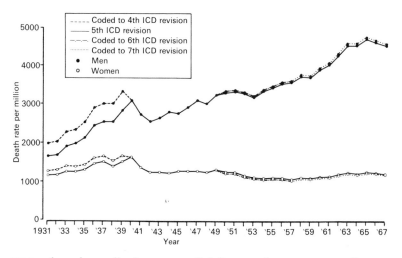

FIG 2—*Annual mortality from myocardial disease and coronary artery disease (ICD 93 and 94) 1931–49 and arteriosclerotic and degenerative heart disease (ICD 420–422) 1950–67 in England and Wales, men and women aged 45–64 with rates adjusted to fifth ICD revision (see text).*

the fifth revision, however, the rates rose until 1940, fell in 1941 and 1942, and thereafter rose almost without interruption until 1963. Among women, the data as published showed a slow rise to a peak in 1936–40, a fall in 1941–2, and little change thereafter. The adjusted rates peaked in 1940.

As would be expected from the data on bronchitis shown in the table, adjustment of the 1931–9 deaths increases the prewar death rates for all respiratory diseases combined (ICD 104–114). Figure 3 shows that even after adjustment there was a striking increase in respiratory deaths among men in 1940. The rise was smaller in women, among whom rates were lower throughout.

There was a similarly abrupt rise in total mortality and infant mortality in 1940 (figs 4 and 5). In both sexes death rates from all causes other than myocardial and coronary arterial disease, and violence (ICD 163–198), rose sharply in 1940 (fig 4). Despite the overall decline in mortality during 1931–49, the 1940 rate for men was the highest during the period. This 1940 peak resulted from an increase in death rates from a range of diseases, including respiratory diseases and infections. Similarly, infant mortality

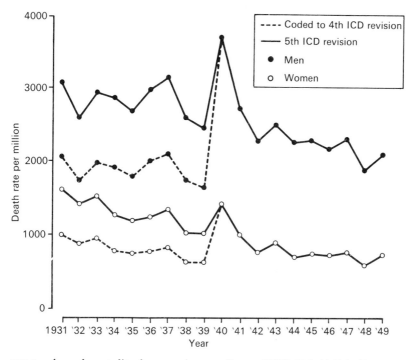

FIG 3—*Annual mortality from respiratory disease (ICD 104–114) in England and Wales, men and women aged 45–64 with 1931–9 rates adjusted to fifth ICD revision (see text).*

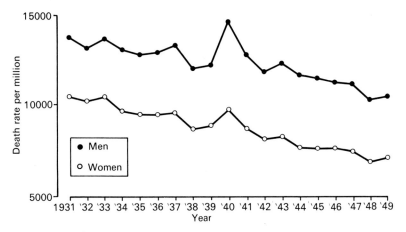

FIG 4—*Annual mortality from all causes, other than myocardial and coronary artery disease and violence, in England and Wales, men and women aged 45–64, 1931–49.*

(fig 5) rose sharply in 1940 and again in 1941 before resuming its downward trend. There were four peaks in deaths attributed to influenza (ICD 11, fourth revision, ICD 33 fifth revision) during 1931–49, of which one was in 1940 (fig 6).

Discussion

Although deaths attributed to coronary heart disease rose steeply and almost without interruption during 1931–49 (fig 1), it was generally agreed that diagnostic transfer between this classification and diseases of the

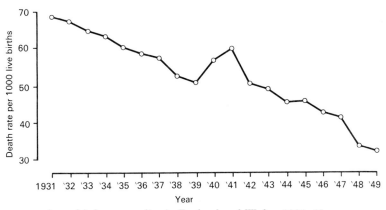

FIG 5—*Annual infant mortality in England and Wales, 1931–49.*

114

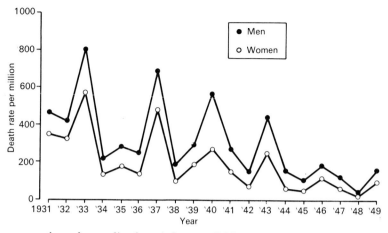

FIG 6—*Annual mortality from influenza (ICD 11, fourth revision, 33 fifth revision) in England and Wales, men and women aged 45–64, 1931–49.*

myocardium had occurred. Hence in the analyses of coronary heart disease trends by Ryle and Russell,[7] Morris,[5] and others, the two causes of death were considered together. The results, based on data coded under the fourth and fifth ICD revisions, led to the conclusions that during the war coronary heart disease mortality fell[4] or that its prewar increase was slowed.[5] These changes have been attributed to a beneficial effect of the wartime diet. Our re-examination of coronary heart disease mortality in middle aged men and women brings into question both the changes that occurred and their relation to diet.

In a review of mortality trends in England and Wales, Campbell noted that revision of the ICD in 1940, and a change in the rules of allocation for deaths with multiple causes, complicated interpretation of the trends at that time.[10] Our adjustment of the 1931–9 data to the fifth ICD revision is based on certain assumptions, including the assumption that a fixed proportion of heart disease deaths was accompanied by respiratory disease throughout the period. Nevertheless the adjusted data shown in fig 2 (continuous lines) seem likely to be more accurate indicators of trends than the data originally published. Adjusting male deaths changes the apparent peak in 1939 to a peak in 1940 and reduces the magnitude of the subsequent decline in relation to prewar levels: the 1942 rate, the lowest during and after the war, is similar to that in 1937–8. In women, there is similarly a 1940 peak in the adjusted data.

We have shown that 1940 was a year of unusually high mortality from a range of diseases, not only among adults (figs 3 and 4) but among infants as well—for whom 1941 was also an unusual year (fig 5). Contributing to this was an influenza epidemic (fig 6) and a cold winter.[4 10] Given this unusual mortality, and the sharp worsening in environmental conditions consequent upon the outbreak of war, it seems reasonable to exclude 1940 when considering trends in coronary heart disease.

Taking the continuous lines in fig 2 as the best estimates of coronary heart disease mortality, and putting aside the 1940 rates, there is no evidence that time trends in coronary heart disease were much influenced by the war. Among men there was a modest fall from 1939 to 1942 such that the 1942 rate was similar to that in 1938. Thereafter the rise in mortality continued steadily until the mid-1960s. Among women there was similarly a fall from 1939 to 1942. Thereafter there was little change.

Wartime and immediate postwar trends in younger and older age groups are similar to those in the middle aged, but their interpretation is less secure because of large scale recruitment of young men into the armed forces and less accuracy of death certification in the elderly.

The wartime dietary changes were large and, because of rationing, widespread. The findings of the Combined Food Board, which compared estimates of consumption during 1943–4 with those during 1934–8, were summarised as follows.[11] "Important increases were: for potatoes 45%, vegetables 34%, milk and milk products 28% and grain products 17%. Important decreases were in tomatoes and citrus fruits 50%, other fruits 44%, poulty and fish 39%, sugar 31%, meat 21% and fats 16%." These large changes did not take place immediately on the outbreak of war. The decline in food importation and increase in home production occurred over one to two years. Not until April 1942 was the extraction rate of flour raised from 68–75% to 85%, with the consequent sharp increase in cereal fibre consumption. Food controls persisted after the war. From 1949 to 1950 they were gradually withdrawn, and rationing finally ended in 1954.

Levels of consumption of fat, fibre, and sugar during the 1940s differed greatly from those in the 1930s and 1950s. Total fat consumption fell from 39% of food energy in 1934–8 to 36% in 1941 and 33% in 1947. It returned to 38% in 1950 and increased thereafter.[2] Wartime levels may be compared with the reduction to 35% recommended by the Committee on Medical Aspects of Food Policy. Using current food tables, the estimated ratio of polyunsaturated to saturated fatty acids was 0·26 and therefore did not reach the Committee on Medical Aspects of Food Policy recommended level of 0·45.[12] Estimated cereal fibre consumption rose from 9 g per person per day in 1938 to 19–25 g in 1944.[3] During the same period vegetable fibre consumption rose from 10·1 g per person per day to 13·2 g. Consumption of both cereal and vegetable fibre fell back after the war, cereal fibre to prewar levels. Sugar consumption fell from 44 kg per person per year in 1938 to 30 kg in 1941. It returned to prewar levels around 1953 and increased thereafter.[2]

These changes in consumption of fat, fibre, and sugar cannot be readily reconciled with the trends in coronary heart disease mortality (fig 2). It could be argued that the decline in mortality from 1939 to 1942 was a response to the changes. The mechanism for so immediate a response would presumably be a change in blood coagulability rather than reduced deposition of atheroma. However, the changes were introduced gradually, over the first one to two years of the war, and food controls persisted throughout the 1940s. There is therefore no evident explanation for the resumed rise after 1942 nor the lack of an acceleration of the rise after the withdrawal of food controls in the 1950s. If it is argued that the wartime dietary changes prevented what would otherwise have been a steeper rise, the lack of response to removal of food controls is similarly unexplained. The proposition of a latent period of some years before dietary change is followed by a reduction in mortality does not lessen the incongruity between the dietary and coronary heart disease mortality trends. If, however, the latent period was about 10 years or more, benefits to middle aged people would be reflected in mortality among the elderly. Figure 2 would reflect the wartime diets of young men, many of whom were in the armed forces.

Comparison of wartime trends in coronary heart disease mortality and changes in estimated per capita consumption of fat, fibre, and sugar cannot give conclusive evidence. Certified cause of death is an important indicator of mortality caused by coronary heart disease. Exposure to other causative influences, dietary and non-dietary, may have changed during the war. Stress, for example, may have increased, but so too may muscular exercise.[11] Cigarette consumption rose to a peak in 1946, fell during 1947–9 and thereafter continued to rise.[13] We conclude that, though our findings do not argue against the Committee on Medical Aspects of Food Policy report, they do not support the view that compliance with the recommendations on fat, fibre, and sugar consumption will lead, by itself, to an appreciable fall in coronary heart disease mortality in middle aged men.

1 Department of Health and Social Security. Report on Health and Social Subjects 28. *Diet and cardiovascular disease.* London: HMSO, 1984.
2 Greaves JP, Hollingsworth DF. Trends in food consumption in the United Kingdom. *World Rev Nutr Diet* 1966;6:34–89.
3 Southgate DAT, Bingham S, Robertson J. Dietary fibre in the British diet. *Nature* 1978;274:51–2.
4 General Register Office. *Registrar general's statistical review of England and Wales for the six years 1940–45: Vol 1, 1940–45.* London: HMSO, 1949.
5 Morris JN. Recent history of coronary disease. *Lancet* 1951;i:69–73.
6 General Register Office. *Registrar general's statistical review of England and Wales.* Part 1. Tables, medical, 1931–49. London: HMSO, 1931–49.
7 Ryle JA, Russell WT. The natural history of coronary disease. *Br Heart J* 1949;11:370–89.
8 *Manual of the International List of Causes of Death: based on the fifth decennial revision by the International Commission, Paris, 1938.* London: HMSO, 1940.
9 Clayton DG, Taylor D, Shaper AG. Trends in heart disease in England and Wales, 1950–73. *Health Trends* 1977;9:1–6.

10 Campbell H. *Changes in mortality trends in England and Wales, 1931–1961*. Washington DC: US Department of Health, Education and Welfare, 1965.
11 Magee HE. Application of nutrition to public health. *BMJ* 1946;i:475–82.
12 Studies in urban household diets 1944–49, second report of the National Food Survey Committee. London: HMSO, 1956.
13 Lee PN, ed. *Statistics of smoking in the United Kingdom*. London: Tobacco Research Council, 1976.

11: Time trends in ischaemic heart disease and stroke in England and Wales predicted by past infant mortality

C OSMOND

This chapter describes a continuous decline in mortality from stroke during the years 1950–84, as predicted by the fall in neonatal death rates at the beginning of the century. It describes the rise and fall of ischaemic heart disease as predicted by the rise in adult exposure to affluence and the decline in adverse influences in early life. The data suggest that the generations of men and women born around 1925 had the highest rates of ischaemic heart disease. Finally, it shows that differences between counties in susceptibility acquired in infancy are strongly associated with differences in subsequent mortality from ischaemic heart disease in the same generation.

Introduction

During the second world war fat and sugar consumption in Britain fell sharply and fibre consumption rose. According to the current hypotheses that link adult diet to ischaemic heart disease, these changes should have been beneficial. There is, however, little to suggest that death rates from ischaemic heart disease among middle aged people were influenced by the wartime diet (chapter 10). We have proposed a model for the cause of ischaemic heart disease which includes a susceptibility component, linked to infant mortality and infant nutrition, in addition to a relation with an affluent diet in adults. Our other proposition relates current mortality from stroke to neonatal and maternal mortality, and hence to prenatal influences, early in this century. Our aim is to see how well national time trends in these adult diseases accord with these suggestions and, in the second half of the chapter, to see whether local changes in susceptibility, as measured by infant mortality, predict subsequent local changes in ischaemic heart disease. Our hypotheses are derived from spatial associations. We hope to deal with time and "space-time".

Infant mortality

Figure 1 shows infant mortality in England and Wales for the years 1883 to 1960.[1] Nationally there has been an enormous and continuous decline in infant mortality throughout this century. It fell from 152 deaths per 1000 births in 1900 to half that many, 76, in the early 1920s. We can also see the progressive decline in both components of infant mortality, neonatal and postneonatal, with the proportion of deaths in the neonatal period increasing from 35% to 70% during the years shown. The infant mortality is the statistic that we use as a measure of susceptibility. In the subsequent discussion the years of greatest interest run from 1890 to 1925.

During 1890–1925 decreases in infant mortality did not occur evenly across the country. Figure 2 shows a selection of nine counties with their

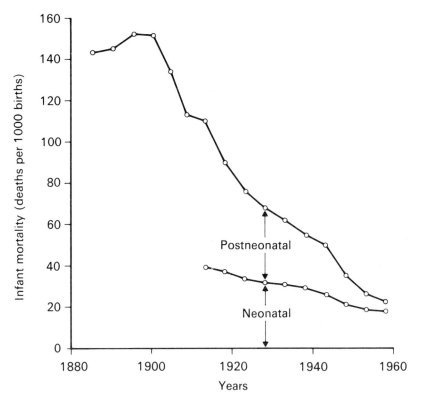

FIG 1—*Infant death rates in England and Wales 1883–1960.*

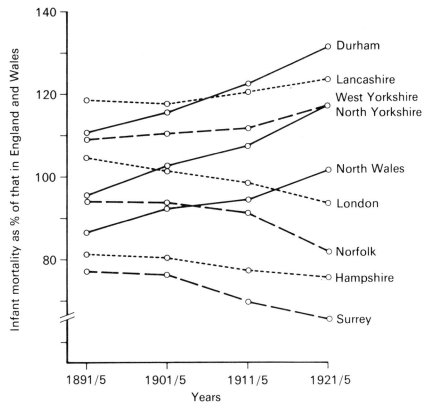

FIG 2—*Infant death rates for selected counties expressed as a percentage of those in England and Wales.*

infant mortality expressed as a percentage of that for England and Wales. Death rates improved most in the south and east (Surrey, Hampshire, Norfolk, London) but worsened relative to England and Wales in northern and western areas (Durham, Lancashire, Yorkshire, North Wales). Thus, the range of percentages increased during the 35 years.

Adult mortality from stroke

Figure 3 shows the age specific mortality from stroke for the period 1950–84 for men and women separately.[12] Both parts of the graph show a consistent and continuous decline, such that the rates had halved for men by the end of the period, and for women they had fallen to three eighths of their 1950 levels; under our hypothesis, the declines in neonatal mortality and maternal mortality suggest that such decreases in stroke should indeed occur.

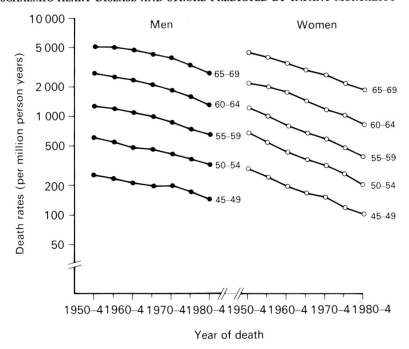

FIG 3—*Age specific mortality from stroke, England and Wales 1950–84 (ICD, 8th revision, Nos 431–438).*

Adult mortality from ischaemic heart disease

How would the hypothesis predict the course of heart disease mortality? Though we do have a measure of the susceptibility factor, the problem is that we do not know what to use for the later harmful exposure—the affluence factor. Perhaps the best we can do is to predict a rise with the advent of the affluence factor and a subsequent decline as susceptibility decreases, and to guess that there will be a worst affected generation— although its timing is impossible to assess.

Figure 4 shows the standardised mortality ratios for heart disease during 1950–84,[1 2] when 1966–70 was the standard period, and so has value 100. We have used ICD codes recommended in a paper by Clayton and others to allow comparison over time.[3] The ages used, 30–69, are chosen for quality of diagnosis. For men the standardised mortality ratios rose to a peak in 1970–4 and subsequently declined. This pattern also occurred in the United States and Australia but with an earlier peak—as would be predicted by the hypothesis, because these countries had lower infant mortality early in the century. For women, for whom current rates are less

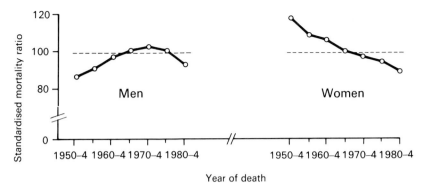

FIG 4—*Standardised mortality ratios from heart disease, England and Wales, 1950–84 relative to 1965–9, ages 30–69 (ICD Nos 400–429).*

than one third as high as those for men, the picture was different, with a continuous decline throughout the period. Closer examination of the age specific rates suggests that although the trends implied by the standard mortality ratios are dominant there are other patterns.

Figure 5 shows the age specific rates for men plotted against year of birth. There is a peak mortality for those born around 1925, which may be seen at all ages that this generation has so far attained.

A similar picture is obtained for women (fig 6), although this time the peak is less clearly defined as 1925, because at younger ages the 1930 generation is worst affected. Thus the prediction of a worst affected generation seems to be justified, as does the prediction of an eventual downturn in the general trend as susceptibility decreases.

Infant mortality related to adult mortality from ischaemic heart disease within counties

Do local changes in infant mortality predict later local changes in ischaemic heart disease mortality in the same generation? We have collated data on ischaemic heart disease for the periods 1957–67 and 1968–78 in 10 year age bands. For example, we start with the age band 65–74 to ensure large numbers of deaths in smaller areas. People who were that age during the two time periods under consideration were born around 1891–5 and 1901–5. Infant mortality data for those periods are only available at a county level, there being only 45 counties at that time. Table I shows observed and expected numbers of deaths and corresponding standardised mortality ratios for both generations and causes with the sexes combined. The question is thus: If infant mortality in an area increases between the two generations, will the same happen for the corresponding ischaemic

123

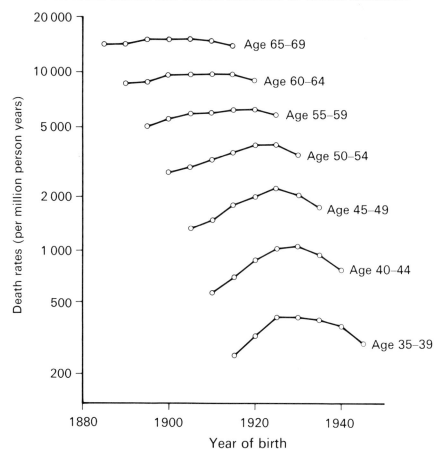

FIG 5—*Mortality from heart disease, men, England and Wales, 1950–84 (ICD Nos 400–429).*

heart disease standardised mortality ratios? In Durham the infant standardised mortality ratio increased by 4%, whereas that for ischaemic heart
disease increased by 5%. Thus Durham fits the hypothesis. Similarly, the
infant mortality decline in Somerset was matched by a subsequent decline
in ischaemic heart disease. On the other hand in Rutland a fall of 7% and a
rise of 8% conflict. Rutland is rather small, however, and estimating the
precision of the ratios shows that neither is close to being significantly
different from unity. In fact a 95% confidence interval for the figure 1·08
runs from 0·87 to 1·34. By contrast the figure for Durham of 1·05 may be
bounded by an interval from 1·03 to 1·07 and is thus significantly different
from unity. Similar precision applies to the infant mortality ratios.

124

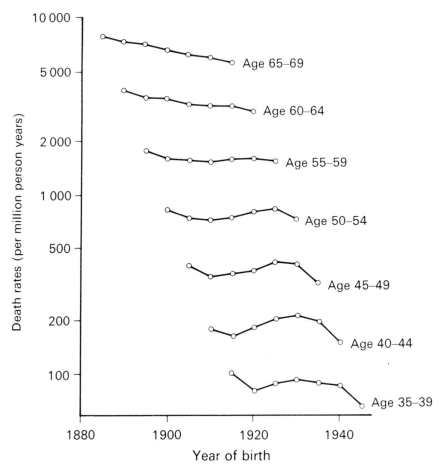

FIG 6—*Mortality from heart disease, women, England and Wales, 1950–84 (ICD Nos 400–429).*

These three counties are representatives of three different groups as far as size is concerned, Somerset being intermediate. The three groups are defined in table II, and the corresponding precision of the infant mortality ratio is stated. In the larger counties the 95% confidence interval for the ratio includes values up to 2·5% on either side of the estimate, for the intermediate counties it extends to 4%, and exceeds this for the remainder.

If these ratios are plotted for the first two groups there is evidence of a positive association. The introduction of the third group obscures this pattern (figure 7). However, as a 95% confidence interval for Rutland in the y direction runs from 0·87 to 1·34 its position is far from secure—similarly in the x direction. Weighting inversely by the combined variance of the

125

TABLE I—*Observed (OBS) and expected (EXP) numbers of deaths and corresponding standardised mortality ratios (SMRs) for two causes of death, both sexes, in three counties.*

	Infant mortality				Ischaemic heart disease			
	1891–5 (age 0) OBS_1 EXP_1 SMR_1		1901–5 (age 0) OBS_2 EXP_2 SMR_2		1959–1967 (age 65–74) OBS_3 EXP_3 SMR_3		1968–78 (age 65–74) OBS_4 EXP_4 SMR_4	
		SMR_2/SMR_1				SMR_4/SMR_3		
Durham	31 990	29 057	34 393	30 012	12 540	11 061	17 258	14 541
	110		115		113		119	
		1·04				1·05		
Somerset	8135	10 768	5193	7549	5236	5702	7282	8445
	76		69		92		86	
		0·91				0·94		
Rutland	303	405	215	307	134	172	214	255
	75		70		78		84	
		0·94				1·08		

estimates yields a correlation coefficient of 0·45, a value which would be exceeded by chance less than one time in one thousand. But how specific is this association to the years used?

Weighted correlation coefficients from this and eight similar exercises are shown in table III. Those in italics represent matchings of the comparison

TABLE II—*Counties in three groups by size*

95% Confidence interval for infant mortality ratio		
Up to 2·5% more/less (n = 14)	Up to 4% more/less (n = 16)	Over 4% more/less (n = 15)
Lancashire	Devonshire	Cornwall
West Yorkshire	Surrey	Cumberland
London	Sussex	Hertfordshire
South Wales	Derbyshire	Berkshire
Durham	Gloucestershire	Shropshire
Staffordshire	Lincolnshire	Wiltshire
Essex	Leicestershire	Buckinghamshire
Warwickshire	East Yorkshire	Dorset
Kent	North Yorkshire	Bedfordshire
Middlesex	North Wales	Cambridgeshire
Cheshire	Norfolk	Oxfordshire
Hampshire	Worcestershire	Herefordshire
Northumberland	Somerset	Huntingdonshire
Nottinghamshire	Monmouth	Westmorland
	Suffolk	Rutland
	Northamptonshire	

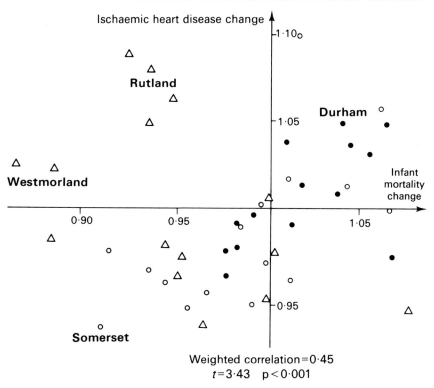

Weighted correlation=0·45
$t=3·43$ $p<0·001$

FIG 7—*Change in infant mortality (1901–5 v 1891–5) and mortality from ischaemic heart disease (ICD 8th v 7th revisions), ages 65–74, plotted for 45 counties in the groups defined in table II.*

generations which are out of phase. The figure of 0·45 exceeds all those at age 65–74 using different infant mortality comparisons (figures of −0·14 and 0·10) and exceeds all those comparing 1891–5 and 1901–5 with other age groups (figures of 0·29 and 0·25). Similarly, the figure of 0·41 is the

TABLE III—*Weighted correlation analysis. Coefficients in italics represent out of phase matchings of comparison generations.*

Infant mortality Comparison years	Mortality from ischaemic heart disease Age of comparison between ICD 7th and 8th revisions		
	65–74	55–64	45–54
1891–5 v 1901–5	0·45	*0·29*	*0·25*
1901–5 v 1911–5	*−0·14*	0·34	*0·35*
1911–5 v 1921–5	*0·10*	0·35	0·41

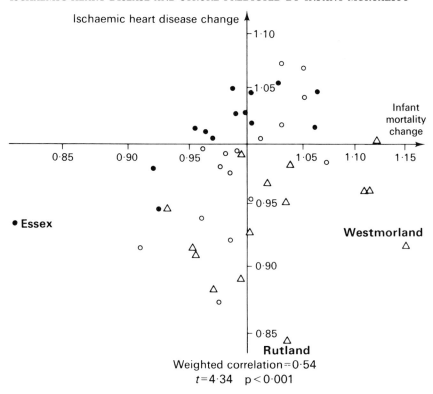

FIG 8—*Change in infant mortality (1911–5 v 1901–5) and mortality from ischaemic heart disease (ages 55–64 v 65–74) (ICD 8th revision), 1968–78, plotted for 45 counties in the groups defined in table II.*

largest obtained at that age or those comparison years; whereas the figure of 0·34 in the centre is twice exceeded but only by values of 0·35. These comparisons encourage the view that we are not looking merely at an association caused by prosperous counties showing the first signs of improvement in both causes, because the effects are focused on the corresponding generations. In addition they encourage the view that the infant mortality and heart disease association is related to events in infancy.

It is also possible to examine the two causes in different ways—for example, entirely within 1968–78. Different generations reach this period at different age groups but otherwise the calculations follow identically.

Plotting the ratios again (figure 8) shows an association, although the counties tend to separate into the groups defined in table II. The weighted correlation is slightly larger at 0·54 and equally significant. It is perhaps important to recall that this test of the association uses only the susceptibility component. The tendency for the county groups to separate could be related to the subsequent affluence factor.

1 *Registrar general's statistical review of England and Wales.* Part 1. Tables, medical. London: HMSO, 1883 and following years.
2 Office of Population Censuses and Surveys. *Mortality statistics: cause.* Series DH2. London: HMSO, 1973 and following years.
3 Clayton DG, Taylor D, Shaper AG. Trends in heart disease in England and Wales, 1950–73. *Health Trends* 1977;**9**:1–6.

PART III
CASE-CONTROL STUDY

12: Childhood risk factors for ischaemic heart disease and stroke

D COGGON, B M MARGETTS, D J P BARKER,
P H M CARSON, J S MANN, K G OLDROYD,
C WICKHAM

To explore the relation between environmental influences in early life and risk of cardiovascular disease in adulthood, case-control comparisons were made on 99 patients with acute myocardial infarction and 55 patients with recent hemisphere stroke. After allowance for smoking habits and current social class, risk of myocardial infarction was higher in subjects of lower social class at birth, smaller stature, and with a history of infant and especially perinatal death in a sibling. Stroke was also associated with infant or perinatal death in a sibling. Although none of these associations was significant at a 5% level, they support other evidence that implicates the prenatal and early postnatal environment in the aetiology of cardiovascular disease.

Introduction

Within England and Wales there is a close relation between current geographical differences in mortality from cardiovascular disease and past differences in infant and maternal mortality (chapters 1 and 2). To test whether this association with an adverse environment in early life applies to individuals as well as communities, we have carried out case-control studies on patients admitted to hospital after acute myocardial infarction or stroke.

Methods

MYOCARDIAL INFARCTION

The study was carried out in Stoke-on-Trent and Newcastle under Lyme county districts. The case group comprised all residents of the study area aged under 65 who were admitted to the local district general hospital with acute myocardial infarction (diagnosed according to WHO criteria)[1] on days when any of three participating medical teams was responsible for emergency admissions. Recruitment began in May 1986 and continued until August 1987. Each patient was paired with a control, who was resident in the study area and of the same age (to within 5 years) and sex. The controls were surgical inpatients and were selected according to a set algorithm.

Patients and controls were interviewed in hospital by a research assistant and asked about their childhood and family background using a tightly structured questionnaire aimed at identifying mortality among siblings. At the time of the interviews, the research assistant was unaware of the study hypothesis.

STROKE

The case group comprised all female patients aged over 65 who were admitted to Southampton hospitals during June 1986–May 1987 with a recent hemisphere stroke. Those with evidence of embolism from a cardiac source or with subarachnoid haemorrhage were excluded. One week after admission, patients were visited in hospital and an interview sought. If they were dysphasic or failed a standard mental function test, information was sought from a visiting relative.[2]

Each patient was paired with two controls, one from admissions to acute surgical wards and one from a list of all patients registered with general practices in the hospitals' catchment area. Each control was age matched to within 5 years of the patient. If information about a patient had been obtained from a relative, information about the hospital control was also sought from a visitor. All community controls were interviewed in person.

Analysis of both studies was by conditional logistic regression for matched sets.[3]

Results

MYOCARDIAL INFARCTION

One hundred and fourteen patients with myocardial infarction satisfied the entry criteria for the study, but six died soon after arriving in hospital, one suffered a stroke and became aphasic, and eight were discharged before they could be interviewed. Of the remaining 99 patients, 74 were men and

25 were women. Their ages ranged from 25 to 64, mean 55·7 and median 57, years.

Table I shows the relation of myocardial infarction to indices of the intrauterine and postnatal environment. Separate risks were calculated for each index independently, and also with allowance for smoking habit and current social class. Risks were higher in people with lower social class at birth, smaller stature (self reported) and a history of infant or perinatal death in one or more siblings. For each of these, the higher risks persisted after adjustment for smoking and current social class, but none was significant at a 5% level.

STROKE

Eighty six patients were identified, but 10 died before interview, 14 were dysphasic and had no relatives who visited, and seven were discharged within a week of admission. Fifty five patients were interviewed, including 21 for whom information was obtained from a relative—usually a sister, daughter, or husband. Hospital controls could not be obtained for two patients aged over 90.

Table II shows the relation of stroke to indices of the early environment. The risk estimates presented were calculated using all controls combined, but findings were similar when the two control groups were analysed

TABLE I—*Risk of myocardial infarction by childhood factors (results of conditional logistic regression)*

	No of cases	No of controls	Relative risk A	95% CI	Relative risk B	95% CI
Social class at birth:						
I, II, III Non-manual	4	9	1		1	
III Manual	34	36	2·0	0·6 to 6·7	1·9	0·6 to 6·5
IV, V	42	46	2·1	0·6 to 7·5	2·0	0·5 to 7·6
Armed forces	12	6	4·7	1·0 to 22·7	3·9	0·8 to 19·2
Unknown	7	2				
Height (cm):						
≤164	26	21	1		1	
165–170	25	23	0·8	0·4 to 1·9	0·9	0·4 to 2·1
171–177	26	23	0·8	0·3 to 2·1	0·8	0·3 to 2·2
≥178	22	29	0·6	0·2 to 1·4	0·6	0·2 to 1·5
Unknown	0	3				
Infant or perinatal death in one or more siblings:						
No	71	77	1		1	
Yes	28	22	1·5	0·7 to 3·0	1·3	0·6 to 2·7
Perinatal death in one or more siblings:						
No	84	89	1		1	
Yes	15	10	1·6	0·7 to 3·9	1·6	0·6 to 3·9

A = adjusted for age and sex; B = adjusted for age, sex, smoking history, and current social class; CI = confidence interval.

135

TABLE II—*Risk of stroke by childhood factors (results of conditional logistic regression)*

	No of cases	No of hospital controls	No of community controls	Relative risk A	95% CI	Relative risk B	95% CI
Social class at birth:							
I, II, III Non-manual	8	9	15	1		1	
III manual	16	14	17	1·3	0·5 to 3·6	1·5	0·4 to 6·3
IV, V	21	26	20	1·1	0·4 to 2·9	0·9	0·2 to 3·3
Armed Forces	1	1	1	0·9	0·1 to 11·3	0·3	0·0 to 5·3
Unknown	9	3	2				
Height (cm):							
≤158	20	23	20	1		1	
159–163	11	11	23	0·7	0·3 to 1·9	0·7	0·2 to 2·6
≥164	18	13	12	1·7	0·7 to 4·1	2·3	0·7 to 7·1
Unknown	6	6	0				
Infant or perinatal death in one or more siblings:							
No	30	38	42	1		1	
Yes	17	14	13	1·9	0·9 to 4·1	1·7	0·7 to 4·3
Unknown	8	1	0				

A = adjusted for age and sex; B = adjusted for age, sex, smoking history, and current social class; CI = confidence interval.

separately. There were no clear trends in relation to social class at birth or height, but risk was higher in women with a history of infant or perinatal death in one or more siblings. The association persisted after adjustment for smoking habits and current social class.

Discussion

The findings of these case-control studies of people with acute myocardial infarction and stroke are consistent with the hypothesis that an adverse environment during early life increases the risk of cardiovascular disease. The associations observed are unlikely to have been strongly influenced by biases in the choice of the control groups. The surgical patients used as controls suffered from a wide range of diseases. Individually, some of these diseases may be related to one or more of the risk factors under examination, but in the control group as a whole, the effects of such selection biases should have been diluted. In the stroke study, the distribution of exposure variables in the hospital and community controls was similar.

Nor are the associations likely to be explained by biases in the recall of patients and controls. We do not know how well middle aged and elderly people remember details of their childhood, but there is no reason to expect that the recall of patients with myocardial infarction or stroke should be more or less accurate than that of surgical patients. Patients and hospital controls were interviewed under similar conditions in hospital wards. Information in the stroke study was obtained by proxy more often for patients than for controls but, if anything, this would be expected to reduce associations.

After allowance for smoking and current social class, the risk of myocardial infarction increased with lower social class at birth (table I). The higher risk of myocardial infarction associated with shorter stature is consistent with this, as height is largely determined during early childhood.

Both myocardial infarction and stroke were associated with an infant or perinatal death in one or more siblings. It was not always easy to distinguish deaths before and after 1 week of age, especially in the study of stroke. Although the reliability of a history of sibling death at an early age may be questioned, our findings support those in the USA, where Rose showed that siblings of ischaemic heart disease patients had stillbirth and infant mortality rates twice those of controls.[4]

Further evidence that the infant environment influences later risk of cardiovascular disease comes from a cohort study carried out in parallel with these case-control investigations (chapter 13). Among 5654 men born in Hertfordshire during 1911–30, those with the lowest weights at birth and at 1 year had the highest death rates from ischaemic heart disease.

As yet, little is known about the processes which could link an adverse environment in childhood with later risk of cardiovascular disease. There is, however, some evidence that aspects of early life can have long term effects on blood pressure (chapter 15) and serum cholesterol (chapter 25), two major cardiovascular risk factors.[5]

We thank the physicians and surgeons at the City General Hospital, Stoke-on-Trent, Southampton General Hospital, and the Royal South Hants Hospital, who allowed us to approach their patients.

1 World Health Organisation. Regional Office for Europe. *Myocardial infarction community registers: results of a WHO international collaborative study coordinated by the regional office for Europe.* Copenhagen: WHO Regional Office for Europe, 1976. (Public Health in Europe 5).

2 Quereshi KN, Hodkinson HM. Evaluation of a ten question mental test in the institutional elderly. *Age Ageing* 1974;3:152–7.

3 Breslow NE, Day NE. *Statistical methods in cancer research. Vol. I. The analysis of case-control studies.* Lyon: International Agency for Research on Cancer, 1980.

4 Rose G. Familial patterns in ischaemic heart disease. *British Journal of Preventive and Social Medicine* 1964;18:75–80.

5 Mott GE. Deferred effects of breast feeding versus formula feeding on serum lipoprotein concentrations and cholesterol metabolism in baboons. In: Filer LJ Jr, Fomon SJ, eds. *The breastfed infant: a model for performance. Report of the 91st Ross Conference on Paediatric Research.* Columbus, Ohio: Ross Laboratories, 1986:144–9.

PART IV
FOLLOW UP STUDIES FROM
BIRTH TO DEATH

13: Weight in infancy and death from ischaemic heart disease

D J P BARKER, P D WINTER, C OSMOND,
B M MARGETTS, S J SIMMONDS

Environmental influences that impair growth and development in early life may be risk factors for ischaemic heart disease. To test this hypothesis, 5654 men born during 1911–30 were traced. They had been born in six districts of Hertfordshire, England, and their weights in infancy had been recorded; 92·4% had been breast fed. Men with the lowest weights at birth and at 1 year had the highest death rates from ischaemic heart disease. The standardised mortality ratios fell from 111 in men who had weighed 18 pounds (8·2 kg) or less at 1 year to 42 in those who had weighed 27 pounds (12·3 kg) or more. Measures that promote prenatal and postnatal growth may reduce deaths from ischaemic heart disease. Promotion of postnatal growth may be especially important in boys who weigh below 7·5 pounds (3·4 kg) at birth.

Introduction

The known causes of ischaemic heart disease explain only part of the differences in risk between populations and between individuals, and do not explain why in Britain the highest rates of the disease are in the poorest areas and lowest income groups.[1 2] The geographical differences in death rates from ischaemic heart disease in England and Wales are related to differences in infant mortality 70 years ago (chapter 1). This relation is with both neonatal mortality (deaths before 1 month of age) and postneonatal mortality (1 month to 1 year) (chapter 4). Impaired growth and development in prenatal and early postnatal life may be an important risk factor for ischaemic heart disease. To investigate this hypothesis, we have studied death rates in men born in Hertfordshire during 1911–30, whose weights at birth and 1 year were recorded.

Subjects and methods

The registration districts of Royston, Bishops Stortford, Ware, Hertford, Hatfield, and Barnet are grouped in east Hertfordshire. At the 1921 census most of the men were employed in agriculture or in trade and services.[3] There were no major industries. The combined population of the districts was 103 211. Infant mortality in the county was below the national average. In 1921–25 the rate was 49 deaths per 1000 births, 27 neonatal and 22 postneonatal.[4] The corresponding figures for England and Wales were 76, 33, and 43.

From 1911 the attending midwife was required to notify every birth to the county medical officer of health within 36 hours. Almost all births occurred at home. The name and address of the mother, the date of birth, and the birth weight were registered. The local health visitor recorded her observations on a form when she visited the home periodically throughout the first year. After a year the form was returned to the county health visitor and data were abstracted on to the register, including weight at 1 year and whether breast fed from birth, bottle fed, or both.

More deaths were expected in men than in women and men are more readily traced because they do not change their surnames. Of 17 464 boys born alive in the six districts in 1911–30, 1477 died during childhood. We excluded twins and triplets, leaving 15 664 singletons of whom 7991 had both birth weight and weight at 1 year recorded. Boys whose weights were recorded at ages other than 1 year but not at 1 year, were excluded. Weights were measured in pounds (2·2 pounds = 1 kg) and were often rounded to the nearest half pound or pound. We therefore used the original units. Where forenames were missing or other data required for tracing were incomplete, we sought additional information from the national birth index, which lists all births in the country, and from local registers of baptisms. For 7613 men identification data were sufficient for submission to the National Health Service central register at Southport: 5654 (74%) were traced, of whom 1186 had died at age 20–74 between 1 January 1951 and 31 December 1987. The average birth weight of men who were not traced was 0·1 pounds less than those who were traced, and the weight at 1 year was 0·2 pounds less.

We analysed cause of death in relation to birth weight, weight at 1 year, and infant feeding. The numbers of deaths were compared with those expected from national rates for men of corresponding age and year of birth.[5] Death rates were expressed as standardised mortality ratios, with the national average as 100. Ischaemic heart disease was defined by the International Classification of Diseases (9th revision) codes 410–414, chronic obstructive lung disease by 491–493 and 496, and lung cancer by 162–164. The social class of all except 22 of the men who had died was derived from the occupation recorded on the death certificate.

Results

Of the 1186 deaths, 434 were due to ischaemic heart disease; 328 occurred below the age of 65. The overall death rate from this condition (standard mortality ratio 82) was below the national average.

The mean (SD) weight at 1 year old was 22·4 (2·6) pounds. Standardised mortality ratios for ischaemic heart disease fell steeply with increasing weight at 1 year (table I). This downward trend was significant ($p < 0.002$, χ^2 for trend). Of the other leading causes of death only chronic obstructive lung disease showed a similar trend (table I). There were only 43 deaths from this cause and the trend was not significant. There was no trend in death rates from lung cancer in relation to weight at 1 year (table I). Death rates from all causes showed a significant downward trend with increasing weight ($p < 0.001$). Exclusion of deaths from ischaemic heart disease and chronic obstructive lung disease abolished this trend.

TABLE I—*Standardised mortality ratios according to weight at 1 year and birth weight. Numbers of deaths in parentheses*

| Weight (lb) | Cause of death | | | |
	Ischaemic heart disease	Chronic obstructive lung disease	Lung cancer	All causes
One year old:				
≤18 (n=324)	111 (37)*	129 (6)	98 (11)	89 (85)
19–20 (n=971)	81 (76)	86 (11)	99 (31)	89 (238)
21–22 (n=1850)	98 (163)	41 (9)	87 (48)	85 (405)
23–24 (n=1464)	71 (98)	61 (11)	57 (26)	68 (265)
25–26 (n=769)	68 (49)	52 (5)	97 (23)	73 (150)
≥27 (n=276)	42 (11)	29 (1)	70 (6)	58 (43)
Birth weight:				
≤5·5 (n=251)	104 (25)	93 (3)	113 (9)	101 (69)
6–6·5 (n=752)	77 (51)	59 (5)	101 (22)	69 (131)
7–7·5 (n=1598)	90 (129)	75 (14)	68 (32)	83 (340)
8–8·5 (n=1757)	85 (141)	50 (11)	85 (47)	80 (380)
9–9·5 (n=868)	62 (53)	69 (8)	67 (19)	70 (170)
≥10 (n=428)	81 (35)	33 (2)	109 (16)	77 (96)
Total (n=5654)	82 (434)	61 (43)	83 (145)	79 (1186)

*2·2 lb = 1 kg.

The mean (SD) birth weight was 7·9 (1·3) pounds. Men who weighed 5·5 pounds or less had the highest standardised mortality ratios for ischaemic heart disease at 104 (table I). The downward trend in standardised mortality ratios with increasing birth weight was not significant. Men who weighed 5·5 pounds or less also had the highest standardised mortality ratios for obstructive lung disease and for all causes of death (trend not significant). There was no trend in standardised mortality ratios for lung cancer.

Of the 5654 men, 429 (7·6%) had been bottle fed. On average they gained 0·4 pounds more between birth and 1 year than did those who were breast fed (p < 0·001, two sample t test). Among the bottle fed men, death rates from ischaemic heart disease did not fall with increasing weight at 1 year (table II). This difference in trend between men who had been breast and bottle fed was not significant. Because of the different weight gain of men who had been bottle fed and the suggestion of a different association with ischaemic heart disease, we restricted analysis of the interrelation of birth weight and weight at 1 to the 5225 men who had been breast fed. The lowest standardised mortality ratios occurred in men who had been above average birth weight or weight at 1 year (table III). The highest standardised mortality ratio (100) was in men for whom both weights had been below average. Men for whom both weights had been lowest, 5·5 pounds or less and 18 pounds or less, respectively, had a standardised mortality ratio of 220 (12 deaths, 95% confidence interval 114–384).

The simultaneous effect of birth weight and weight at 1 on standardised mortality ratios is shown in fig 1, derived with Cox's proportional hazards method.[6] The lines join points with equal risk of ischaemic heart disease and are truncated to define an area within which lie 95% of the weights. The values are risks relative to the value of 100 for those with average birth weight and weight at 1. Fig 2 shows the percentiles of weight at one year according to birth weight.[7] Fewer men with lower birth weights attained

TABLE II—*Standardised mortality ratios for ischaemic heart disease according to weight at 1 year and method of feeding. Numbers of deaths in parentheses*

Weight (lb)	Breast fed	Bottle fed
≤18	112 (33)	105 (4)
19–20	81 (71)	79 (5)
21–22	100 (154)	72 (9)
23–24	69 (85)	97 (13)
25–26	61 (40)	144 (9)
≥27	38 (9)	89 (2)
Total	81 (392)	94 (42)

TABLE III—*Standardised mortality ratios for ischaemic heart disease according to birth weight and weight at 1 year in men who had been breast fed. Numbers of deaths in parentheses*

Weight (lb) at 1 year	Weight at birth (lb)			
	Below average ($\leqslant 7$)	Average 7·5–8·5	Above average ($\geqslant 9$)	Total
Below average ($\leqslant 21$)	100 (80)	100 (77)	58 (17)	93 (174)
Average (22–23)	86 (34)	87 (67)	80 (29)	85 (130)
Above average ($\geqslant 24$)	53 (14)	65 (42)	59 (32)	60 (88)
Total	88 (128)	85 (186)	65 (78)	81 (392)

the heaviest weights at 1 year and hence the lowest risks of ischaemic heart disease (fig 1). For example, only 10% of men whose birth weight had been 5 pounds attained the median weight at 1 for those whose birth weight had been 10 pounds.

Among the men who died, mean birth weight was not related to social class at death (table IV). There was no downward trend in mean weight at 1 year with lower social class, but men in social class V had a lower than average mean weight ($p < 0.05$). The standard deviations in each social class were similar.

Discussion

We traced a population of men born in one part of Hertfordshire during 1911–30 whose weights in infancy were recorded. Hertfordshire is a prosperous part of England, and rates of ischaemic heart disease in the population are 18% below the national average. Weight at 1 year of age

TABLE IV—*Mean birth weight and weight at 1 year according to social class at death*

Social class	Mean (SD) weight at birth (lb)	Mean (SD) weight at 1 year (lb)
I (n = 38)	7·7	21·9
II (n = 177)	7·8	22·2
III non-manual (n = 125)	7·8	22·4
III manual (n = 430)	7·9	22·3
IV (n = 264)	7·8	21·9
V (n = 130)	7·8	21·6
Total (n = 1164)	7·9 (1·3)	22·1 (2·7)

145

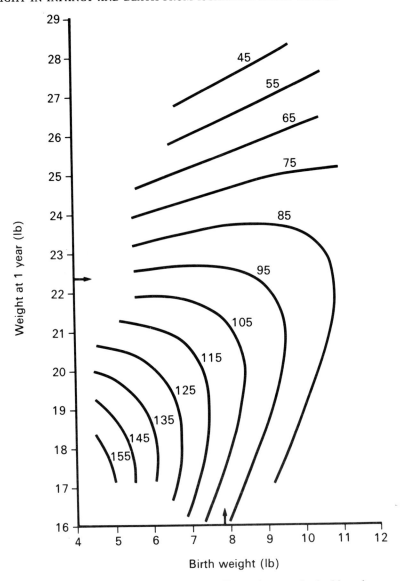

FIG 1—*Relative risks for ischaemic heart disease in men who had been breast fed, according to birth weight and weight at 1 year. Lines join points with equal risk. Arrows = mean weights.*

predicted death from ischaemic heart disease. Among those whose weights were 18 pounds or less, death rates were almost three times greater than those who attained 27 pounds or more. These large differences were reflected in differences in deaths from all causes and hence life expectancy.

146

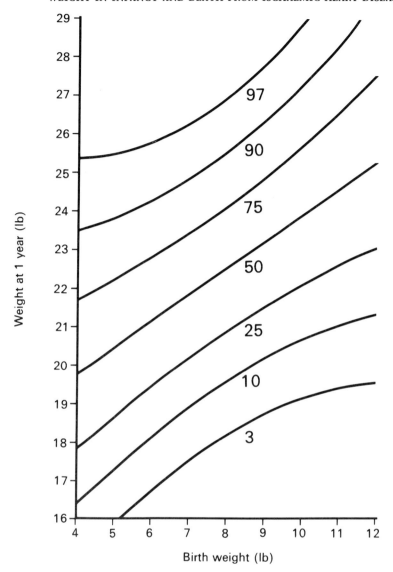

FIG 2—*Percentiles of weight at 1 year according to birth weight in men who had been breast fed.*

As 92·4% of the men had been breast fed, these results cannot be extrapolated to bottle fed populations.

Of all 15 664 singleton boys born in the area during the study period, 7991 were weighed both at birth and at 1 year. Those who were not weighed at these ages may have differed from those who were. However, our analysis was based on internal comparisons and bias would be introduced only if the relation between infant growth and death from ischaemic heart disease differed in the two groups; this is unlikely. We traced 71% of the 7991 men, despite the lapse of more than 60 years. Again bias from exclusion of those untraced is unlikely because the comparisons were internal. The variation within the data enabled us to make comparisons across a wide range of weights. Birth weights below 5·5 pounds had been recorded for 251 men. They had the highest death rates from ischaemic heart disease and chronic obstructive lung disease, and from all causes combined. Other evidence linking child growth with ischaemic heart disease comes from the inverse relation between adult height and cardiovascular mortality in England,[8] Norway,[9] and Finland.[10] Average height is also inversely related to cardiovascular mortality in the counties of England and Wales and in social classes (chapter 7).

From our findings it could be argued that an environment which produces poor fetal and infant growth is followed by an adult environment that determines high risk of ischaemic heart disease. The adult influence is a matter of speculation. It is unlikely to be cigarette smoking, as early growth is unrelated to death from lung cancer; nor is growth related to any other leading cause of death except obstructive airways disease. We have information on social class only for a selected group of men, namely those who had died. Among those men birth weight was unrelated to social class at death. Although average weight at 1 year was lower in men in social class V, the difference was small and there was no downward trend through all the social classes. These results argue against persistence of an adverse environment from intrauterine life to death.

The relation between weight at 1 year and death from ischaemic heart disease is strong: it spans more than 60 years, and it is graded. Among other leading causes of death only chronic obstructive lung disease shows a similar relation. Both prenatal and postnatal growth were important in determining weight at 1 year, as few infants with below average birth weights reached the heaviest weights at 1. The combination of poor prenatal and postnatal growth led to the highest death rates from ischaemic heart disease. We conclude that processes linked to growth and acting in prenatal or early postnatal life strongly influence risk of ischaemic heart disease. Birth weight is inversely related to adult blood pressure, and fetal growth can therefore be linked with hypertension, a known risk factor (chapter 15). Experiments on animals have shown that infant feeding programmes lipid metabolism throughout life.[11]

Our results suggest that greater early growth will reduce deaths from ischaemic heart disease. In England and Wales past trends in infant mortality, an indicator of infant growth and health, correlate with subsequent trends in ischaemic heart disease in the same generations (chapter 11). The large falls in cardiovascular mortality in the United States, Canada, Australia, and New Zealand during the past 20 years may also have resulted from improved child growth and health, reflected in the fall in infant mortality 60 and more years ago.

The benefits associated with postnatal growth are greatest for babies with below average birth weight (fig 1): heavier weight at 1 year is accompanied by large reductions in death rates. Promotion of infant growth in babies of below average birth weight may therefore be a priority. Among babies with above average birth weight the risk of ischaemic heart disease is below average, irrespective of infant growth. Measures that promote infant growth may have additional benefit. Birth weight is strongly influenced by maternal height,[12] which is itself largely determined by growth in early childhood.[13] Increased growth of infant girls may lead to improved prenatal growth in their babies and may further reduce deaths from ischaemic heart disease.

We are grateful to Hertfordshire County Archives, who preserved the records and allowed us to use them and to the University of Southampton Archives, who stored the records during data abstraction. Maire Dudleston, Carol Mincher, Sunita Parhar, and Julie Stevens computerised the data. The Milk Marketing Board gave a grant to assist tracing.

1 Gardner MJ, Crawford MD, Morris JN. Patterns of mortality in middle and early old age in the county boroughs of England and Wales. *Br J Prev Soc Med* 1969;**23**:133–40.
2 Office of Population Censuses and Surveys. *Registrar general's decennial supplement, occupational mortality in England and Wales 1970–72.* London: HMSO, 1978.
3 Registrar general for England and Wales. *Census of England and Wales 1921: county report for Hertfordshire.* London: HMSO, 1923.
4 General Register Office. *Registrar general's statistical review of England and Wales.* Part 1. Tables, medical. London: HMSO, 1921 and following years.
5 Berry G. The analysis of mortality by the subject–years method. *Biometrics* 1983; **39**:173–84.
6 Cox DR. Regression models and life-tables. *J R Stat Soc Ser B* 1972;**34**:187–220.
7 Cole TJ. Fitting smoothed centile curves to reference data. *J R Stat Soc Ser A* 1988;**151**:385–418.
8 Marmot MG, Shipley MJ, Rose G. Inequalities in death—specific explanations of a general pattern? *Lancet* 1984;i:1003–6.
9 Waaler HT. Height, weight and mortality: the Norwegian experience. *Acta Med Scand* 1984;**679** (suppl):1–56.
10 Notkola V. *Living conditions in childhood and coronary heart disease in adulthood.* Helsinki: Finnish Society of Science and Letters, 1985.
11 Mott GE. Deferred effects of breastfeeding versus formula feeding on serum lipoprotein concentrations and cholesterol metabolism in baboons. In: Filer LJ Jr, Fomon SJ, eds. *The breastfed infant: a model for performance. Report of the 91st Ross conference on paediatric research.* Columbus, Ohio: Ross Laboratories, 1986:144–49.
12 Butler N, Alberman E. *Perinatal problems: the second report of the 1958 British perinatal mortality survey.* Edinburgh: Livingstone, 1969.
13 Tanner J, Healy M, MacKenzie J, Whitehouse R. Aberdeen growth study I: the prediction of adult body measurements from measurements taken each year from birth to 5 years. *Arch Dis Child* 1956;**31**:372.

14: Relation of birth weight and childhood respiratory infection to adult lung function and death from chronic obstructive airways disease

D J P BARKER, K M GODFREY, C FALL,
C OSMOND, P D WINTER, S O SHAHEEN

A total of 5718 men born in Hertfordshire, England during 1911–30 was followed up. Their birth weights, weights at 1 year, and childhood illnesses had been recorded at the time by health visitors.

Fifty five of the men had died of chronic obstructive airways disease. The standardised mortality ratios were progressively lower with higher weights at birth and 1 year. In a subgroup of 825 men born in the county during 1920–30 and still living there the mean forced expiratory volume in one second (FEV_1) at age 59 to 70, adjusted for height and age, rose by 0·06 litre (95% confidence interval 0·02 to 0·09) with each pound (1 lb = 450 g) increase in birth weight, independent of smoking habit and social class. Bronchitis or pneumonia in infancy was associated with a 0·17 litre (0·02 to 0·32) lower adult FEV_1 and with a higher odds ratio of wheezing and persistent sputum production in adult life, independently of birth weight, smoking habit, and social class. Whooping cough in infancy was associated with a 0·22 litre (0·02 to 0·42) lower adult FEV_1.

It was concluded that lower birth weight was associated with

150

worse lung function. Intrauterine influences which retard fetal weight gain may irrecoverably constrain the growth of the airways. Bronchitis, pneumonia, or whooping cough in infancy further reduced adult lung function. They also retarded infant weight gain. Consistent with this, death from chronic obstructive airways disease in adult life was associated with lower birth weight and weight at 1 year. Promoting lung growth in fetuses and infants and reducing the incidence of lower respiratory tract infection in infancy may reduce the incidence of chronic obstructive airways disease in the next generation.

Introduction

Evidence from several sources suggests that infection of the lower respiratory tract in early childhood may impair lung function in adult life and lead to respiratory symptoms. Follow up studies of infants and young children who have had bronchitis, bronchiolitis, or pneumonia show that there are persisting abnormalities of lung function up to the age of 10 years.[1-3] In a sample of British children born in 1946 and followed up to age 36 years those reported as having had one or more lower respiratory infections before 2 years of age had a higher prevalence of cough during the day or night in winter and a lower peak expiratory flow rate.[4]

Though there is no direct evidence that childhood respiratory infection is linked with clinically significant obstructive lung disease, the findings of geographical studies point to such a link. Differences in death rates from chronic bronchitis and emphysema in the 212 local authority areas in England and Wales are strongly related to differences in infant mortality from bronchitis and pneumonia 70 years ago and before (chapter 3). The distributions of respiratory disease in childhood and late adult life internationally are also similar.[5] Studies of British born men who emigrated to other parts of the country or to the United States show that the prevalence of obstructive lung disease is associated with the place of birth independently of the place of current residence (chapter 6).[6]

Lower respiratory tract infections are more common among infants with low birth weight.[7] In later childhood these infants have a higher prevalence of cough and worse lung function than infants with normal birth weight.[8] We do not yet know whether birth weight relates to adult lung function or obstructive lung disease. Such a relation could result either from the association between lower birth weight and infant respiratory infection or an association between birth weight and lung size, as growth of the airways is largely completed in utero.[9]

In Hertfordshire, England, the birth weights of all babies born in the county have been recorded since 1911. From 1923 onwards information on illnesses up to the age 5 years has also been recorded. These data allow birth weight and childhood respiratory infection to be related to adult lung function and death from chronic obstructive airways disease.

Subjects and methods

As described in chapter 13, from 1911 onwards all births in Hertfordshire were notified by the attending midwife. Health visitors saw the children at home periodically throughout infancy (the first year of life). From 1923 onwards the health visitors continued to see the child up to the age of 5 years. They followed the child's development and noted the occurrence of illnesses. Illnesses occurring up to the age of 1 year and between the ages of 1 and 5 years were recorded in separate sections of each child's record, but the precise age at which each illness occurred was not generally recorded.

The health visitors' records have been preserved. We are tracing all singleton babies born in the county during 1911–30 who had birth weight and weight at 1 year recorded. Because tracing of women is complicated by change of name at marriage the present study is limited to men. In the six registration districts of east Hertfordshire tracing has been completed and the whereabouts of 5718 men (74%) is known. We analysed deaths from chronic obstructive airways disease (ICD (ninth revision) codes 491–493 and 496) and lung cancer (ICD codes 162–164) in relation to birth weight and weight at 1 year. Most of the deaths had occurred in men born before 1923, for whom childhood illnesses were not recorded. The numbers of deaths were compared with those expected from national rates for men of corresponding age and year of birth. Death rates were expressed as standardised mortality ratios, with the national average being taken as 100.

Of the men born in the six districts during 1920–30, 1157 still live there. They are an accessible and not too elderly sample; 845 (73%) of them agreed to be visited at home. They were interviewed by one of our four fieldworkers, who had not seen the health visitors' records. Each man was asked about his medical and social history, including standard questions approved by the Medical Research Council on respiratory symptoms.[10] Father's occupation was used to define social class at birth, and current social class was derived from the man's occupation. Before starting the study the procedures for the measurements were standardised and the fieldworkers trained. Lung function was measured with a hand-held turbine microspirometer (Micro Medical). After practice blows, and once reproducibility in an individual subject had been obtained, forced expiratory volume in one second (FEV_1) and forced vital capacity (FVC) were measured three times. The highest of the three values was analysed.[11 12]

Height was measured with a portable stadiometer. Statistical analysis was carried out using multiple regression; odds ratios were calculated by logistic regression.[13]

Results

Of the 5718 men, 55 had died from chronic obstructive lung disease. The death rate was below the national average, the standardised mortality ratio being 66. Table I shows that standardised mortality ratios fell progressively from 111 in men who had weighed $\leqslant 18$ lb at 1 year to 25 in men who weighed $\geqslant 27$ lb (χ^2 for trend $= 4.5$, p $= 0.03$). There was a weak trend of falling standardised mortality ratios with increasing birth weight (χ^2 for trend $= 2.6$, p $= 0.11$). There were no similar trends for lung cancer.

Complete data were obtained from 825 of the 845 men visited at home; their ages ranged from 59 to 70 (mean 64) years. FEV_1 fell by 0.05 litre for each year of age and rose by 0.03 litre for each centimetre of height. We therefore standardised all volumes for age and height with regression. The mean adjusted FEV_1 was 2.48 (SD 0.59) litres. Mean FEV_1 rose progressively with increasing birth weight, rising by 0.06 litre (95% confidence interval 0.02 to 0.09, p $= 0.0007$) with each pound increase in birth weight (table II). One standard deviation increase in birth weight was associated with a 0.07 litre increase in FEV_1. The corresponding increase for current height was 0.17 litre.

TABLE I—*Standardised mortality ratios (numbers of deaths in parentheses) for chronic obstructive airways disease and lung cancer in 5718 men, according to birth weight and weight at 1 year*

Weight (lb)	Chronic obstructive airways disease	Lung cancer
At 1 year		
$\leqslant 18.0$	111 (6)	87 (11)
− 20.0	87 (13)	99 (35)
− 22.0	65 (17)	91 (58)
− 24.0	60 (13)	59 (31)
− 26.0	44 (5)	96 (26)
$\geqslant 27.0$	25 (1)	61 (6)
At birth:		
$\leqslant 5.5$	131 (5)	110 (10)
− 6.5	69 (7)	96 (24)
− 7.5	80 (18)	73 (40)
− 8.5	46 (12)	86 (54)
− 9.5	79 (11)	67 (22)
> 9.5	28 (2)	103 (17)
All	66 (55)	83 (167)

TABLE II—*Mean forced expiratory volume in one second adjusted for height and age among men aged 59–70, according to birth weight*

Birth weight (lb)	No of men	Forced expiratory volume (l)
≤5·5	33	2·28
−6·5	103	2·41
−7·5	258	2·44
−8·5	242	2·52
−9·5	132	2·55
>9·5	57	2·57
All	825	2·48*

*Standard deviation = 0·59.

Table III shows the mean FEV_1 values of the 639 men born from 1923 onwards, when childhood illnesses were recorded. Fifty nine men were recorded as having had an attack of bronchitis or pneumonia during infancy. Their mean birth weight was 7·5 lb compared with 7·9 lb in all other men (difference 0·4 lb (0·1 to 0·8)). At each birth weight their mean FEV_1 was lower than that of men not recorded as having had bronchitis or pneumonia. After allowing for the birth weight distribution their mean FEV_1 was 0·17 litre lower (table IV). Sixty three men were recorded as having had an attack of bronchitis or pneumonia between 1 and 5 years of age. Their mean FEV_1 after adjustment for birth weight was similar to that of all other men (table IV).

Thirty one men were recorded as having had whooping cough during infancy, only four of whom had also had bronchitis or pneumonia. Table III shows that the mean FEV_1 of those who had had whooping cough in infancy tended to be lower than that of other men who had the same birth

TABLE III—*Mean forced expiratory volume in one second (litres) adjusted for height and age among men aged 59–67, according to birth weight and bronchitis or pneumonia and whooping cough in infancy. Numbers of men in parentheses*

Birth weight (lb)	Bronchitis or pneumonia in infancy		Whooping cough in infancy	
	Absent	Present	Absent	Present
≤5·5	2·39 (22)	1·81 (4)	2·30 (26)	
−6·5	2·40 (70)	2·23 (10)	2·38 (78)	2·39 (2)
−7·5	2·47 (163)	2·38 (25)	2·47 (175)	2·29 (13)
−8·5	2·53 (179)	2·33 (12)	2·53 (183)	2·40 (8)
−9·5	2·54 (103)	2·36 (5)	2·56 (103)	2·00 (5)
>9·5	2·57 (43)	2·36 (3)	2·57 (43)	2·30 (3)
All	2·50 (580)	2·30 (59)	2·49 (608)	2·28 (31)

TABLE IV—*Difference in lung volumes adjusted for height, age, and birth weight between men who had had recorded childhood illnesses and other men*

Childhood illness	Age (years)	No of men	Differences (l) (95% confidence interval)	
			Mean forced expiratory volume	Mean forced vital capacity
Bronchitis or pneumonia	<1	59	−0·17 (−0·32 to −0·02)	−0·24 (−0·40 to −0·07)
	1–4	63	−0·04 (−0·19 to 0·11)	−0·06 (−0·22 to 0·11)
Whooping cough	<1	31	−0·22 (−0·42 to −0·02)	−0·31 (−0·54 to −0·09)
	1–4	124	0·11 (−0·22 to 0·00)	−0·09 (−0·22 to 0·03)
Measles	<1	20	0·17 (−0·09 to 0·42)	0·10 (−0·18 to 0·38)
	1–4	134	−0·06 (−0·17 to 0·05)	−0·04 (−0·16 to 0·08)

weight. After allowing for the distribution of birth weight their mean FEV_1 was 0·22 litre lower (table IV). One hundred and twenty four men were recorded as having an attack of whooping cough from 1 to 5 years of age. Their mean FEV_1 after adjustment for birth weight was only 0·11 litre lower than that of other men.

Twenty men were recorded as having had measles during infancy, three of whom had also had bronchitis or pnuemonia in infancy. In contrast with the findings for whooping cough, the mean FEV_1 of these men was 0·17 litre higher than that of all other men, after allowing for birth weight (table IV). The mean volume of the 134 men recorded as having had measles between 1 and 5 years was similar to that of all other men.

Mean FEV_1 rose progressively by 0·02 litre for each pound increase in weight at 1 year (0·00 to 0·03). This trend was greatly weakened after simultaneous adjustment for birth weight whereas the trend in forced expiratory volume with birth weight remained strongly significant. The mean weight at 1 year of the 59 men who had bronchitis or pneumonia during infancy was 0·7 lb less than that of all other men. After allowing for birth weight, the mean reduction of weight at 1 year associated with bronchitis or pneumonia was 0·3 lb (−0·3 to 1·0).

One hundred and twenty seven of the men had never smoked cigarettes, 462 were ex-smokers, and 236 were current smokers. Mean FEV_1 fell from 2·69 litres in never smokers to 2·52 litres in ex-smokers and 2·29 litres in current smokers. Table V shows that this trend of increasing forced expiratory volume with increasing birth weight occurred within each smoking group. Analysis of covariance showed there was no significant difference in the relation of birth weight and FEV_1 between the groups. The reductions in FEV_1 associated with bronchitis or pneumonia and whooping cough (tables III, IV) were little changed by adjustment for smoking habits.

The social class at birth could be determined in 781 men. Birth weight, infant bronchitis or pneumonia, or whooping cough were not related to social class at birth and neither was adult FEV_1. The associations in tables

II, III, and IV were found within each social class. FEV_1, however, was lower in men with lower current social class. This relation partly depended on the higher prevalence of cigarette smoking in men with lower current social class, though there was a residual relation after allowing for smoking habit.

FVC fell by 0·03 litre for each year of age and rose by 0·04 litre for each centimetre of height. Mean FVC adjusted for age and height showed a weak positive trend with birth weight, which was not significant (table VI). At each birth weight, however, mean FVC was lower in the 59 men recorded as having had bronchitis or pneumonia during infancy. After allowing for the distribution of birth weight, the overall mean FVC of the 59 men was 0·24 litre lower (table IV). The mean FVC of the men recorded as having had an attack of bronchitis or pneumonia between 1 and 5 years of age was similar to that of all other men. The mean FVC of the 31 men recorded as having had whooping cough in infancy was 0·31 litre below that of the remaining men (table IV). Recording of measles in infancy or childhood was not associated with differences in FVC (table IV). The mean FVC rose progressively by 0·02 litre for each pound increase in weight at 1 year (0·00 to 0·03). The mean FVC fell from 3·16 litres in non-smokers to 2·99 in ex-smokers and 2·84 in current smokers. There was no trend in FVC with social class at birth. It was lower in men with lower current social class. Similarly to FEV_1 this relation partly depended on cigarette smoking. The associations with bronchitis or pneumonia and whooping cough were found in each current social class group.

At interview 226 of the men said that they had had wheezing at some time during the past year; 95 brought up sputum first thing on most mornings during three or more months of the year, and 155 usually coughed first thing in the morning. The odds ratio of wheezing was increased in association with lower birth weight and with bronchitis or pneumonia in infancy, though the trend with birth weight was not significant (table VII). Persistent production of sputum was not associated with birth weight but was associated with bronchitis or pneumonia in infancy. Cough was not associated with either birth weight or bronchitis or pneumonia in infancy. None of the three symptoms was associated with whooping cough in infancy.

Discussion

We examined death rates from chronic obstructive airways disease in a group of 5718 men born in Hertfordshire during 1911–30. We also studied respiratory function in 825 of the men who still live in the county. Their infant weights and childhood illnesses were recorded at the time, and these records allow early growth and illness to be related to death from obstructive airways disease, adult lung function, and respiratory symptoms.

TABLE V—*Mean forced expiratory volume in one second (litres) adjusted for height and age among men aged 59–70, according to birth weight and smoking habit. Numbers of men in parentheses*

Birth weight (lb)	Smoking habits			
	Never smoker	Ex-smoker	Current smoker	All
≤5·5	2·53 (4)	2·34 (16)	2·14 (13)	2·28 (33)
6·5	2·48 (20)	2·46 (52)	2·29 (31)	2·41 (103)
7·5	2·65 (37)	2·49 (154)	2·21 (67)	2·44 (258)
8·5	2·77 (39)	2·53 (134)	2·35 (69)	2·52 (242)
9·5	2·83 (19)	2·60 (75)	2·30 (38)	2·55 (132)
>9·5	2·79 (8)	2·60 (31)	2·43 (18)	2·57 (57)
All	2·69 (127)	2·52 (462)	2·29 (236)	2·48 (825)

TABLE VI—*Mean forced vital capacity (litres) adjusted for height and age among men aged 59–67, according to birth weight and bronchitis or pneumonia in infancy. Numbers of men in parentheses*

Birth weight (lb)	Bronchitis or pneumonia in infancy		
	Absent	Present	All
≤5·5	2·91 (22)	2·88 (4)	2·91 (26)
−6·5	3·02 (70)	2·81 (10)	3·00 (80)
−7·5	2·94 (163)	2·74 (25)	2·91 (188)
−8·5	3·03 (179)	2·76 (12)	3·01 (191)
−9·5	3·01 (103)	2·75 (5)	3·00 (108)
>9·5	3·11 (43)	2·57 (3)	3·08 (46)
All	3·00 (580)	2·76 (59)	2·98* (639)

*Standard deviation = 0·65.

TABLE VII—*Odds ratios (95% confidence intervals) of respiratory symptoms in men aged 59–67, according to birth weight and bronchitis or pneumonia in infancy*

	Symptom		
	Wheezing	Persistent sputum production	Cough
Birth weight (lb):			
≤6·5	1·38 (0·88 to 2·17)	1·04 (0·56 to 1·92)	1·04 (0·63 to 1·72)
−8·5	1·11 (0·73 to 1·69)	0·79 (0·44 to 1·43)	1·04 (0·66 to 1·65)
>8·5	1·00	1·00	1·00
Bronchitis or pneumonia			
Present	1·83 (1·05 to 3·20)	1·73 (0·83 to 3·61)	1·06 (0·54 to 2·07)
Absent	1·00	1·00	1·00

Mean FEV_1 fell with decreasing birth weight (table II). This trend was strongly significant and remained so after regression adjustment for current height, age, smoking habit, and social class. The effect of birth weight on FEV_1 was independent of the effect of current height, and nearly half as strong. This is remarkable given the imprecise nature of birth weight measurements made over 60 years ago. The association between birth weight and FEV_1 is unlikely to result from processes in the selection of our sample as comparisons are made within the sample and the relations are consistent across different levels of social class and smoking habit.

One possible explanation for the association between birth weight and FEV_1 is that babies with lower birth weight are more susceptible to lung damage during infancy resulting from adverse influences such as lower respiratory tract infection. However, the trend of falling FEV_1 with decreasing birth weight was largely independent of the occurrence of lower respiratory tract infection in infancy recorded by health visitors (table III). Furthermore, such adverse influences might be expected to retard infant growth. This is known to occur with lower respiratory tract infection,[14] and was again shown in our data. FEV_1 did not, however, fall with decreasing weight at 1 year, independently of birth weight. This suggests that reduced FEV_1 is related to lower birth weight independently of an adverse postnatal environment.

We suggest that the association between birth weight and FEV_1 reflects a direct relation between fetal lung growth and adult lung function. Growth of the airways,[9] as opposed to growth and expansion of the alveoli,[15] is largely completed in utero. We conclude that the relation between birth weight and adult FEV_1 may be a consequence of an adverse environment in utero which retards the weight gain of the fetus and irrecoverably constrains the growth of the airways. Such a long term effect of an adverse environment during a critical period of growth is a form of "programming."[16] Experiments in rats have shown that malnutrition around the time of birth permanently reduces lung size and DNA content.[17]

We found that men whom health visitors, during periodic visits in infancy, had recorded as having had an attack of bronchitis or pneumonia had a lower mean FEV_1 and FVC (table IV). This observation was independent of birth weight, smoking habit, and social class. Follow up studies of infants with acute lower respiratory tract infection showed that symptoms and abnormal lung function may persist into adolescence.[1-3] In a national sample of 3261 children born in 1946 and followed up to the age of 36 those whose mothers recalled, at interview two years after the birth, an episode of lower respiratory tract infection had a higher prevalence of winter cough and a lower peak expiratory flow rate.[4] We found no association between FEV_1 and lower respiratory tract infection between the ages of 1 and 5 years. The simplest explanation of these observations is that infection of the lower respiratory tract during a critical period in infancy has persisting deleterious effects.

Several studies have reported that whooping cough is not followed by persisting symptoms or abnormalities of lung function during childhood or early adult life.[18 19] In one study, however, persisting effects were found in those infected during infancy.[20] We found that men recorded as having whooping cough in infancy had a lower mean FEV_1 (table III) and FVC (table IV) independently of a history of bronchitis or pneumonia and independently of birth weight, smoking habit, and social class. The occurrence of whooping cough from 1 to 5 years was associated with smaller reductions in FEV_1 and FVC (table IV).

Measles infection was not related to a reduction in either FEV_1 or FVC (table IV). This is surprising as measles was a common antecedent of bronchitis and pneumonia 70 years ago.[21] Futhermore, the geographical distribution of infant deaths from measles in England and Wales 70 years ago was similar to the present distribution of deaths from obstructive lung disease (chapter 3). Given the difficulty of diagnosing measles during infancy, some infants with little or no rash may have been recorded as having bronchitis or pneumonia. Alternatively, measles tends to affect infants at an older age than does whooping cough, and the lungs may therefore be infected at a time when they are growing less rapidly.

Measurements taken with a turbine pocket spirometer are as repeatable as those taken with a Vitalograph, although the values given are slightly lower.[22 23] Previous studies with turbine pocket spirometers (as opposed to pneumotachograph microspirometers) did not show any significant downward drift in readings with time. We found no drift in recordings of FEV_1, although a small downward drift occurred in recordings of FVC during the study. In our study FVC was not related to birth weight but was reduced in men who had had a lower respiratory tract infection in infancy (table IV), in those with lower weight at 1 year, and in those who smoked. These relations were unaltered by adjustment for the drift in readings of FVC with regression. Notwithstanding the difficulties in measuring, an interpretation of these findings is that the components of lung behaviour which determine FVC, as opposed to FEV_1, are programmed in infancy rather than intrauterine life. This interpretation is supported by a study of 250 children aged 7 years whose FVC was not related to birth weight but whose FEV_1 was.[8]

In keeping with the results for forced expiratory volume, men who were of lower birth weight or had had bronchitis or pneumonia in infancy were more likely to report wheezing (table VII). Persistent sputum production, however, was not associated with lower birth weight but with bronchitis or pneumonia in infancy. This is consistent with the hypothesis that chronic airflow obstruction, indicated by a reduced FEV_1 and wheezing, and mucus hypersecretion, indicated by sputum production, are different diseases that often coexist.[11] A follow up study of men whose lung function and respiratory symptoms had been assessed in adult life showed that the risk of death from chronic obstructive airways disease was strongly correlated with the initial FEV_1. Symptoms of mucus hypersecretion were, however, a poor predictor of death from chronic obstructive airways disease.[12]

Death rates from chronic obstructive airways disease but not from another disease related to smoking, lung cancer, fell with increasing birth weight and weight at 1 year (table I). This is consistent with the strong relation between birth weight and forced expiratory volume and the relation between infant bronchitis or pneumonia and lower weight at 1 year. There were, however, only 55 deaths. Continued follow up and extension of the study to the entire county will bring greater statistical power.

One interpretation of our findings could be that the association of lower birth weight and infant respiratory infection with adult lung function merely reflects maternal smoking. The men in our sample, however, were born at a time when maternal smoking was uncommon. Although paternal smoking was common at the time, much disagreement still surrounds the issue of whether paternal smoking is associated with low birth weight,[24 25] and the magnitude of the effect, if any, is likely to be small. Earlier this century mothers' physique, nutrition, and health were the major determinants of fetal growth, and infant respiratory infection was linked with poor housing, large families, and overcrowding. Prevention of chronic obstructive airways disease may partly depend on promotion of fetal and infant lung growth and reduction in the incidence of lower respiratory tract infection in infancy.

We thank the men in Hertfordshire who gave us their time; Hertfordshire County Archives, who preserved the records; and Dr I Clarke, district community physician, who helped with the survey.

1 Pullan CR, Hey EN. Wheezing, asthma, and pulmonary dysfunction 10 years after infection with respiratory syncytial virus in infancy. *BMJ* 1982;**284**:1665–9.
2 Kattan M, Keens TG, Lapierre J-G, Levison H, Bryan C, Reilly BJ. Pulmonary function abnormalities in symptom-free children after bronchiolitis. *Pediatrics* 1977;**59**:683–8.
3 Mok JYQ, Simpson H. Outcome for acute bronchitis, bronchiolitis and pneumonia in infancy. *Arch Dis Child* 1984;**59**:306–9.
4 Britten N, Davies JMC, Colley JRT. Early respiratory experience and subsequent cough and peak expiratory flow rate in 36 year old men and women. *BMJ* 1987;**294**:1317–20.
5 Reid DD. The beginnings of bronchitis. *Proc R Soc Med* 1969;**62**:311–6.
6 Reid DD, Fletcher CM. International studies in chronic respiratory disease. *Br Med Bull* 1971;**27**:59–64.
7 McCall MG, Acheson ED. Respiratory disease in infancy. *J Chronic Dis* 1968;**21**:349–59.
8 Chan KN, Noble-Jamieson CM, Elliman A, Bryan EM, Silverman M. Lung function in children of low birth weight. *Arch Dis Child* 1989;**64**:1284–93.

9 Bucher U, Reid L. Development of the intrasegmental bronchial tree: the pattern of branching and development of cartilage at various stages of intrauterine life. *Thorax* 1961;**16**:207–18.

10 Medical Research Council. *Questionnaire on respiratory symptoms.* London: MRC, 1986.

11 Fletcher CM, Peto R. The natural history of chronic airflow obstruction. *BMJ* 1977;i:1645–8.

12 Peto R, Speizer FE, Cochrane AL, Moore F, Fletcher CM, Tinker CM *et al.* The relevance in adults of air-flow obstruction, but not of mucus hypersecretion, to mortality from chronic lung disease. *Am Rev Respir Dis* 1983;**128**:491–500.

13 Breslow NE, Day NE. *Statistical methods in cancer research.* Vol 1. *The analysis of case control studies.* Lyons: International Agency for Research on Cancer, 1980.

14 Rowland MGM, Rowland SGJG, Cole TJ. Impact of infection on the growth of children from 0 to 2 years in an urban west African community. *Am J Clin Nutr* 1988;**47**:134–8.

15 Thurlbeck WM. Postnatal human lung growth. *Thorax* 1982;**37**:564–71.

16 Bock GR, Whelan J, eds. *The childhood environment and adult disease.* Chichester: Wiley, 1991. (Ciba Foundation Symposium No 156.)

17 Winick M, Noble A. Cellular response in rats during malnutrition at various ages. *J Nutrition* 1966;**89**:300–6.

18 Johnston IDA, Lambert HP, Anderson HR, Patel S. Respiratory morbidity and lung function after whooping cough. *Lancet* 1983;ii:1104–8.

19 Britten N, Wadsworth J. Long term respiratory sequelae of whooping cough in a nationally representative sample. *BMJ* 1986;**292**:441–4.

20 Swansea Research Unit of the Royal College of General Practitioners. Respiratory sequelae of whooping cough. *BMJ* 1985;**290**:1937–40.

21 Halliday JL. *An inquiry into the relationship between housing conditions and the incidence and fatality of measles.* London: Medical Research Council, 1928. (MRC Special Report Series No 120.)

22 Gunawardena KA, Houston K, Smith AP. Evaluation of the turbine pocket spirometer. *Thorax* 1987;**42**:689–93.

23 Hosie HE, Nimmo WS. Measurement of FEV$_1$ and FVC. Comparison of a pocket spirometer with the Vitalograph. *Anaesthesia* 1988;**43**:233–8.

24 Chen Y, Pederson LL, Lefoe NM. Passive smoking and low birth weight. *Lancet* 1989;ii:54–5.

25 Davis DL. Paternal smoking and fetal health. *Lancet* 1991;**337**:123.

PART V
BLOOD PRESSURE

15: Growth in utero, blood pressure in childhood and adult life, and mortality from cardiovascular disease

D J P BARKER, C OSMOND, J GOLDING, D KUH,
M E J WADSWORTH

In national samples of 9921 children aged 10 and 3259 adults in Britain systolic blood pressure was inversely related to birth weight. The association was independent of gestational age and may therefore be attributed to reduced fetal growth. This suggests that the intrauterine environment influences blood pressure during adult life. It is further evidence that the geographical differences in average blood pressure and mortality from cardiovascular disease in Britain partly reflect past differences in the intrauterine environment.

Within England and Wales 10 year olds living in areas with high cardiovascular mortality were shorter and had higher resting pulse rates than those living in other areas. Their mothers were also shorter and had higher diastolic blood pressures. This suggests that there are persisting geographical differences in the childhood environment that predispose to differences in cardiovascular mortality.

Introduction

Blood pressure has been suggested as being one link between the intrauterine environment and risk of cardiovascular disease (chapter 2). We have therefore examined the relations among blood pressure, pulse rate, and intrauterine influences, as measured by birth weight, gestational period, mother's height, and mother's blood pressure. To do this we have used data from two large national samples, one of children aged 10 and another of adults aged 36.

We used geographical comparisons within England and Wales to examine the relation between intrauterine influences and cardiovascular disease. We compared geographical variations in mothers' heights and blood pressures, and in the birth weights of their children, with differences in cardiovascular mortality.

Subjects and methods

1970 Cohort—Roughly 97·5% of all births in Great Britain during one week in April 1970 were included in the British births survey.[1-3] Information recorded at around the time of birth included birth weight, gestational period, and mother's blood pressure at first attendance at the antenatal clinic. Social class at birth was derived from father's occupation. Surviving children were followed up at 10 years when they were examined by clinical medical officers. Their heights, weights, blood pressures, and pulse rates were measured by standardised procedures. Mothers' heights were also recorded. Blood pressure was measured towards the end of the examination by using a sphygmomanometer. The cuff size, which was recorded, was sufficient to encircle the upper arm completely and cover two thirds of its length. Diastolic pressure was recorded at the fourth Korotkoff sound. Recordings were usually rounded to the nearest 10 mm Hg. Pulse rate was recorded over one minute at the beginning and end of the examination after the child had been left to settle for two minutes. We took the lower of the two recordings as the resting rate. Our analysis of these data is based on the 9921 children born in England and Wales for whom there were complete data.

1946 Cohort—The Medical Research Council's national survey of health and development is a follow up study from birth of 5362 people born in 1946.[4] The sample was taken from births in England, Wales, or Scotland during the week 3–9 March and comprises all single, legitimate births to wives of non-manual and agricultural workers and a randomly selected one in four sample of single, legitimate births to manual workers. Information on birth weight and mother's height was obtained from maternity records and by health visitors eight weeks after the birth. At the last data collection, when the study population was aged 36, contact was made with 3259 men and women, representing 86% of the sample still alive and resident in England, Wales, or Scotland. At that time heights, weights, blood pressures, and pulse rates were measured by specially trained nurses. Blood pressure was measured at the end of an interview, during which the subject had been seated for a median of 100 minutes. Measurements were taken on the left arm by using the Hawksley random zero sphygmomanometer and a regular size (12×23 cm) upper arm cuff. Systolic and diastolic (phase V) pressures were recorded and corrected for arm circumference.

Cardiovascular mortality—Our analysis is based on cardiovascular mortality during 1968–78 at ages 35–74 in both sexes combined, as described in chapter 1.

Results

BLOOD PRESSURE AND PULSE RATE

Among the 10 year old children in the 1970 cohort both systolic blood pressure and diastolic blood pressure were positively related to pulse rate. Regression analysis showed that an increase of 10 mm Hg in systolic pressure was associated with an increase in pulse rate of 0·7 beat/min in boys (95% confidence interval 0·4 to 0·9) and 0·9 beat/min in girls (0·6 to 1·1). There was a similar relation among the 36 year old adults from the 1946 cohort, the corresponding figures being an increase of 1·2 beats/min in men (95% confidence interval 0·9 to 1·6) and 0·9 beat/min in women (0·6 to 1·2). The mean pulse rate was higher in girls (79·4 beats/min) than boys (76·3 beats/min) and higher in women (73·0 beats/min) than men (70·9 beats/min).

BLOOD PRESSURE, PULSE RATE, AND BIRTH WEIGHT

There was an inverse relation between systolic blood pressure at age 10 and birth weight. Systolic pressure was also related to current weight but in the opposite direction. These relations are shown in table I, which gives

TABLE I—*Mean systolic blood pressures (mm Hg) of 9921 children aged 10 stratified by thirds of current weight and birth weight*

Birth weight*	Boys Current weight (kg)				Girls Current weight (kg)			
	<29·7	29·7–33·9	>33·9	All boys	<29·7	29·7–34·6	>34·6	All girls
Lowest	95·8	98·0	101·4	98·5	96·0	98·6	101·2	98·6
Middle	96·2	97·4	100·9	98·1	95·4	97·7	100·9	98·0
Highest	95·7	97·7	100·8	98·1	94·7	97·3	99·8	97·3
All	95·9	97·7	101·0	98·2	95·3	97·9	100·6	98·0

*Boys: Lower tertiles of birth weight 3030, 3230, and 3320 g; upper tertiles 3430, 3630, and 3710 g. *Girls:* Lower tertiles of birth weight 2980, 3090, and 3180 g; upper tertiles 3350, 3490, and 3540 g.
Numbers of subjects in each cell within table ranged from 499 to 584; standard errors ranged from 0·42 to 0·51.

mean systolic pressures with subjects divided into three roughly equal groups by birth weight within each third of body weight. Among boys within each body weight group mean systolic pressure fell by around 0·38 mm Hg from the lowest to the highest birthweight group (95% confidence interval −0·04 to 0·80). Among girls the fall was 1·32 mm Hg (95% confidence interval 1·03 to 1·61). There was no similar trend for diastolic pressure.

There was a stronger inverse relation between systolic pressure at age 36 and birth weight. As before, systolic pressure was also related to current weight. These relations are shown in table II, which gives mean systolic pressures with men and women divided into three roughly equal groups by birth weight within each third of body weight. Because birth weight was recorded only to the nearest quarter of a pound (113 g) there is some variation in the numbers of subjects in each cell within table II. Among men within each body weight group mean systolic pressure fell by 2·57 mm Hg from the lowest to the highest birthweight group (95% confidence interval 0·98 to 4·16). Among women the fall was 1·83 mm Hg (0·28 to 3·39). There was no similar trend for diastolic pressure.

Both at 10 and 36 years of age pulse rate was weakly inversely related to birth weight. At neither age was this significant at the 5% level.

Table III shows mean systolic blood pressures at 10 years of age stratified by completed weeks of gestation. Mean pressures were similar at all gestational periods. Hence the inverse relation with birth weight was not the result of a shortened gestational period. There were no data on length of gestation for the adults.

TABLE II—*Mean systolic blood pressures (mm Hg) of 1625 men and 1634 women at age 36 stratified by thirds of current weight and birth weight*

Birth weight*	Men Current weight (kg)				Women Current weight (kg)			
	<71·1	71·1–80·0	>80·0	All men	<56·6	56·6–64·5	>64·5	All women
Lowest	123·2	124·2	124·6	124·0	118·7	117·3	120·2	118·6
Middle	122·2	121·2	125·6	122·8	117·5	115·0	117·1	116·7
Highest	121·3	119·8	123·2	121·5	116·8	115·3	118·6	116·7
All	122·4	122·0	124·4	122·9	117·8	116·1	118·6	117·4

Men: Lower tertiles of birth weight 3180, 3200, and 3410 g; upper tertiles 3520, 3770, and 3750 g. *Women:* Lower tertiles of birth weight 3070, 3180, and 3180 g; upper tertiles 3410, 3520, and 3640 g.
Numbers of subjects in each cell within table ranged from 121 to 236; standard errors ranged from 0·96 to 1·38.

TABLE III—*Mean systolic blood pressures of 10 year olds stratified by gestational age*

	Gestation (weeks)				
	≤36	37-	39-	≥41	All
Mean systolic pressure (mm Hg)	98·1	98·4	98·2	98·1	98·2
No of children	304	1119	4035	2645	8103

BLOOD PRESSURE, PULSE RATE, AND MOTHER'S HEIGHT

Table IV shows the mean systolic blood pressures and pulse rates of the adults with subjects divided into three roughly equal groups according to maternal height. Between the groups with the shortest and tallest mothers systolic pressure fell by 2·2 mm Hg (95% confidence interval 0·4 to 4·1) among men and by 1·0 mm Hg (95% confidence interval −0·9 to 3·0) among women. Standardisation to allow for the subjects' weight increased the differences. Falls in diastolic pressure between the groups were smaller than falls in systolic pressure. Mean pulse rates showed small differences with maternal height, and these disappeared after allowing for the subjects' height. Among the 10 year olds blood pressure and mother's height were not related.

BLOOD PRESSURE, PULSE RATE, AND MOTHER'S BLOOD PRESSURE

Mothers' blood pressures were not recorded for the 36 year olds. Among the 10 year olds mean systolic pressure and pulse rates varied with mothers' systolic and diastolic pressures measured at first attendance at the antenatal

TABLE IV—*Mean systolic blood pressures and pulse rates of men and women at age 36 stratified by mothers' heights*

	Mother's height		
	≤62 in (157 cm)	63–64 in (160–163 cm)	≥65 in (165 cm)
Men:			
Systolic pressure (mm Hg)	123·8	123·4	121·6
(adjusted for weight)	(124·0)	(123·4)	(121·3)
Pulse rate (beats/min)	71·2	71·3	70·3
(adjusted for height)	(71·0)	(71·3)	(70·6)
Women:			
Systolic pressure (mm Hg)	118·0	116·7	117·0
(adjusted for weight)	(118·0)	(116·7)	(117·0)
Pulse rate (beats/min)	73·1	73·3	72·4
(adjusted for height)	(72·8)	(73·4)	(72·6)

TABLE V—*Mean systolic blood pressures and pulse rates of 10 year olds stratified by mothers' diastolic blood pressures*

	Mother's diastolic pressure (mm Hg)			
	< 70	70	71–80	> 80
Systolic pressure (mm Hg)	97·4	97·9	98·5	99·5
(adjusted for weight)	(97·8)	(98·0)	(98·4)	(99·2)
Pulse rate (beats/min)	77·5	77·8	77·8	78·5
(adjusted for height)	(77·5)	(77·9)	(77·9)	(78·6)

clinic. Table V gives the results for diastolic pressure, with mothers divided into four groups. Rounding of results led to many pressures being recorded as 70 mm Hg. Between the groups of mothers with the lowest and highest pressures the children's systolic pressure rose by 2·0 mm Hg (95% confidence interval 1·0 to 3·0) and pulse rate by 1·0 beat/min (95% confidence interval 0·1 to 1·9). The results were similar for boys and girls. Adjustment for mothers' blood pressure made little difference to the relation between birth weight and children's blood pressure.

CARDIOVASCULAR MORTALITY

The number of adult subjects was too small to allow examination of differences in their variables among the 154 areas of England and Wales. To examine the geographical distribution of variables in the 1970 cohort we ordered the 154 areas according to standardised mortality ratios from cardiovascular disease. We derived five groups of areas with increasing cardiovascular mortality and roughly similar population size. Areas in the lowest cardiovascular mortality group were mostly in the south and east of the country, around London. Those in the highest mortality group were mostly in the north and west. Table VI shows the distribution of variables in the five groups. All values were adjusted to take account of the differing social class distributions in each group.

Among mothers heights fell from the lowest mortality group to the highest. There was no trend in systolic blood pressure but diastolic pressure rose from the lowest to the highest groups. Among children there was no significant trend in systolic pressure. There was, however, a clear trend of increasing pulse rate from the lowest to the highest mortality groups. This trend was little affected by adjustment for height, which fell from the lowest to the highest groups.

Discussion

Our analysis was based on two large samples of children and adults born in Britain and followed up from birth. These provide unique data for

TABLE VI—*Mean values of variables in 10 year olds and their mothers (adjusted for social class) in areas of England and Wales grouped according to cardiovascular mortality (ages 35–74, both sexes, 1968–78)*

	Group of areas					
	1 (Lowest mortality)	2	3	4	5 (Highest mortality)	χ^2 For trend (df = 1)
Mothers:						
Height (cm)	162·0	162·2	161·4	161·2	160·7	29·0**
Diastolic blood pressure (mm Hg)	71·0	71·1	71·2	72·2	71·8	9·0*
Children:						
Systolic blood pressure (mm Hg)	97·8	97·9	98·5	97·8	98·4	1·0
Pulse rate (beats/min)	77·0	77·2	77·5	78·5	78·3	13·4**
Height (cm)	138·9	139·2	138·6	138·5	138·0	14·6**
Weight (kg)	32·9	33·1	32·7	32·8	32·6	2·0
Birth weight (g)	3333	3334	3318	3335	3316	0·4

* $p < 0.01$; ** $p < 0.001$.

examining the relation between intrauterine influences and subsequent blood pressure and pulse rate.

Blood pressure and pulse rate correlated with each other both at 10 and 36 years of age. Blood pressure was higher in men than women but little different in boys and girls. Pulse rates were on average 2·1 beats/min higher in women than men and 3·1 beats/min higher in girls than boys. Blood pressure showed the well known association with body weight.[5] Pulse rate was inversely related to height, as might be expected from the general inverse relation between heart rate and body size in mammals.[6]

Both at 10 years of age (table I) and more strongly at age 36 (table II) systolic blood pressure was inversely related to birth weight. This was independent of current weight. Systolic blood pressure was also inversely related to maternal height (table IV) and positively related to maternal blood pressure (table V). Our data may underestimate the association of blood pressure and birth weight. Blood pressure measurements were not automated and were therefore subject to observer variation, and results were often rounded to the nearest 10 mm Hg. The spread of diastolic pressures was less than that of systolic pressures and rounding had a greater effect. This may explain the lack of associations with diastolic pressure. At both 10 and 36 years pulse rate was only weakly related to birth weight and was not related to maternal height (table IV). It was, however, positively related to maternal blood pressure (table V).

An inverse relation between blood pressure and birth weight had been recorded previously in two groups of children. Among 143 children in

Aberdeen who weighed between 2001 and 2500 g at birth the systolic and diastolic pressures at age 10 were higher than in a group of controls.[7] Among 692 children born in Dunedin, New Zealand, systolic pressure at 7 years was inversely related to birth weight.[8] To our knowledge the relation of birth weight to adult blood pressure has not been examined in any other set of data, except for a small retrospective study of 77 young men.[9] This inverse relation was not due to shortened gestation (table III) and may therefore be attributed to reduced fetal growth. Though the differences in mean systolic pressures were only 2 mm Hg between adults in the lowest and highest birthweight groups (table II), small differences in the population distribution of risk factors may have large effects on disease mortality. Available data suggest that a lowering of the blood pressure distribution by 10 mm Hg would correspond to a 30% reduction in total attributable mortality.[10] Birth weight is an indicator of many intrauterine influences. The magnitude of the intrauterine effect on blood pressure cannot be deduced from the size of the relation of blood pressure with birth weight.

The inverse association between blood pressure and maternal height (table IV) is consistent with the known relation between shorter maternal stature and reduced fetal growth.[11] The relation of blood pressure with birth weight was independent of the relation between blood pressure and maternal blood pressure (table V). This is consistent with the known lack of an association between maternal blood pressure and birth weight other than in severe pre-eclampsia.[11 12] A relation between blood pressure and maternal blood pressure has been recorded before.[13] The relation between blood pressure and other maternal variables known to influence fetal growth—for example, age and parity—is being examined.

Analyses on blood pressure at age 36 showed that the relation with birth weight was independent of two possible confounding variables—namely, cigarette smoking and the subjects' parity.[4] Other than current weight, which our analysis took into account, we know of no variables which might confound the relation of birth weight with blood pressure in childhood. We conclude that this relation is evidence that the intrauterine environment influences blood pressure and pulse rates in later life. Further studies being carried out in different areas of Britain will clarify the role of other variables in this relation.

There are several possible mechanisms linking an adverse intrauterine environment with higher blood pressure through an effect on fetal growth. Pressure in the fetal circulation might be raised as a method of maintaining placental perfusion, and the raised pressures may persist after birth.[9] Retardation of intrauterine growth may lead to accelerated postnatal growth that is accompanied by an accelerated increase in blood pressure.[14]

A link between the intrauterine environment and adult blood pressure might explain part of the geographical variation in death rates from cardiovascular disease within Britain. These variations are known to correlate with differences in mean systolic pressure in middle aged men.[15] The evidence that past differences in the intrauterine environment contributed to them rests on the close geographical relation between current cardiovascular mortality throughout England and Wales and past neonatal and maternal mortality 60 and more years ago (chapters 1, 2 and 4). Recent comparison of birth weights during 1912–38 in Preston and London— areas with high and low neonatal and maternal mortality in the past— supports considerable anecdotal evidence that fetal growth was less in the areas with higher mortality. Mean birth weight in Preston was 289 g below that in London (unpublished data).

Our analysis of children born during 1970 shows that there are no longer large geographical differences in birth weight. Among the mothers, however, those living in areas with high cardiovascular mortality were on average shorter and had higher diastolic pressures at first attendance at the antenatal clinic (table VI). Children in areas with high mortality were shorter and had higher pulse rates. These differences between areas were independent of social class. Only small geographical differences in children's blood pressures were recorded. In a recent survey in nine British towns, however, the mean pressures of children aged 5 to 7, measured with an automated recorder, were higher in towns with higher cardiovascular mortality.[16]

It may be expected that despite general improvements in the growth and development of girls, differences in the intrauterine environment from place to place will take several generations to disappear. The stability of fetal growth rates through successive generations has been shown by the positive correlation between the birth weight of mothers and their babies.[17 18] The geographical differences in the heights of mothers who had babies in 1970 and the differences in the pulse rates of their children at 10 years of age suggest that differences in the intrauterine environment predisposing to differences in blood pressure and cardiovascular mortality persist in Britain.

1 Chamberlain R, Chamberlain G, Howlett BC, Claireaux A. *British births*. Vol 1. *The first week of life*. London: Heinemann, 1975.
2 Butler NR, Golding J. *From birth to five: a study of the health and behaviour of Britain's five year olds*. Oxford: Pergamon Press, 1986.
3 Butler NR, Golding J. Haslum M, Stewart-Brown S. Recent findings of the 1970 child health and education study: preliminary communication. *J R Soc Med* 1982;75:781–4.
4 Wadsworth MEJ, Cripps HA, Midwinter RE, Colley JRT. Blood pressure in a national birth cohort at the age of 36 related to social and familial factors, smoking and body mass. *BMJ* 1985;291:1534–8.
5 Szklo M. Epidemiologic patterns of blood pressure in children. *Epidemiol Rev* 1979;1:143–69.
6 Schmidt-Nielsen K. *Scaling. Why is animal size to important?* Cambridge: Cambridge University Press, 1984.

7 Cater J, Gill M. The follow-up study: medical aspects. In: Illsley R. Mitchell RG, eds. *Low birth weight, a medical psychological and social study*. Chichester: Wiley, 1984;191–205.
8 Simpson A, Mortimer JG, Silva PA, Spears G, Williams S. In: Onesti G, Kim KE, eds. *Hypertension in the young and old*. New York: Grune and Stratton, 1981:153–63.
9 Gennser G, Rymark P, Isberg PE. Low birth weight and risk of high blood pressure in adulthood. *BMJ* 1988;**296**:1498–9.
10 Rose G. Sick individuals and sick populations. *Int J Epidemiol* 1985;**14**:32.
11 Butler N, Alberman ED. *Second report of the 1958 British perinatal mortality survey*. Edinburgh and London: Livingstone, 1969.
12 Baird D, Thomson AM, Billewicz WZ. Birth weight and placental weight in pre-eclampsia. *Journal of Obstetrics and Gynaecology of the British Empire* 1957;**64**:370–2.
13 Zinner SH, Rosner B, Oh W, Kass EH. Significance of blood pressure in infancy: familial aggregation and predictive effect on later blood pressure. *Hypertension* 1985;**7**:411–6.
14 Ounsted MK, Cockburn JM, Moar VA, Redman CWG. Factors associated with the blood pressures of children born to women who were hypertensive during pregnancy. *Arch Dis Child* 1985;**60**:631–5.
15 Shaper AG, Pocock SJ, Walker M, Cohen NM, Wale CJ, Thomson AG. British regional heart study: cardiovascular risk factors in middle-aged men in 24 towns. *BMJ* 1981;**283**:179–86.
16 Whincup PH, Cook DG, Shaper AG, MacFarlane DJ, Walker M. Blood pressure in British children: associations with adult blood pressure and cardiovascular mortality. *Lancet* 1988;ii:890–3.
17 Ounsted MK. Familial trends in low birth weight. *BMJ* 1974;iv:163.
18 Little RE. Mother's and father's birth weight as predictors of infant birth weight. *Paediat Perinat Epidemiol* 1987;**1**:19–31.

16: Fetal and placental size and risk of hypertension in adult life

D J P BARKER, A R BULL, C OSMOND,
S J SIMMONDS

To study the effect of intrauterine growth and maternal physique on blood pressure in adult life, infants born during 1935–43 in Preston, Lancashire were followed up. Their measurements at birth had been recorded in detail. The blood pressures of 449 men and women aged 46 to 54, who still lived in Lancashire, were measured.

In both sexes systolic and diastolic pressures were strongly related to placental weight and birth weight. Mean systolic pressure rose by 15 mm Hg as placental weight increased from 1 lb (0·45 kg) or less to more than 1·5 lb and fell by 11 mm Hg as birth weight increased from 5·5 lb or less to more than 7·5 lb. These relations were independent so that the highest blood pressures occurred in people who had been small babies with large placentas. Higher body mass index and alcohol consumption were also associated with higher blood pressure, but the relations of placental weight and birth weight to blood pressure and hypertension were independent of these influences.

These findings show for the first time that the intrauterine environment has an important effect on blood pressure and hypertension in adults. The highest blood pressures occurred in men and women who had been small babies with large placentas. Such discordance between placental and fetal size may lead to circulatory adaptation in the fetus, altered arterial

175

structure in the child, and hypertension in the adult. Prevention of hypertension may depend on improving the nutrition and health of mothers.

Introduction

The follow up study described in chapter 13 gave the first indication that the association between poor fetal growth and cardiovascular disease, found in geographical studies, exists for individual people. Among 5654 men born in Hertfordshire during 1911–30 those who had the lowest weights at birth and at the age of 1 year subsequently had the highest death rates from ischaemic heart disease. Differences in death rates according to early weight were large and were reflected in differences in life expectancy.

These findings raise the question of what processes link intrauterine life with risk of cardiovascular disease. Blood pressure, a known risk factor for both ischaemic heart disease and stroke, is one possibility. Geographical differences in the incidence of cardiovascular disease in Britain correlate with differences in mean blood pressure of men and women.[1] The persistence of rank order of blood pressure among people examined at intervals (tracking) has been repeatedly observed in longitudinal studies of children and adults.[2,3] Factors in adult life that are known to influence blood pressure, such as body mass, alcohol consumption, and intake of salt, account for only a small part of the differences in pressure between individual people and populations.[4]

To study the relation between intrauterine growth and blood pressure in adults we examined a group of middle aged men and women whose measurements at birth had been recorded in unusual detail.

Subjects and methods

From 1932 a standardised record was kept for each woman admitted to the labour ward at Sharoe Green Hospital, Preston, Lancashire. The record contained details of the mother's previous pregnancies and external measurements of her pelvis, including the conjugate diameter (distance between the symphysis pubis and the fifth lumbar vertebra). The baby's birth weight, placental weight, length from crown to heel, and head circumference were also recorded. Weights were measured in pounds (1 lb = 0·45 kg) and lengths and head circumferences in inches (1 inch = 2·54 cm). Measurements had often been rounded and we therefore preserved the original units.

Our first sample was of 259 men and women born during 1935–40 and the second, which was taken to test the strong associations found in the first, was of 190 people born up to 1944. The total sample came from 1298 singleton infants who were born to married mothers during 1935–43 and had complete records. We traced 1122 (86%) through the NHS central register; 503 were living in Lancashire at addresses known to their general practitioners and were asked to take part in the study. Of these, 449 (89%) agreed to do so.

Each subject was visited at home by one of four fieldworkers. The fieldworkers had not seen the obstetric data recorded for the subjects. Height was measured with a portable stadiometer and weight with a portable Seca scale. Blood pressure and pulse rate were measured with an automated recorder (Dinamap) when the subjects were sitting down. Readings were taken on the left arm with the cuff size recommended for the arm circumference. The room temperature was also measured. The subjects, who remained seated, were asked about their medical history, current medication, smoking habits, alcohol consumption, and family history of cardiovascular disease. Alcohol consumption was converted to the total number of grams consumed each week. According to criteria in general use, consumption was categorised as low (men $\leqslant 168$ g, women $\leqslant 112$ g), moderate (169–280 g, 113–168 g), and high (> 280 g, > 168 g).[5] The father's occupation was used to define social class at birth,[6] and current social class was derived from the subject's or her husband's occupation. After the interview the subject's blood pressure was measured again. The average of the two readings was used in the analysis. Before starting the study the procedures for measurements were standardised and the fieldworkers trained. No important interobserver variation was found during checks at intervals throughout the survey, in which repeat measurements were made on subjects selected from outside the study population.

Results

Systolic and diastolic blood pressures were strongly related to placental weight. In the first sample of 259 subjects the mean systolic pressure was 148 mm Hg in those who had had placental weights of $\leqslant 1.5$ lb and 159 mm Hg in those who had had weights of > 1.5 lb (difference 11, 95% confidence interval, 4 to 18). A second sample of 190 subjects was taken to test this relation. Among them the mean systolic pressure was 148 mm Hg for those whose placentas had weighed $\leqslant 1.5$ lb and 155 mm Hg for those whose placentas had weighed > 1.5 lb (7, 0 to 14). When the two samples were combined the difference was 9 (4 to 14).

Because the two samples were similar we combined them for further analysis. The ages of the 236 men and 213 women ranged from 46 to 54 (mean 50) years. The mean (SD) systolic pressures were 154 (20) mm Hg in men and 146 (23) mm Hg in women, and the mean diastolic pressures were 89 (11) mm Hg in men and 83 (11) mm Hg in women. Systolic pressure rose by 1·3 mm Hg for each year of age, and diastolic pressure rose by

1·0 mm Hg. We adjusted all pressures to age 50. One fieldworker took 55% of the blood pressure measurements, and the small, non-significant differences in the mean values obtained by the three other fieldworkers were adjusted for. The mean placental weight for the men was 1·4 lb and for the women 1·3 lb; mean birth weights were 7·0 and 6·9 lbs respectively. Placental weight and birth weight were strongly correlated (r = 0·52)

Table I shows the mean systolic and diastolic pressures according to placental weight and birth weight. For each birth weight systolic and diastolic pressures rose with placental weight, and for each placental weight both pressures fell with increasing birth weight. Simultaneous adjustment by regression for systolic pressure showed a rise of 15 mm Hg (95% confidence interval 8 to 23) from adults who had had placental weights of ≤ 1 lb to those who had had weights > 1·5 lb, and a fall of 11 mm Hg (3 to 19) from those who had had birth weights of ≤ 5·5 lb to those who had weighed > 7·5 lb. Similar patterns were found in men and women (table II). When birth weights were grouped at intervals of 0·5 lbs from ≤ 5·0 lb to > 9·5 lb systolic pressure in each group was higher in those who had had placental weights > 1·5 lb. The figure shows the simultaneous effect of placental weight and birth weight on systolic pressure. The highest pressures were among people who had been small babies with large placentas and the lowest were among people who had been large babies with small placentas. Multiple regression analysis for diastolic pressure showed a rise of 6 mm Hg (2 to 10) from subjects who had had placental weights of ≤ 1 lb to those who had had weights > 1·5 lb, and a fall of

TABLE I—*Mean systolic and diastolic blood pressures (mm Hg) of men and women aged 46 to 54, according to placental weight and birth weight. Number of subjects in parentheses*

Birth weight (lb)	Placental weight (lb)				
	≤1·0	−1·25	−1·5	>1·5	All
Systolic pressure					
≤5·5	152 (26)	154 (13)	153 (5)	206 (1)	154 (45)
−6·5	147 (16)	151 (54)	150 (28)	166 (8)	151 (106)
−7·5	144 (20)	148 (77)	145 (45)	160 (27)	149 (169)
>7·5	133 (6)	148 (27)	147 (42)	154 (54)	149 (129)
All	147 (68)	149 (171)	147 (120)	157 (90)	150 (449)
Diastolic pressure					
≤5·5	84	87	87	97	86
−6·5	84	88	85	93	87
−7·5	84	84	84	90	85
>7·5	78	85	85	88	86
All	84	86	85	89	86

TABLE II—*Mean systolic pressure (mm Hg) among adults, according to birth weight, placental weight, and sex. Number of subjects in parentheses*

Birth weight (lb)	Placental weight (lb)				
	$\leqslant 1 \cdot 0$	$- 1 \cdot 25$	$- 1 \cdot 5$	$> 1 \cdot 5$	All
	Men				
$\leqslant 6 \cdot 5$	150	159	152	161	155 (79)
$- 7 \cdot 5$	152	154	147	164	154 (85)
$> 7 \cdot 5$	132	149	153	154	153 (72)
All	149 (26)	155 (88)	151 (66)	158 (56)	154 (236)
	Women				
$\leqslant 6 \cdot 5$	150	143	149	191	149 (72)
$- 7 \cdot 5$	141	141	143	155	144 (84)
$> 7 \cdot 5$	133	148	139	152	145 (57)
All	146 (42)	143 (83)	143 (54)	157 (34)	146 (213)

2 mm Hg (-2 to 7) from subjects who had had birth weights of $\leqslant 5 \cdot 5$ lb to those who had weighed $> 7 \cdot 5$ lb.

In both men and women mean systolic and diastolic pressures were higher with higher body mass index (weight/height^2). When the sexes were combined those in the lowest quarter of the distribution ($\leqslant 24$ kg/m^2) had a mean systolic pressure of 145 mm Hg and mean diastolic pressure of 84 mm Hg and those in the highest quarter (> 28 kg/m^2) had mean pressures of 156 mm Hg and 87 mm Hg respectively. Among the 78 subjects with moderate or high intakes of alcohol, the mean systolic pressure was 4 mm Hg higher than that among those with low intakes (-1 to 10) and the mean diastolic pressure was also 4 mm Hg higher (2 to 7). Blood pressure was not consistently related to smoking or room temperature. Adjusting for body mass index and intake of alcohol made little difference to the values in table I. The simultaneous trends in systolic pressure with placental weight, birth weight, body mass index, intake of alcohol, and sex were calculated by multiple regression. Table III shows that the size of the trends in systolic pressure with placental weight and birth weight was only slightly changed by adjustment for the three other variables. The findings for diastolic pressure were similar.

Thirty six of the subjects (21 men, 15 women) were being treated for hypertension. Table IV shows the relative risk of hypertension according to placental weight. Risks were estimated by odds ratios. The trend of increase in risk up to 3·0 was significant (p = 0·01). There was no corresponding trend with birth weight. Table IV also shows the trend of increasing risk of hypertension defined by a systolic pressure of > 160 mm Hg, which was found in 124 subjects (75 men, 49 women). Risk

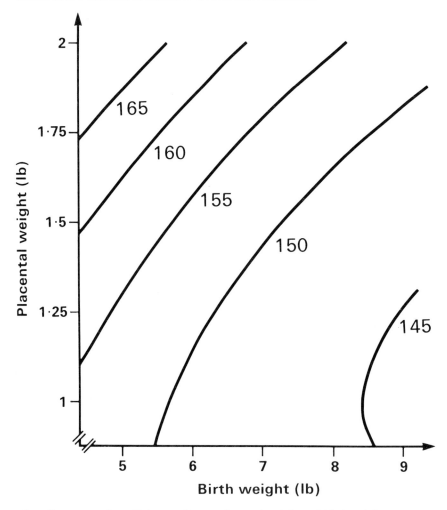

Systolic pressure (mm Hg) according to placental weight and birth weight.

rose to 2·5 in those who had had the heaviest placentas and fell to 0·7 in those who had had the heaviest birth weights. With body mass index risk rose to 2·3 in those with values in the highest quarter.

The duration of gestation of 370 subjects could be estimated because the date of onset of the mother's last menstrual period had been recorded. The simultaneous trends in systolic pressure with placental weight, birth weight, length of gestation, and sex were calculated by multiple regression. Adjusting for gestation had little effect on the trends in systolic pressure with placental weight and birth weight (table V). Findings for diastolic

TABLE III—*Mean change (95% confidence interval) in systolic pressure associated with placental weight, birth weight, body mass index, alcohol consumption, and sex*

	Systolic pressure (mm Hg)
Placental weight (lb):	
$\leqslant 1$	0
$-1 \cdot 25$	4 (-2 to 10)
$-1 \cdot 5$	1 (-5 to 8)
$> 1 \cdot 5$	12 (5 to 20)
Birth weight (lb):	
$\leqslant 5 \cdot 5$	0
$-6 \cdot 5$	-5 (-12 to 3)
$-7 \cdot 5$	-8 (-15 to -1)
$> 7 \cdot 5$	-10 (-18 to -2)
Body mass index (kg/m^2):	
$\leqslant 24$	0
-26	3 (-2 to 8)
-28	3 (-3 to 8)
> 28	10 (4 to 15)
Alcohol consumption:	
Low	0
Moderate	5 (-2 to 12)
High	5 (-2 to 12)
Sex:	
Men	0
Women	-6 (-10 to -2)

pressure were similar. Length of gestation had no significant effect on either systolic or diastolic pressure.

The parity of all except nine mothers had been recorded. The systolic and diastolic pressures were related to placental weight in the children of the 353 primiparous mothers and the 87 multiparous ones (table VI). The difference in systolic pressures associated with placental weights $> 1 \cdot 5$ lb and $\leqslant 1 \cdot 5$ lb was, however, greater in children of multiparous mothers. The inverse relation between pressure and birth weight was similar in children of primiparous and multiparous mothers.

TABLE IV—*Relative risk (95% confidence interval) of being treated for hypertension or having a systolic pressure > 160 mm Hg, according to placental weight*

	Placental weight (lb)			
	$\leqslant 1 \cdot 0$	$-1 \cdot 25$	$-1 \cdot 5$	$> 1 \cdot 5$
Treated for hypertension (n = 36)	1·0	1·3 (0·4 to 5·0)	2·4 (0·7 to 8·9)	3·0 (0·8 to 11·3)
Systolic pressure > 160 mm Hg (n = 124)	1·0	1·1 (0·6 to 2·2)	1·2 (0·6 to 2·5)	2·5 (1·2 to 5·0)

TABLE V—*Mean change (95% confidence interval) in systolic pressure associated with placental weight, birth weight, length of gestation, and sex*

	Systolic pressure (mm Hg)
Placental weight (lb):	
≤1	0
−1·25	4 (−2 to 10)
−1·5	3 (−4 to 9)
>1·5	13 (6 to 21)
Birth weight (lb):	
≤5·5	0
−6·5	−4 (−11 to 4)
−7·5	−7 (−15 to 0)
>7·5	−10 (−18 to −2)
Length of gestation (weeks):	
≤37	0
38	−2 (−9 to 5)
39	−2 (−8 to 3)
40	−3 (−9 to 20)
41	1 (−6 to 7)
≥42	−1 (−8 to 6)
Sex:	
Men	0
Women	−7 (−11 to −3)

All except 25 of the subjects could be classified according to social class at birth. In each social class there was a similar relation between systolic and diastolic pressures and placental weight (table VI). The results were similar when subjects were classified by current social class. In each social class there was also an inverse relation between pressure and birth weight.

TABLE VI—*Mean systolic pressure (mm Hg) by parity and social class at birth and at age 46–54.* Number of subjects in parentheses*

	Placental weight (lb)		
	≤1·5	>1·5	All
Parity:			
Primiparous	149 (289)	156 (64)	150 (353)
Multiparous	146 (65)	162 (22)	150 (87)
Social class at birth:			
I, II, III Non-manual	147 (101)	156 (20)	148 (121)
III Manual	150 (143)	160 (36)	152 (179)
IV, V	148 (94)	155 (30)	150 (124)
Social class at age 46–54:			
I, II, III Non-manual	147 (140)	158 (37)	149 (177)
III Manual	150 (131)	154 (34)	151 (165)
IV, V	149 (86)	164 (18)	152 (104)

* Parity of nine mothers not known and social class of 25 subjects at birth and of three at age 46–54 not classifiable.

Ninety four subjects said that their mothers had suffered from high blood pressure. These subjects' mean systolic pressure was 8 mm Hg higher than that of the other subjects (3 to 13). The 58 subjects whose fathers had high blood pressure did not themselves have higher pressure, the difference from the other subjects being −1 mm Hg (−7 to 5). The mean placental weight of those whose mothers had high blood pressure was the same as that of the remainder at 1·3 lb.

The mean circumference of the head at birth was 13·6 (SD 0·7) inches and the mean length was 20·4 (1·1) inches. Circumference of the head and length increased with birth weight. For any birth weight head circumference increased with placental weight whereas length decreased, so that the ratio of length to head circumference was strongly inversely related to placental weight. A 0·5 lb increase in placental weight was associated with a decrease of 0·23 SD (p < 0·01) in the ratio of length to head circumference.

Birth weight increased progressively with mothers' external conjugate diameter. The mean birth weight rose from 6·6 lb among those with mothers with conjugates of ⩽7·25 inches, to 7·5 among those with mothers with conjugates >8·25 inches. Placental weight was not related to the external conjugate diameter independently of birth weight.

Discussion

We found that blood pressure and risk of hypertension among men and women aged around 50 are predicted by a combination of placental weight and birth weight. The highest blood pressures and risk of hypertension were among people who had been small babies with large placentas. Because the strong relation with placental weight was unexpected we repeated our first study and found similar results. Higher body mass index and alcohol consumption were also associated with higher blood pressure, in agreement with the results of many other studies,[4] but the relation of placental weight and birth weight to blood pressure and hypertension was independent of these influences and stronger (table III). Two routine measurements taken at birth were better predictors of blood pressure than any current measurement. To our knowledge this has not been observed before.

The 449 people in our study had been born in hospital. In Preston 50 years ago only a small proportion of babies were born in hospital, and most of them were firstborn children. The correspondence attached to the maternity records showed that many mothers booked a bed at an early stage of pregnancy. Medical problems were not an important reason for the women choosing to have their babies in hospital. As the analysis was based on comparisons within the sample, bias would have been introduced only if the relations of blood pressure to placental weight and birth weight were different among people born in and outside hospital. Such bias seems unlikely because we showed that the relations were similar for first and later born children (table V). The similar results seen in people in each social class, whether defined at birth or currently, suggest that the findings were not biased by selective migration according to socioeconomic state. Weights recorded routinely at birth, especially placental weights, are subject to error. This would tend to reduce the strength of relations with later blood pressure, as would the inclusion of people whose blood pressures were being lowered by treatment (tables I–III).

In the only previous follow up study relating birth weight to blood pressure in adults there were no data on placental weight (chapter 15). There was a small difference of 2 mm Hg in mean systolic pressure between the 36 year old adults in the highest and lowest thirds of the distribution of birth weight. The differences by birth weight among all subjects in table I are consistent with this. The large, independent, and opposing effects of a fall in systolic pressure of 10 mm Hg associated with increasing birth weight and a rise of 12 mm Hg (table III) associated with increasing placental weight were not seen when all pressures at a given birth weight are combined.

The strength and gradation of the relation between blood pressure and placental weight and birth weight make it less likely that it depends on some unknown confounding variable. Findings in children, among whom there are fewer possible confounding variables, support this. Two recent surveys in Britain of children aged 5 to 10 found that blood pressure was inversely related to birth weight (chapter 15).[7] These associations in children are, however, weaker than those we found in adults.

Our data point to a possible mechanism for the relation between placental weight and blood pressure. Studies of fetal blood flow in animals have shown that in response to hypoxia there is a redistribution of fetal cardiac output, which favours the perfusion of the brain.[8 9] In our data greater placental weight at any birth weight was associated with a decrease in the ratio of length to head circumference. This disproportionate growth is consistent with diversion of blood away from the trunk in favour of the brain. Reduced blood flow to the trunk induced in a fetus that is small in relation to its placenta could have irreversible consequences, perhaps by influencing arterial structure.

There is evidence in animals and humans that changes in the haemodynamic load in early life can alter the structure and compliance of larger arteries.[10] In rats made hypertensive four weeks after birth the wall of the aorta thickens rapidly. This partly reverses if the hypertension is relieved. In young children born with a single umbilical artery the common iliac artery that gave rise to it is elastic whereas the other, which had lower blood flow, is thin walled and muscular.[11] These differences are reflected in differences in compliance, as measured by Doppler ultrasonography.[12] Compliance determines pulse pressure, and changes in pulse pressure produce changes in vessel wall scleroprotein, which in turn change compliance. This feedback could perpetuate high systolic pressure from infancy to old age. This is, however, only one possible mechanism by which fetal circulatory changes could change the structure of blood vessels in adults.[13]

Mothers' blood pressures are related to those of their children,[14] and it could be argued that placental weight is linked to adult blood pressure through a genetic mechanism that determines both the blood pressure of the child and the growth of the placenta. The blood pressure of pregnant women at their first antenatal attendance was studied in 5161 consecutive first births in Oxford during 1987–8. The pressures were unrelated to either birth weight or placental weight (C W G Redman, unpublished data). In our survey people who reported that their mothers had high blood pressure had higher blood pressure themselves, but their placental weights were similar to those of the remainder. People who reported that their fathers had high blood pressure did not themselves have higher blood pressure.

A question arising from our findings is, What environmental influences act on the mother and determine placental weight and birth weight? In particular, what determines the discordance between placental and fetal size which leads to high blood pressure? Little is known about maternal factors that influence placental growth. In our data the mothers' smoking habit and alcohol consumption were not recorded. The data show, however, that the mothers' external conjugate diameter is strongly related to birth weight. This is consistent with the known relation between maternal height and birth weight.[15] A woman's physique depends partly on her nutrition in childhood. The nutrition of girls may therefore be linked to blood pressure in the next generation.

The customary explanation for differences in blood pressure is that they depend on the environment during adult life.[16] Our findings, however, suggest that the intrauterine environment has a dominant effect on blood pressure. Research into the adult environment and hypertension has focused on salt.[4 17] A recent cross cultural study in 52 centres concluded that lowering the daily intake of sodium from 170 mmol to 70 mmol corresponded to a 2 mm Hg reduction in systolic blood pressure.[4] This is a small effect compared with those associated with placental weight and birth weight, which range over 25 mm Hg (table III). Differences of this order may have large effects on mortality from cardiovascular disease. Available data suggest that lowering the distribution of blood pressure among a population by 10 mm Hg would correspond to a 30% reduction in total attributable mortality.[18]

The decrease in mortality from stroke in Britain during the past 40 years is consistent with past improvements in maternal physique and health (chapter 11). Reducing blood pressure in a population may partly depend on improving the environment of girls and women, including improving their nutrition. This will reduce discordance between placental and fetal growth, which leads in turn to circulatory adaptation in the fetus, altered arterial structure in the child, and hypertension and cardiovascular disease in the adult.

We thank Mrs F Foden and the medical records staff at Sharoe Green Hospital, who preserved the records and allowed us to use them, and general practitioners throughout Lancashire, who helped us trace the subjects.

1 Shaper AG, Pocock SJ, Walker M, Cohen NM, Wade CJ, Thomson AG. British regional heart study: cardiovascular risk factors in middle-aged men in 24 towns. *BMJ* 1981;**283**:179–86.
2 de Swiet M. Fayers P, Shinebourne EA. Value of repeated blood pressure measurements in children—the Brompton study. *BMJ* 1980;i:1567–9.
3 Clarke WR, Schrott H, Leaverton PE, Connor WE, Laver RM. Tracking of blood lipids and blood pressure in school age children: the muscatine study. *Circulation* 1978;**58**:626–34.
4 Intersalt Cooperative Research Group. Intersalt: an international study of electrolyte excretion and blood pressure. Results for 24 hour urinary sodium and potassium excretion. *BMJ* 1988:**297**:319–28.
5 Royal College of Physicians. *A great and growing evil: the medical consequences of alcohol abuse*. London: Tavistock Publications, 1987.
6 Office of Population Censuses and Surveys. *Classification of occupations 1980*. London: HMSO, 1980.
7 Whincup PH, Cook DG, Shaper AG. Early influences on blood pressure: a study of children aged 5 to 7 years. *BMJ* 1989;**299**:587–91.
8 Campbell AGM, Dawes GS, Fishman AP, Hyman AI. Regional redistribution of blood flow in the mature fetal lamb. *Circ Res* 1967;**21**:229–35.
9 Rudolph AM. The fetal circulation and its response to stress. *J Dev Physiol* 1984;**6**:11–9.
10 Berry CL. Hypertension and arterial development: long-term considerations. *Br Heart J* 1978;**40**:709–17.
11 Meyer WW, Lind J. Iliac arteries in children with a single umbilical artery: structure, calcification and early atherosclerotic lesions. *Arch Dis Child* 1974;**49**:671–9.
12 Berry CL, Gosling RG, Laogun AA, Bryan E. Anomalous iliac compliance in children with a single umbilical artery. *Br Heart J* 1976;**38**:510–5.
13 Folkow B. Physiological aspects of primary hypertension. *Physiol Rev* 1982;**62**:347–504.
14 Zinner GH, Rosner B, Oh W, Kass EH. Significance of blood pressure in infancy, familial aggregation and predictive effect of later blood pressure. *Hypertension* 1985;**7**:411–6.
15 Butler N, Alberman ED. *Second report of the 1958 British perinatal mortality survey*. Edinburgh: Churchill Livingstone, 1969.
16 Elford J, Phillips A, Thomson AG, Shaper AG. Migration and geographic variations in blood pressure in Britain. *BMJ* 1990;**300**:291–5.
17 Anonymous. Diet and hypertension. [Editorial.] *Lancet* 1984;ii:671–3.
18 Rose G. Sick individuals and sick populations. *Int J Epidemiol* 1985;**14**:32.

17: Relation of fetal length, ponderal index, and head circumference to blood pressure and risk of hypertension in adult life

D J P BARKER, K M GODFREY, C OSMOND,
A R BULL

The blood pressure of 327 men and women aged 46 to 54 was related to birth weight, placental weight, length, ponderal index, and head circumference at birth. All the subjects were born after 38 completed weeks of gestation. There were strong trends of higher blood pressure in adult life with lower birth weight (p = 0·04) and greater placental weight (p = 0·002). In subjects with placental weights of 1·25 lb or less, mean blood pressure, and the risk of hypertension, rose as ponderal index at birth fell (p = 0·0001). Mean systolic pressure rose by 13 mm Hg as ponderal index fell from more than 14·75 to 12 or less. In those with placental weights above 1·25 lb, mean blood pressure, and the risk of hypertension, rose as length decreased and as the ratio of head circumference to length increased (p = 0·02). Mean systolic pressure rose by 14 mm Hg as the ratio of head circumference to length increased from less than 0·65 to 0·7 or more. These findings characterise the birth measurements of two groups of babies who are at increased risk of hypertension in adult life.

Introduction

Low birth weight in relation to placental weight is associated with hypertension in later life. Among 449 men and women followed up from birth, hypertension at age 50 was strongly related to lower birth weight and higher placental weight (chapter 16). This study was based on births in a maternity hospital in Preston, England, where from 1932 onwards routine obstetric data were recorded in unusual detail. Mean systolic pressure fell by 11 mm Hg as birth weight increased from less than 5·5 lb (1 lb = 454 g) to more than 7·5 lb, and rose by 15 mm Hg as placental weight increased from less than 1 lb to more than 1·5 lb. The highest blood pressures were in people who had had heavy placentas and whose birth weights were lower than expected from their placental weight. These strong and highly significant relations were apparent in babies of all gestational ages. They were independent of the two major adult influences on blood pressure— body mass index and alcohol consumption.

The processes which link low birth weight for placental weight with adult hypertension are unknown. To elucidate this further, we have examined the distributions of birth length, ponderal index, and head circumference in relation to adult blood pressure in the same Preston men and women. We have also analysed how placental weight is related to two maternal variables—social class and pelvic size.

Methods

The methods are described in chapter 16.

Results

Because the proportionate relations of head circumference, length, and birth weight differ between babies born prematurely and those born around term, we restricted the analysis to the 327 men and women known to have been born after 38 completed weeks of gestation: 255 of these babies were firstborn. The mean (SD) placental weights were 22·1 oz (5·3) for boys and 21·1 oz (4·6) for girls (16 oz = 1 lb). Mean (SD) birth weights were 113·9 oz (16·1) and 113·2 oz (16·0). Mean (SD) lengths were 20·5 inches (1·0) and 20·4 inches (0·8), and mean (SD) head circumferences were 13·7 inches (0·6) in both sexes.

In table I we have used the same groupings of birth weights and placental weights as in our previous analysis of babies of all gestational ages. Systolic pressure rose with increasing placental weight (p = 0·002) and fell with increasing birth weight (p = 0·04). Systolic pressure rose as the ratio of placental weight to birth weight increased (p = 0·004).

Birth weight, length, and head circumference were strongly positively associated with placental weight. We therefore analysed their relation to systolic blood pressure within two placental weight groups, dividing the subjects roughly equally into those with weights of 1·25 lb or less, and those with weights above 1·25 lb. The trends of systolic blood pressure with length contrasted sharply in the two groups (table II). At placental weights of 1·25 lb or less, systolic pressure rose as length increased (p = 0·06). At placental weights above 1·25 lb, systolic pressure fell as length increased (p = 0·06).

We used the ponderal index (weight/length³) to examine the trends in systolic pressure with length in relation to weight. Table III shows that at placental weights of 1·25 lb or less systolic pressure fell with increasing ponderal index. Mean systolic pressure fell from 154 mm Hg to 141 mm Hg as the index increased from 12 or less to more than 14·75 (p = 0·0001). At placental weights above 1·25 lb there was a trend in the opposite direction, though this did not achieve significance (p = 0·11).

The trends of systolic pressure with head circumference (table IV) differed from those with length. At low placental weights pressure fell as head circumference increased, though this did not achieve significance (p = 0·2). At high placental weight there was no trend. At low placental

TABLE I—*Mean systolic blood pressure (mm Hg) of men and women aged 46 to 54, born after 38 completed weeks of gestation, according to placental weight and birth weight (numbers of subjects in parentheses)*

Birth weight (lb)	Placental weight (lb)				
	≤ 1·0	− 1·25	− 1·5	> 1·5	All
≤ 5·5	153(10)	141 (5)	147 (4)	− (0)	149 (19)
− 6·5	146(14)	153 (41)	152(14)	167 (6)	152 (75)
− 7·5	139(16)	148 (63)	146(35)	159(23)	148 (137)
> 7·5	131 (3)	143 (23)	148(30)	153(40)	149 (96)
All	144(43)	148(132)	148(83)	156(69)	149*(327)

* Standard deviation = 20·4.

TABLE II—*Mean systolic pressure (mm Hg) of men and women aged 46 to 54, born after 38 completed weeks of gestation, according to length at birth and placental weight (numbers of subjects in parentheses)*

Placental weight (lb)	Length (inches)				
	< 20	20	− 21	> 21	All
≤ 1·25	142(33)	146 (72)	150(46)	153(23)	147(174)
> 1·25	159(11)	153 (77)	149(38)	147(26)	152(152)
All	146(44)	150(149)	149(84)	150(49)	149(326)

TABLE III—*Mean systolic pressure (mm Hg) of men and women aged 46 to 54, born after 38 completed weeks of gestation, according to ponderal index at birth and placental weight (numbers of subjects in parentheses)*

Placental weight (lb)	Ponderal index $(oz/inch^3) \times 1000$				
	$\leqslant 12$	$-13 \cdot 25$	$-14 \cdot 75$	$> 14 \cdot 75$	All
$\leqslant 1 \cdot 25$	154(53)	147 (54)	142(42)	141(25)	147(174)
$> 1 \cdot 25$	148(27)	149 (27)	152(48)	154(50)	152(152)
All	152(80)	148 (81)	147(90)	150(75)	149(326)

TABLE IV—*Mean systolic pressure (mm Hg) of men and women aged 46 to 54, born after 38 completed weeks of gestation, according to head circumference at birth and placental weight (numbers of subjects in parentheses)*

Placental weight (lb)	Head circumference (inches)				
	$\leqslant 13 \cdot 25$	$-13 \cdot 75$	-14	> 14	All
$\leqslant 1 \cdot 25$	149(67)	146 (37)	147 (52)	144(19)	147(175)
$> 1 \cdot 25$	151(26)	145 (31)	155 (61)	152(34)	152(152)
All	149(93)	146 (68)	151(113)	149(53)	149(327)

weights head circumference was positively associated with ponderal index ($p = 0 \cdot 0002$).

Analysis by multiple regression of the simultaneous effects of head circumference and ponderal index on systolic pressure showed that head circumference had no significant effect independently of ponderal index. At high placental weights the fall in systolic pressure with increasing length (table II) but the lack of any trend with head circumference was reflected in a trend of rising pressure with an increasing ratio of head circumference to length (table V). Mean systolic pressure rose from 142 mm Hg to 156 mm Hg as the ratio increased from less than 0·65 to 0·7 or above ($p = 0 \cdot 02$).

The predictors of adult blood pressure therefore differed with placental weight. At placental weights of 1·25 lb or less, a low ponderal index predicted high adult blood pressure (table III); at placental weights above 1·25 lb a high ratio of head circumference to length predicted high blood pressure (table V). These relations were similarly strong in boys and girls, and in firstborn and subsequent children. They were independent of any residual effects of gestational age at delivery. They were also independent of placental weight within each placental weight group. Defining hypertension as a systolic pressure above 160 mm Hg, among people with placental

190

TABLE V—*Mean systolic pressure (mm Hg) of men and women aged 46 to 54, born after 38 completed weeks of gestation, according to ratio of head circumference to length at birth and placental weight (numbers of subjects in parentheses)*

| Placental weight (lb) | Ratio of head circumference to length | | | | |
	<0·65	0·65 − <0·675	0·675 − <0·7	≥0·7	All
≤1·25	152(47)	149(48)	145(37)	142 (42)	147(174)
>1·25	142(30)	152(32)	152(29)	156 (61)	152(152)
All	148(77)	150(80)	148(66)	150(103)	149(326)

weights of 1·25 lb or less the relative risk of hypertension rose from 1·0 at a birth ponderal index above 14·75 to 2·1 (95% confidence interval 0·6–7·1) at an index of 12 or less. At placental weights above 1·25 lb, the risk rose from 1·0 at a ratio of head circumference to length of less than 0·65 to 2·3 (95% confidence interval 0·8–6·4) at a ratio of 0·7 or above.

From these analyses we can characterise the birth measurements of babies who had higher mean blood pressure in adult life. At placental weights of 1·25 lb (20 oz) or less, the highest mean systolic pressure, 154 mm Hg, was seen in the 53 subjects, 30 men and 23 women whose ponderal index had been 12 or less (table III). Their mean birth weight had been below the average for all babies born after 38 weeks or more of gestation (6·3 compared with 7·1 lb). However, though their mean head circumference had also been below average, 13·4 compared with 13·7 inches, their mean length had been above average, 20·9 compared with 20·4 in. At placental weights above 1·25 lb (20 oz), the highest mean systolic pressure, 156 mm Hg, was seen in the 61 subjects, 38 men and 23 women, whose ratio of head circumference to length had been 0·7 or above (table V). Their mean birth weight had been above average at 7·3 lb. Though their mean head circumference had also been above average at 14·2 inches, their length had been below average, at 20·0 inches.

The trends in diastolic pressure with birth weight, placental weight, length, ponderal index, and head circumference were similar to those of systolic pressure but smaller. The trends of systolic pressure were little changed by adjustment for the subject's current body mass index and alcohol consumption and all remained significant.

The social class of 310 of the mothers could be classified from the father's occupation. Table VI shows mean systolic pressure according to mother's social class and placental weight. There was no trend in systolic pressure with mother's social class. Nor was there a trend with the man or woman's current social class. In each social class group, however, mean systolic pressure rose with increasing placental weight and the highest pressure was in subjects with placental weight above 1·5 lb (table VI). The distribution of placental weight varied with social class. Out of 254 subjects whose

191

TABLE VI—*Mean systolic pressure (mm Hg) of men and women aged 46 to 54, born after 38 completed weeks of gestation, according placental weight and mother's social class (numbers of subjects in parentheses)*

Social class	Placental weight (lb)				
	$\leqslant 1\cdot0$	$-1\cdot25$	$-1\cdot5$	$>1\cdot5$	All
I,II	142 (5)	150 (29)	146(18)	160 (4)	148 (56)
III	145(13)	149 (68)	149(43)	157(42)	151(166)
IV,V	145(19)	146 (29)	148(20)	156(20)	148 (88)
All	143(37)	148(126)	148(81)	157(66)	149(310)

mothers were in social classes III, IV, and V, 62 (24%) had placentas weighing more than 1·5 lb. This compared with four (7%) out of 56 subjects whose mothers were in social classes I and II. The relative risk of a baby having a placenta weighing more than 1·5 lb was 4·2 (95% confidence interval 1·5 to 12·1) in social classes III, IV, and V compared with 1·0 in social classes I and II.

Mean systolic pressure increased with mother's external conjugate diameter ($p = 0\cdot05$). Mean mother's external conjugate fell from 7·83 inches in social classes I and II combined to 7·79 inches in social class III and 7·72 inches in social classes IV and V. Increasing external conjugate diameter was associated with heavier placental weight, independently of social class and of parity ($p < 0\cdot01$). Among the 138 mothers with external conjugate diameters of 8 inches or more, the relative risk of a placenta weighing more than 1·5 lb was 1·9 (95% confidence interval 1·1 to 3·2). The relation between external conjugate and systolic pressure was no longer significant after allowing for placental weight.

Discussion

We have examined the relation between birth measurements and adult blood pressure in 327 men and women aged around 50 who were born after 38 completed weeks of gestation. We have previously described the strong trends of higher blood pressure with lower birth weight and greater placental weight (chapter 16). In the present analysis we have examined the relations of blood pressure with weight, length, and head circumference within two groups of placental weight. In men and women whose placental weights were 1·25 lb or less, mean blood pressure, and the risk of hypertension, rose as ponderal index fell (table III). In those whose placental weights were more than 1·25 lb, mean blood pressure, and risk of hypertension, rose as the ratio of head circumference to length increased (table V).

Both these trends were strongly significant. They can be used to characterise two groups of babies who developed higher mean blood pressure as adults. The first had placental weights of 1·25 lb or less, were thin (ponderal index of 12 or less), had below average birth weight and head circumference but above average length. The second had placental weights above 1·25 lb, were short in relation to their head size, with above average birth weight and head circumference but below average length. Only 9% of babies in these two groups had low birth weights, as defined by the customary criterion of 5·5 lb or less. However, in a group of people born 50 years ago, it is likely that a disproportionate number of those with low birth weights would have died in infancy.

The results of clinical observation and animal studies give only a limited insight into the processes which could result in the two groups of babies we have characterised. Babies with a low ponderal index, born at term, have been labelled as having fetal malnutrition.[1] Their scanty subcutaneous fat, and below average head circumference are regarded as additional signs of malnutrition. Maternal influences associated with reduction in weight but preservation of length include energy restriction and low weight gain in pregnancy.[2] Babies born after the Dutch "hunger winter" of 1944–5 had a disproportionate reduction in birth weight in relation to length.[3] The processes which link a low ponderal index and later high blood pressure remain a matter for conjecture. Impaired blood vessel growth at a critical period in intrauterine life is one possibility.

To our knowledge, babies with large placental weight, whose length is disproportionately small in relation to their above average weight and head circumference, have not previously been studied. In these babies, blood flow may have been directed away from the trunk in favour of the brain, thereby retarding trunk and limb growth. This is known to occur in animals in response to hypoxia.[4] Little is known about maternal influences which lead to this response in humans. In our data, large placental weight was associated with low social class. Several studies have shown that large placental weight is associated with maternal anaemia.

A recent survey of 8684 pregnant women in Oxford showed that heavy placental weight was associated with a fall in maternal mean cell volume as well as with low haemoglobin concentration (chapter 27). This suggests that the association with low haemoglobin partly results from iron deficiency, which in the past was more common in women of low social class.[5][6] Mothers with larger external conjugate diameters tended to have babies with heavy placentas. Larger conjugate diameter was associated with higher social class. This association therefore opposes that between low social class and heavier placental weight and may partly explain the absence of a strong relation between social class and adult blood pressure.[7]

Our data contained no information about maternal smoking. It seems unlikely, however, that this is an important influence. Most studies have shown that maternal smoking is associated with a proportionate reduction in birth weight and length.[8] Smoking is not associated with increased placental weight.[9]

An inverse relation between birth weight and blood pressure has now been shown in three separate studies of adults: in the present study in Preston, in a national sample of men and women aged 36 in Britain (chapter 15) and in a study of 597 men aged 64 in Hertfordshire (chapter 20). Studies in progress will show whether the strong relations of blood pressure to low ponderal index, heavy placental weight, and a high ratio of head circumference to length, which are described in this paper, are present in other groups of adults. The strength of these associations, their occurrence in men and women within each social class and in firstborn and subsequent children, and their independence from current body mass index and alcohol consumption suggests that they will be. If the associations are found in other adults research can be focused on the intrauterine processes that lead to particular birth measurements and hence on the maternal influences that determine hypertension in the next generation.

1 Miller HC, Hassanein K. Fetal malnutrition in white newborn infants: maternal factors. *Pediatrics* 1973;**52**:504–12.
2 Naeye RL, Blanc W, Paul C. Effects of maternal nutrition on the human fetus. *Pediatrics* 1973;**52**:494–503.
3 Stein Z, Susser M, Saenger G, *et al*. Famine and human development. In: *The Dutch hunger winter of 1944–5*. New York: Oxford University Press, 1975: 119–48.
4 Dawes GS, Borruto F, Zacutti A, *et al*. *Fetal autonomy and adaptation*. Chichester: Wiley, 1990.
5 Doyle GD, McGrath J. Pregnancy anaemia survey. Coombe lying-in hospital, Dublin, 1953. *Irish Journal of Medical Science* 1954;**345**:414–24.
6 Reid WJS, Mackintosh JM. Incidence of anaemia in pregnancy; influence of social circumstances and other factors. *Lancet* 1937;i:43–5.
7 Shaper AG, Pocock SJ, Walker M, *et al*. British Regional Heart Study: cardiovascular risk factors in middle-aged men in 24 towns. *BMJ* 1981;**283**:179–86.
8 Miller HC, Hassanein K. Maternal smoking and fetal growth of full term infants. *Paediatric Research* 1974;**8**:960.
9 Spira A, Spira N, Goujuard J, *et al*. Smoking during pregnancy and placental weight: a multivariate analysis on 3759 cases. *J Perinat Med* 1975;**3**:327–41.

18: Maternal and fetal influences on blood pressure

C M LAW, D J P BARKER, A R BULL, C OSMOND

To study maternal and fetal influences on blood pressure in childhood 405 children aged 4 years who were born and still resident in the Salisbury health district were visited at home for blood pressure and growth measurements. Information on the pregnancy, delivery, and baby was abstracted from the routine obstetric notes.

Similarly to recent findings in adults, the child's systolic pressure was inversely related to birth weight and positively related to placental weight. Systolic pressure at 4 years increased by 1·2 mm Hg for every standard deviation decrease in the ratio of head circumference to length at birth, and by 1·1 mm Hg for every standard deviation decrease in ponderal index at birth. Mothers whose haemoglobin concentrations fell below 100 g/l during pregnancy had children whose systolic pressures were on average 2·9 mm Hg higher than the children of mothers with higher haemoglobin concentrations.

Patterns of placental weight, birth weight, head circumference, and length that are associated with high blood pressure in adults are also associated with higher blood pressure in 4 year old children. Identification of the intrauterine influences that lead to these patterns of fetal growth could lead to the primary prevention of hypertension.

Introduction

Among men and women aged 50 in Preston, England, systolic and diastolic blood pressure were strongly predicted by birth weight and placental weight, which had independent and opposing effects (chapter 16). Mean systolic pressure fell by 11 mm Hg as birth weight increased from less than 2475 g to more than 3375 g and rose by 15 mm Hg as placental weight increased from less than 450 g to more than 675 g. The highest pressures and risk of hypertension were among people who had been small babies with large placentas. These associations, which were highly significant, were independent of gestational age, current body mass index, and alcohol intake.

These findings raise the question of whether the opposing relations of blood pressure with birth weight and placental weight are apparent in children today, and if so what is the timing and nature of the intrauterine influences. To examine this we have measured the blood pressures of 405 children aged 4 who were born in a city in southern England, and related them to measurements at birth.

Methods

All singleton children born in hospital in the Salisbury health district between July 1984 and February 1985, and still resident in the district at the age of 4 years, were eligible for inclusion in the study. (All hospital deliveries in this health district are at a single hospital.) Four hundred subjects was estimated as being the sample size needed to give 95% power to detect a difference in systolic pressure of 4 mm Hg between two subgroups of equal size, using a test at the 5% level.

Information on the pregnancy and measurements at birth was abstracted from the haematology and maternity records, including parity, first and maximum systolic and diastolic blood pressures recorded, routine haematology, gestation (estimated from the last menstrual period or, if absent, ultrasound scan), birth length, weight, head circumference, and placental weight.

Children were visited at home by one of two field workers: neither had seen the obstetric data. The children's ages ranged from 4·0 to 4·9 years (median 4·2 years): 93% were visited between the ages of 4 and 4·5 years. The child's social and medical history was recorded on a questionnaire. Social class was allocated according to occupation of the father, or if absent, the mother.[1] Members of the armed forces and housewives were not allocated to a social class. The blood pressure, height, and weight of the child and both parents were measured. After the subjects had rested for five minutes, blood pressure was measured on the left arm at the level of the heart, using an automated blood pressure recorder (Dinamap model 18465X). Cuff size was chosen according to recommendations based on those of the American Heart Association:[2] three measurements were taken at one minute intervals. Weight was measured on digital scales to the nearest 0·1 kg. Height was measured in the Frankfurt plane on a portable stadiometer to the nearest mm. Before starting the study, the procedures for measurements were standardised and the fieldworkers trained. No important interobserver variation was found during checks at intervals throughout the study, in which repeat measurements were made on subjects selected from outside the study population.

Results

Of 638 eligible children, 206 (32%) could not be traced at their last known address, or their parents did not reply to the letters of invitation, and 20 (3%) declined to take part in the study. Seven children reported as having renal or cardiac disorders or other congenital abnormalities were excluded. There remained 405 mothers and children, 205 boys and 200 girls. Of these 395 (98%) had haematological records and 376 (93%) had obstetric information, although this was not complete in all cases. Altogether 347 (86%) fathers were studied: 37 fathers (9%) had never or no longer lived in the same household, 10 (2%) were working away, and 11 (3%) did not wish to participate.

The children's systolic pressure fell by a mean of 5·5 mm Hg (95% confidence interval 4·2 to 6·9) from the first to the third reading. The within child standard deviation was 9·2 mm Hg. We present the analysis of the average of the three systolic pressure measurements. Neither age or sex of child, room temperature, month and time of day, or time since last meal, had a consistent effect on mean systolic pressure. The mean systolic pressure and weight at 4 years, and the mean gestation, placental weight, and size at birth are given in table I.

SIZE AT BIRTH, PLACENTAL WEIGHT, GESTATION, AND WEIGHT AT 4 YEARS

Placental weight and weight, length, and head circumference at birth were adjusted for gestational age by linear regression. The simultaneous effects of weight at 4 years and adjusted birth weight and placental weight on systolic pressure were examined by multiple regression (table II).

TABLE I—*Characteristics of 405 children aged 4 by sex*

	Boys		Girls	
	No	Mean (SD)	No	Mean (SD)
Birth weight (g)	205	3391 (576)	200	3342 (495)
Placental weight (g)	185	662 (192)	181	653 (149)
Length at birth (cm)	181	51·5 (2·6)	180	50·8 (2·4)
Head circumference at birth (cm)	183	34·8 (1·4)	182	54·3 (1·4)
Gestation (weeks)	205	40·1 (1·7)	198	40·2 (1·6)
Weight at 4 years (kg)	205	17·8 (2·2)	200	17·3 (2·2)
Systolic blood pressure (mm Hg)	205	105·7 (9·7)	200	105·0 (9·9)

TABLE II—*Simultaneous effects of weight at 4 years, birth weight,* and placental weight* on systolic pressure, expressed as mean difference (95% confidence interval) from the baseline*

	No	Systolic pressure (mm Hg)
Weight at 4 years (kg):		
≤16·5	108	0·0 (baseline)
−17·5	92	0·1 (−2·6 to 2·9)
−18·5	66	0·3 (−2·7 to 3·4)
>18·5	98	3·7 (0·8 to 6·5)
Birth weight (g):		
≤3000	75	0·0 (baseline)
−3300	102	−0·8 (−3·7 to 2·2)
−3600	82	−0·9 (−4·1 to 2·4)
>3600	105	−2·6 (−6·0 to 0·8)
Placental weight (g):		
≤550	96	0·0 (baseline)
−650	102	−0·1 (−3·0 to 2·7)
−750	83	0·6 (−2·5 to 3·7)
>750	83	2·6 (−0·8 to 6·0)

* Birth weight and placental weight are adjusted for gestational age.

Variables were grouped into approximate fourths so that we could explore non-linear variation of systolic pressure with each variable. The lowest fourth was set as the baseline and the systolic pressure in each group is given as its difference from this. Systolic pressure rose with increasing weight at 4 years with a pronounced rise in the heaviest group. Pressure fell with increasing birth weight and rose with placental weight: the average systolic pressure in children whose birth weight exceeded 3600 g was 2·6 mm Hg (95% confidence interval −0·8 to 6·0) below that of children whose birth weights were 3000 g or less. Children whose placental weights were greater than 750 g had average pressures of 2·6 mm Hg (95% confidence interval −0·8 to 6·0) above those whose placental weights were 550 g or less.

We further examined the association of systolic blood pressure with size at birth by analysing length and head circumference at birth after adjustment for gestational age. Children whose head circumferences had been in the lowest fourth (≤33·5 cm) had pressures which were 1·3 (95% confidence interval −2·1 to 4·7) mm Hg above those whose head circumferences had been in the highest fourth (>35·5 cm). Children whose lengths had been in the lowest fourth (≤49·5 cm) had pressures that were 1·4 (95% confidence interval −1·8 to 4·6) below those whose lengths had been in the highest fourth (>52·5 cm). Because of the opposing relations of systolic pressure to head circumference and length, mean systolic pressure rose as the ratio of head circumference to length decreased. A decrease in the ratio of 1 standard deviation (0·03) was associated with a 1·2 mm Hg (95%

confidence interval 0·1 to 2·2) increase in systolic pressure. We examined the relations of systolic pressure to birth weight and length using the ponderal index (weight/length³). Systolic pressure fell as the ponderal index at birth increased. An increase in ponderal index of 1 standard deviation (3·1 kg/m³) was associated with a 1·1 mm Hg (95% confidence interval 0·1 to 2·1) decrease in systolic pressure.

MATERNAL BLOOD PRESSURE, HEIGHT, HAEMOGLOBIN CONCENTRATION, AND SMOKING

The mean (SD) systolic pressure of mothers, measured when the child was aged 4 years, was 120·1 (13·5) mm Hg. The children's mean systolic pressure rose as the mother's systolic pressure increased (table III). There was a similar relation with the mothers' maximum systolic pressure during

TABLE III—*Mean children's systolic pressure (mm Hg) unadjusted and adjusted both for children's weight at 4 years and for mother's systolic pressure*

	No	Unadjusted*	Adjusted*
Total	405	105·3	105·2
Mother's systolic pressure when child aged 4 (mm Hg):			
≤110	99	103·3	
−120	128	104·9	
−130	96	105·1	
>130	82	108·7	
Mother's height (cm):			
≤159	103	105·9	106·0
−163	106	104·5	104·7
−167	99	104·9	104·9
>167	94	105·8	104·9
Lowest haemoglobin during pregnancy (g/l):			
<100	36	108·1	108·1
−109	88	105·8	105·9
−119	164	104·8	104·7
≥120	106	105·2	104·6
Cigarettes smoked/day during pregnancy:			
0	323	105·1	105·0
−10	34	106·2	105·9
−20	28	106·1	105·6
>20	19	105·2	106·1
Parity:			
First born	152	105·0	104·9
Later born	253	105·5	105·3
Mother's age at birth of child (years):			
≤25	92	105·2	104·9
−28	106	105·9	106·3
−31	92	105·2	104·8
>31	115	104·9	104·5

* Standard deviation of unadjusted values is 9·8 and of adjusted values is 9·4.

pregnancy. As would be expected the mothers' blood pressure at the time of the survey and during pregnancy were strongly related.

Table III shows the relation of maternal variables to the children's systolic pressure which is given both unadjusted and adjusted (by linear regression) for its two main correlates, child's weight and mother's systolic pressure. The mean (SD) maternal height was 162·6 (5·9) cm. Although the children of the smallest mothers had the highest blood pressures, there was no overall trend with mother's height (table III).

We examined the lowest haemoglobin concentrations and mean corpuscular volumes for each mother during pregnancy. We defined anaemia by a commonly used clinical definition of a haemoglobin value below 100 g/l. We also divided haemoglobin concentrations at 110 g/l; this is the World Health Organisation's defining concentration for pregnancy anaemia.[3] The children of anaemic mothers (haemoglobin below 100 g/l) had unadjusted systolic pressures which were, on average, 2·9 mm Hg (95% confidence interval −0·4 to 6·3) higher than those of other children (table III). The adjusted systolic pressures were also highest in children of anaemic mothers. The children of mothers with mean corpuscular volumes of 80 fl or less (n = 33) had systolic pressures which were, on average, 2·2 mm Hg (95% confidence interval −1·3 to 5·7) higher than those of other children.

Birth weight fell from an average of 3377 g in mothers who did not smoke during pregnancy to 3178 g in mothers who smoked more than 20 cigarettes a day. However, the children's systolic pressures were not associated with their mother's smoking history, parity, or age (table III).

MOTHERS' AND FATHERS' BLOOD PRESSURES

The mean (SD) of the fathers' systolic pressure at the time of the study was 131·8 (14·0) mm Hg. Where both parents' blood pressures were recorded, we examined the separate relation of the child's pressure with those of its parents. The children's mean systolic pressure, adjusted for weight, rose by 1·2 mm Hg (95% confidence interval 0·5 to 1·9) for every 10 mm Hg increase in mothers' systolic pressure, and by 0·7 mm Hg (95% confidence interval 0·0 to 1·4) for every 10 mm Hg increase in fathers' systolic pressure. The corresponding figures for firstborn children were 1·8 (95% confidence interval 0·6 to 2·9) and 1·9 (95% confidence interval 0·7 to 3·1) and for subsequent children were 0·8 (95% confidence interval −0·1 to 1·7) and 0·1 (95% confidence interval −0·8 to 0·9).

SOCIAL CLASS

Children in social classes I and II had lower systolic pressures (table IV). Haemoglobin concentration during pregnancy was highest in social class I and II. Mean corpuscular volume was highest in mothers of social class I, II and III non-manual (table IV).

TABLE IV—*Children's systolic pressure and mother's lowest haemoglobin concentration and mean corpuscular volume during pregnancy, by social class*

Social class	No	Mean (unadjusted) children's pressure (mm Hg)	Lowest* haemoglobin concentration (g/l)	Mean* corpuscular volume (fl)
I	34	103·6	115	86·8
II	100	104·7	114	86·8
III non-manual	43	105·4	111	87·0
III manual	121	106·0	113	85·3
IV and V	51	105·8	111	85·2
Total	349	105·3	113	86·1
(SD)		9·6	10	4·6

*Haematological indices were not known for 10 subjects.

SIMULTANEOUS EFFECT OF FETAL SIZE AND MATERNAL INFLUENCES

Table V shows the simultaneous effects of child and fetal size and maternal variables on the children's systolic pressure. Weight at 4 years, placental weight, ponderal index at birth, mother's systolic pressure, and haemoglobin concentration during pregnancy all had independent relations with systolic pressure. We examined the relation of mean diastolic pressure to the variables shown in table V. The relations were similar to those with systolic pressure but the mean differences were smaller and none reached significance.

When systolic pressure was regressed on the same variables expressed continuously, rather than in groups, the results were comparable (table VI).

Discussion

We have examined the relations of systolic pressure to maternal and fetal influences in a series of 4 year old children born in a maternity unit which provides all hospital obstetric care for one health district. The children were selected only by their continuing residence in the health district. Blood pressure was measured with an automated recorder in the child's home by a standardised procedure. Efforts were made to minimise stress and disturbance to the child before and during measurement, but there was still considerable within child variation in systolic pressure, including a pronounced order effect. The mean (SD) of the third reading, 102·7 mm Hg (11·6), was 5·4 mm Hg above the 50th centile in the British standards, which were measured with a sphygmomanometer.[4] In keeping with other studies we have used the average of the readings in our analysis. Average systolic pressure was positively related to weight at 4 years; this is

TABLE V—*Simultaneous effects of weight at 4 years, size at birth,* and maternal influences on systolic pressure, expressed as mean difference (95% confidence interval) from the baseline*

	No	Systolic pressure (mm Hg)
Weight at 4 years (kg):		
≤16·5	103	0·0 (baseline)
−17·5	85	−0·1 (−3·0 to 2·7)
−18·5	60	0·0 (−3·2 to 3·1)
>18·5	95	2·6 (−0·2 to 5·4)
Placental weight (g):		
≤550	90	0·0 (baseline)
−650	97	0·3 (−2·6 to 3·1)
−750	77	1·2 (−1·9 to 4·3)
>750	79	2·3 (−0·8 to 5·3)
Ponderal index (kg/m³):		
<23	79	0·0 (baseline)
−25	86	−0·8 (−3·8 to 2·3)
−27·5	94	−2·4 (−5·4 to 0·5)
>27·5	84	−3·9 (−7·0 to −0·9)
Mother's systolic pressure (mm Hg):		
<110	81	0·0 (baseline)
−120	109	1·6 (−1·2 to 4·4)
−130	81	−0·9 (−2·2 to 3·9)
>130	72	5·0 (1·9 to 8·1)
Lowest haemoglobin (g/l):		
<100	30	2·8 (−3·4 to 1·7)
−109	77	0·3 (−2·7 to 3·3)
−119	141	−0·9 (−1·3 to 6·8)
≥120	95	0·0 (baseline)

* Birth weight, length, and placental weight are adjusted for gestational age.

TABLE VI—*Simultaneous effects of weight at 4 years, size at birth,* and maternal influences, expressed as continuous variables, on systolic pressure*

	Regression slope	95% CI	p Value
Weight at 4 years (kg)	0·65	0·17 to 1·13	<0·01
Placental weight (g)	0·003	−0·003 to 0·009	0·4
Ponderal index (kg/m³)	−0·41	−0·74 to −0·09	<0·05
Mother's systolic pressure (mm Hg)	0·12	0·04 to 0·19	<0·002
Lowest haemoglobin (<100 g/l v ≥100 g/l)	−3·1	−6·7 to 0·5	0·09

* Birth weight, length, and placental weight are adjusted for gestational age.
CI = Confidence interval.

in agreement with other studies in Britain (chapter 15)[45] and North America.[6]

The opposing relations of systolic pressure to birth weight and placental weight shown in 50 year old men and women in Preston were present in 4 year old children, though weaker. Systolic pressure at age 4 was inversely related to birth weight. This was independent of gestation and implies an association with reduced fetal growth, which is consistent with findings in 10 year old children (chapter 15). However, birth weight is a summary measure of fetal growth, which includes head size, length, and fatness. Further examination showed that systolic pressure was related to failure of head growth in relation to length and to a low ponderal index. Analysis of the Preston data has shown the same associations in adults (chapter 17). To our knowledge neither of these associations with children's blood pressure has been described before. Both were significant. The nature of intrauterine influences that cause reduced head circumference and weight in relation to length are unknown and require further study.

The highest systolic pressures were found in children who had been small babies with large placentas, although the magnitude of the relations between pressure and placental and fetal size were smaller than in adults, even allowing for the smaller variation in children's blood pressure. Furthermore these relations were at the margin of significance and require confirmation in other samples of children. The causes of high placental weight and discordance between placental and birth weight are mostly unknown. Smoking during pregnancy is associated with reduced placental weight, though with a relatively greater decrease in birth weight than placental weight, and thus discordance between the two (chapter 27). We found no relation between maternal smoking and the children's blood pressure (table III).

The children's blood pressure was more closely related to the mothers' than the fathers' systolic pressure. This has been found before and has been ascribed to X linked genes.[78] Another possibility is that higher blood pressure in a mother reflects her own fetal experience, which in turn influences the intrauterine environment she provides for her children. Studies of the Dutch famine have shown that women whose mothers were malnourished during pregnancy themselves had babies with retarded intrauterine growth.[9] The relation between the child's and father's pressure was found only in firstborn children, which suggests that in subsequent children the genetic contribution of the father's pressure is overridden by other factors. Our data do not allow further resolution of this.

We found that a maternal haemoglobin concentration below 100 g/l was associated with higher systolic pressure in the child, though this was not significant (table III). Although haemoglobin may fall in pregnancy as a result of haemodilution, there is evidence that a haemoglobin concentration below 100 g/l is usually associated with iron deficiency.[10] The lower mean corpuscular volumes and haemoglobin concentrations in the lower social classes in our study are consistent with this (table IV). Although Salisbury has a relatively high socioeconomic status, 31% of mothers had haemoglobin concentrations below 110 g/l, the WHO definition of anaemia in pregnancy.[3]

Anaemia is associated with increased placental size,[11] but this did not appear to be the sole mechanism of its relation with increased blood pressure, which was still present when considered simultaneously with the effects of placental weight (table V). The rise in a child's blood pressure that is associated with anaemia could be a response to reduced maternal oxygen carrying capacity or a consequence of nutritional deficiency causing both anaemia and raised blood pressure. Findings in a rural community in the Gambia, West Africa, support a link between maternal nutrition and children's blood pressure. Failure of mothers to gain weight during the last trimester was associated with increased blood pressure in the child at 8 to 10 years (chapter 19). Better maternal nutrition could explain the lower pressures recently found in 5 to 7 year old children in Guildford, a British town with relatively high socioeconomic status.[12]

Patterns of placental weight, birth weight, head circumference, and length that are associated with high blood pressure in adults are also associated with higher blood pressure in 4 year old children. We are carrying out a further study in another part of Britain to confirm this. Identification of the intrauterine influences which lead to these patterns of fetal growth could lead to the primary prevention of hypertension.

We are grateful to the obstetric and community health departments, Odstock Hospital, and the medical records department, Salisbury General Infirmary, for their cooperation.

1 Office of Population Censuses and Surveys. *Classification of occupations*. London: HMSO, 1980.

2 Prineas RJ, Gillum RF, Horobe H, Hanna PJ. The Minneapolis children's blood pressure study. Part I: standards of measurement for children's blood pressure. *J Hypertens Suppl* 1980;2:(suppl 1):18–24.

3 World Health Organisation Technical Report Series. *Nutrition anaemias*. Geneva: World Health Organisation, 1968, No 405.

4 de Swiet M, Fayers P, Shinebourne E. Blood pressure in four and five year old children. The effects of environment and other factors in its measurement. *J Hypertens* 1984;2:501–5.

5 Whincup PH, Cook DG, Shaper AG. Early influences on blood pressure: a study of children aged 5–7 years. *BMJ* 1989;**299**:587–91.

6 Voors AW, Webber LS, Frerichs RR, Berenson GS. Body height and body mass as determinants of basal blood pressure in children—the Bogalusa heart study. *Am J Epidemiol* 1977;**106**:101–8.

7 Bengtsson B, Thulin T, Schersten B. Familial resemblance in casual blood pressure—a maternal effect? *Clin Sci* 1979;**57**:279–94.

8 Gerson LW, Fodor JG. Family aggregation of high blood pressure groups in two Newfoundland communities. *Can J Public Health* 1975;**66**:294–9.

9 Lumey H. *Obstetric performance of women after in utero exposure to the Dutch famine (1944–1945)*. New York: Columbia University, 1988. (PhD thesis.)

10 de Leeuw NKM, Lowenstein L, Hsieh YS. Iron deficiency hydremia in normal pregnancy. *Medicine* 1966;**45**:291–315.

11 Beischer NA, Sivasamboo R, Vohra S, Silpisornkosal S, Reid S. Placental hypertrophy in severe pregnancy anaemia. *Journal of Obstetrics and Gynaecology of the British Commonwealth 1970;*77:398–409.

12 Whincup PH, Cook DG, Shaper AG, MacFarlane DJ, Walker M. Blood pressure in British children: associations with adult blood pressure and cardiovascular mortality. *Lancet* 1988;i:890–3.

19: Relation of maternal weight to blood pressures of Gambian children

B M MARGETTS, M G M ROWLAND, F A FOORD,
A M CRUDDAS, T J COLE, D J P BARKER

The objective of the study was to relate blood pressure levels in children to their mother's weight in pregnancy. The blood pressures of 675 children aged from 1 to 9 years in three villages in rural Gambia were measured. They were matched to antenatal clinic data which had been collected from all pregnant women in the three villages since 1980.

Among children aged under 8 those born in the dry season had the highest blood pressures and were heavier. Their blood pressures were positively related to body weight and to mothers' weight at six months of pregnancy. These relations were independent of mothers' age and parity, birth weight, gestational age, and placental weight. Among older children, aged 8 and 9, those born in the rainy season had the highest blood pressures. Their blood pressures were not related to their mothers' weight at six months of pregnancy. Rather they were inversely related to mothers' weight gain in the last trimester.

An interpretation of these findings is that among young children differences in blood pressure are largely determined by rates of maturation. However, the long term effects of adverse intrauterine influences that raise pressure become apparent in older children.

Introduction

Among 449 men and women aged 50 who had been born in one hospital in Preston, England, the highest blood pressures occurred in those who had been small babies with large placentas (chapter 16). These findings raise the question of what maternal influences determine the discordance between fetal and placental weight that leads to high blood pressure. Poor maternal nutrition is one obvious possibility.

We measured the blood pressures of children in a rural community in west Africa where seasonal variations in food intake and energy expenditure lead to large variations in the nutritional status of pregnant women, and in the birth weights of their babies. During the wet summer months food stocks from the previous year's harvest become low. Energy expenditure remains high. Food intakes are so low that some pregnant women lose weight in the last trimester. The objective of this study was to relate blood pressure levels in young children to their mother's nutritional state, as indicated by weight in pregnancy.

Methods

All children born in three villages, Keneba, Manduar, and Kanton Kunda in Gambia since January 1980, and their mothers, were asked to participate in the study. The survey was carried out during February and March 1989. Children aged under 1 and over 9 were not included.

Since 1979, maternal anthropometry and blood pressure and the birth weight of the child have been recorded for each pregnant woman in the three villages. For each child, growth and morbidity data have been collected during the first 18 months after the birth. In addition, at all clinic visits after 18 months the weight, height, diagnosis, and treament have been recorded for each child. We related these data to those collected at interview and examination during the present survey.

In addition to recording all births and deaths in the three villages, the Medical Research Council conducts periodic censuses. Before the study the census list was checked by house to house visits, and additional births and deaths, and departures from the household, were noted. The census was used to form the population base for the study.

Before the study its purpose was explained to the village elders and their permission was sought. On the evening before each survey day all women and their children in specified compounds were visited and asked to attend next morning at the community centre. On arrival each mother and child had their height, weight, and blood pressures measured.

For children under about 900 mm, length was measured using a Harpenden infantometer. All adults and children over 900 mm had their height measured using a Raven Maximeter. Weight was measured using a Seca model 727 (5 g gradations) for small children or Soehnle digital bathroom scales (10 g gradations) for heavier children and mothers. These were checked each day for accuracy by comparison to a standard weight. Before starting each day's survey the accuracy of the equipment was checked using standard measures. To reduce observer variation blood pressure was measured by use of a Dinamap (model 18465X). The Dinamap is a microprocessor controlled automatic device that measures blood pressure using the oscillometric technique. The cuff is deflated one step each time the device detects two pulsations of relatively equal amplitude; this reduces artefact error due to subject movement. The relative validity of the Dinamap has been assessed previously by comparison with the Hawksley random zero sphygmomanometer. Group mean levels of both instruments were virtually identical and the correlation between the measures was 0·98 for systolic and 0·96 for diastolic pressure.[1] Blood pressure was measured twice, in the sitting position on the right arm, after five minutes seated at rest. For young children the blood pressure was measured with the child on the mother's knee. Usually measurements were made on the mother and all her children at the same time.

Subjects were asked when they had last had something to eat and whether they were well. Of the children, 19 were found on examination to be suffering from a febrile illness and were excluded from the analysis. Ambient temperatures were recorded at the time of measuring blood pressures.

To assess the effect of the observer on blood pressure, a subset of 50 subjects was measured on two occasions, once by BMM and once by FF, the midwife in the villages whom the subjects all know well. A cross section of ages was included. Mean systolic blood pressure measured by BMM was 98·5 mm Hg and by FF was 98·2. The mean difference of 0·27 had a standard error of 1·36. Diastolic pressure and pulse rate were also closely similar for the two observers.

We classified the month of birth into three periods: August to November, encompassing most of the rainy season; December to March the cool season; and April to July, which is mostly hot and dry. This division of the year into three seasons has been used in previous studies in Gambia. During the rainy season the incidence of malaria rises sharply. Of first attacks of malaria in children, for example, some 85% occur during this season.

Because of the variable dates at which mothers were weighed in the last trimester of pregnancy, and because of the collinearity between weight and weight gain, we restricted our analysis of mother's weight to those weighed within 15 days of six months of pregnancy and 30 days of birth. We have used these weights to derive a value for 7·5 months by linear interpolation. The slope over the period between the weights was used as a measure of weight gain.

Results

We measured the blood pressures of 675 children, 346 boys and 329 girls, aged 1 to 9 years, and the blood pressures of 315 mothers. This represented 98% of the study population. Some 211 mothers had more than one child in the survey. We divided the children into three age groups: 1–4 years, 5–7 years, and 8–9 years. Those aged 1–4 were born after malaria prophylaxis with Daraprim began to be given routinely to pregnant women. For those aged 8 to 9 mothers' blood pressures had been measured in pregnancy in the lying position. Thereafter they were measured in the sitting position. Mothers' blood pressures are therefore not comparable between older and younger children.

Systolic and diastolic pressures rose progressively with children's age. Mean systolic pressure rose from 89·3 mm Hg in those aged 1 to 102·7 mm Hg in those aged 9; diastolic pressure rose from 56·2 mm Hg to 63·9 mm Hg. Blood pressure increased with body weight and decreased with the time since the last meal. Pressures were unrelated to ambient temperature, which ranged from 21°C to 38°C. Blood pressure was adjusted where indicated for age, body weight, and time since eating, and weight was transformed so that it was independent of age using a procedure based on Cole's LMS method for calculating centile curves.[2] There were no important sex differences in blood pressure and we analysed the sexes together.

SEASONAL CHANGES

Table I shows mean systolic pressures by season of birth. Among children in the two younger groups mean pressure was lowest among those

TABLE I—*Mean children's systolic pressure (mm Hg) according to season of birth, with number of children and 95% confidence interval*

Age (years)	Season			
	Rainy (August to November)	Cold (December to March)	Dry (April to July)	All seasons
1–4	92·8 (n=107) (CI 90·8 to 94·8)	93·2 (n=111) (CI 91·0 to 95·4)	96·5 (n=93) (CI 94·2 to 98·8)	94·0 (n=311) (CI 92·8 to 95·3)
5–7	98·1 (n=77) (CI 96·1 to 100·1)	98·6 (n=79) (CI 96·4 to 100·8)	100·5 (n=69) (CI 97·8 to 103·2)	99·0 (n=225) (CI 97·7 to 100·3)
8–9	104·2 (n=39) (CI 101·8 to 106·6)	100·3 (n=57) (CI 98·3 to 102·3)	102·5 (n=43) (CI 100·2 to 104·8)	102·1 (n=139) (CI 100·8 to 103·3)
All ages	96·6 (n=223) (CI 95·3 to 98·0)	96·6 (n=247) (CI 95·2 to 97·9)	99·1 (n=205) (CI 97·6 to 100·6)	97·3 (n=675) (CI 96·5 to 98·1)

CI = 95% Confidence intervals.

209

born in the rainy season. Among the older children, aged 8 to 9, pressures were highest among those born during the rains. The seasonal variation adjusted for age, body weight, and time since eating was significant in the two younger age groups combined ($F = 3.8$, p = 0.02), and those aged 8 to 9 ($F = 3.0$, p = 0.05). In each age group the current weights of children born in the dry season were greater than those of children born in the other two seasons, though the differences were not significant.

Mothers' weight gain over the last three months of pregnancy was derived from 351 pregnancies. Mothers' weight gain varied greatly with the season, being lowest in the rainy season (p < 0.001) (table II).

MOTHERS' BLOOD PRESSURES

Mothers' maximum systolic blood pressures during pregnancy were recorded for 648 pregnancies. They correlated with those recorded at the time of the survey. Excluding pregnancies eight or more years ago, when measurements of blood pressure were not comparable to those taken more recently, and using the most recent pregnancy for each mother, the correlation coefficient between mothers' pregnancy and survey systolic pressures was 0.44. Mothers' ages at the time of survey varied from 17 to 53 years; blood pressures increased slightly with age (0.2 mm Hg per year of age: t = 2.64; p = 0.01).

Mothers' maximum systolic pressures during pregnancy were strongly related to the blood pressures of children aged under 8. Every 10 mm Hg rise in a mother's systolic pressure was associated with a 1 mm Hg rise in the child's adjusted systolic pressure (p = 0.008). Adjusting for maternal age did not alter this relation. No similar relation was found in children

TABLE II—*Mean weight gain (kg) of mothers in the last trimester of pregnancy, in relation to season of birth, with numbers of children and 95% confidence intervals*

Age (years)	Rainy (August to November)	Cold (December to March)	Dry (April to July)	All seasons
		Season		
1–4	1.8 (n=60) (CI 1.1 to 2.5)	3.7 (n=67) (CI 3.1 to 4.3)	3.6 (n=49) (CI 2.8 to 4.4)	3.0 (n=176) (CI 2.6 to 3.4)
5–7	1.1 (n=42) (CI 0.3 to 1.9)	3.2 (n=47) (CI 2.2 to 4.0)	3.0 (n=39) (CI 2.4 to 3.7)	2.4 (n=128) (CI 1.9 to 2.9)
8–9	2.3 (n=11) (CI 0.8 to 3.9)	3.8 (n=21) (CI 2.9 to 4.7)	2.9 (n=15) (CI 0.6 to 5.1)	3.1 (n=47) (CI 2.3 to 4.0)
All ages	1.6 (n=113) (CI 1.1 to 2.1)	3.5 (n=135) (CI 3.1 to 4.0)	3.3 (n=103) (CI 2.7 to 3.8)	2.8 (n=351) (CI 2.5 to 3.1)

CI = 95% Confidence intervals.

aged 8 to 9. Exclusion of four women diagnosed as having pre-eclampsia did not alter the findings.

MOTHERS' WEIGHTS

Among children aged under 8, the mother's weight at 7·5 months was positively related to the child's adjusted systolic blood pressure (p = 0·003). This was independent of mother's maximum systolic pressure. Table III shows children's mean systolic pressure with the children divided into thirds according to mothers' weight. Among children aged 1 to 4, mean pressure rose by 3·2 mm Hg from the lowest to the highest maternal weight group (95% confidence interval: −0·8 to 7·2). Among children aged 5 to 7 the rise was 6·2 mm Hg (95% confidence interval: 1·9 to 10·4). There was no similar trend in the children aged 8 to 9.

Table IV shows mean systolic pressures with children divided into thirds by mothers' weight gain in the last three months of pregnancy. At ages 8 and 9 mean pressure fell by 5·2 mm Hg from the lowest to the highest weight gain group (95% confidence interval: −0·5 to 10·8). Among the younger children blood pressure was not related to mothers' weight gain. The relation between children's adjusted systolic pressure at ages 8 and 9 and mothers' weight gain (p = 0·02) was independent of weight at 7·5 months and was also independent of mother's height and blood pressure. There was no difference in mean children's systolic pressure between those with and without complete information on maternal weight.

BIRTH WEIGHT

Table V shows that mean birth weights were lower during the rainy season, though the differences were not significant. Similarly, there were

TABLE III—*Mean blood pressure (mm Hg) of children stratified into thirds by mother's weight during the last trimester of pregnancy, with numbers of children and 95% confidence intervals*

| Age (years) | Mother's weight at 7·5 months (kg) | | | |
	<54·1	54·1–59·2	>59·2	All weights
1–4	92·1 (n = 57) (CI 89·3 to 94·9)	94·1 (n = 58) (CI 91·6 to 96·6)	95·4 (n = 61) (CI 92·4 to 98·3)	93·9 (n = 176) (CI 92·3 to 95·5)
5–7	95·5 (n = 45) (CI 92·3 to 98·7)	97·8 (n = 40) (CI 94·7 to 100·8)	101·7 (n = 43) (CI 98·8 to 104·5)	98·3 (n = 128) (CI 96·4 to 100·0)
8–9	102·5 (n = 15) (CI 96·6 to 108·4)	103·7 (n = 15) (CI 99·8 to 107·6)	101·1 (n = 17) (CI 98·1 to 103·9)	102·3 (n = 47) (CI 100·0 to 104·6)
All ages	94·8 (n = 117) (CI 92·7 to 96·8)	96·7 (n = 113) (CI 94·9 to 8·5)	98·4 (n = 121) (CI 96·5 to 100·3)	96·6 (n = 351) (CI 95·5 to 97·7)

CI = 95% Confidence intervals.

211

TABLE IV—*Mean systolic blood pressure (mm Hg) of children stratified into thirds by mothers' weight gain in last trimester of pregnancy, with numbers of children and 95% confidence intervals*

Age (years)	Weight gain (kg)			All weight gains
	≤1·85	1·85–3·80	>3·80	
1–4	93·3 (n=53) (CI 90·6 to 96·0)	93·4 (n=64) (CI 90·8 to 96·1)	95·0 (n=59) (CI 92·1 to 97·8)	93·9 (n=176) (CI 92·3 to 95·5)
5–7	98·0 (n=54) (CI 95·2 to 100·7)	99·6 (n=34) (CI 95·1 to 104·0)	97·7 (n=40) (CI 95·3 to 100·0)	98·3 (n=128) (CI 96·4 to 100·0)
8–9	104·5 (n=11) (CI 98·7 to 110·2)	104·1 (n=18) (CI 99·9 to 108·2)	99·3 (n=18) (CI 96·2 to 102·4)	102·3 (n=47) (CI 100·0 to 104·6)
All ages	96·5 (n=118) (CI 94·6 to 98·4)	96·9 (n=116) (CI 94·7 to 99·0)	96·6 (n=117) (CI 94·8 to 98·3)	96·6 (n=351) (CI 95·5 to 97·7)

CI = 95% Confidence intervals.

no significant seasonal differences in placental weight. Mean duration of gestation was higher in the cold season. Birth weight was unrelated to adjusted systolic blood pressure at any age. Birth weight was strongly postively related to mother's height, mother's weight at 7·5 months of pregnancy, and weight gain in the last trimester (p = 0·005). The effect of mothers' weight at 7·5 months on the blood pressure of children aged under 8 was independent of birth weight, gestational age, parity, and placental weight.

TABLE V—*Mean birth weight (kg) placental weight (kg) and gestation (weeks) of children according to season of birth, with numbers of children and 95% confidence intervals*

	Season			All seasons
	Rainy (August to November)	Cold (December to March)	Dry (April to July)	
Birth weight	2·96 (n=188) (CI 2·90 to 3·01)	2·98 (n=196) (CI 2·93 to 3·04)	3·02 (n=171) (CI 2·96 to 3·08)	2·99 (n=555) (CI 2·95 to 3·02)
Placental weight	0·50 (n=117) (CI 0·48 to 0·51)	0·50 (n=106) (CI 0·48 to 0·51)	0·52 (n=87) (CI 0·50 to 0·53)	0·50 (n=310) (CI 0·49 to 0·51)
Gestation period	38·8 (n=168) (CI 38·6 to 39·0)	39·2 (n=188) (CI 39·0 to 39·4)	38·7 (n=143) (CI 38·4 to 38·9)	38·9 (n=499) (CI 38·8 to 39·0)

CI = 95% Confidence intervals.

Discussion

This study of children in a rural area of Gambia was based on the detailed recording of antenatal attendances over 10 years in three villages in which censuses are regularly carried out for medical research purposes. It showed that children's blood pressures were related to mothers' weight in pregnancy and weight gain during the last trimester. The findings differed, however, in children under and over 8 years of age.

There have been few studies measuring blood pressures in a similarly aged rural African population. Compared with children aged 5 to 9 in Nigeria the blood pressures of children in our study were higher.[3] They were similar to those of somewhat older children in Uganda.[4] The children in our study had higher blood pressures than children in Europe and America (chapter 15).[5,6] The reasons for these differences are unknown. Maternal blood pressures in the present study were similar to previously published data from rural Africa.[4,7] Our results show a relatively small difference in blood pressure levels between the children aged 9 and the mothers. It is not clear whether the apparently higher levels in younger children is part of a secular trend of increasing blood pressures in Gambia.

Among children aged under 8 those born in the dry season had the highest blood pressures (table I) and were heavier. In this age group blood pressure was strongly related to body weight and to mothers' weight at six months of pregnancy (table III). These relations were independent of birth weight. Other surveys have shown that children's blood pressures are strongly related to their current weight. One interpretation of this is that both variables rise with maturation and the association is indirect.

The findings in older children contrasted with those in children aged under 8. Their blood pressures were not related to their mothers' weight at six months of pregnancy (table III). Rather, they were strongly inversely related to mothers' weight gain in the last trimester (table IV).

In a survey of 449 men and women who had been born in a hospital in Preston, England, around 50 years previously and whose measurements at birth had been recorded in unusual detail, current blood pressure was strongly related to birth and placental weight (chapter 16). The highest pressures occurred in people who had been small babies with large placentas. It was concluded that this discordance between placental and fetal size reflected impaired fetal growth, itself a consequence of adverse maternal factors. The nature of these adverse factors is as yet unknown but we suggest that they include poor maternal nutrition. Impaired fetal growth may be associated with circulatory adaptation in the fetus and altered blood vessel structure and higher blood pressure in the child. The inverse relation between maternal weight gain in pregnancy and blood pressures in older children in Gambia is consistent with a relation between poor maternal nutrition and higher blood pressure in the child. The nutritional factors that determine low weight gain of mothers, which occurs most often in the rainy season (table II), and which are thereby associated with high blood pressure in the children, are unknown.

A possible explanation of our findings is that among younger children blood pressure levels are largely determined by rates of maturation, which are themselves determined by, among other factors, maternal size. Among older children, however, the long term effects of adverse intrauterine influences become apparent. We will test this interpretation by surveying the Gambian children again to assess whether among those aged 6 and 7 at the time of our survey the effects of maternal weight gain in pregnancy will have become evident.

We would like to thank Doctors Rob and Barbara Downes, Dr Sally Poppit, and the Keneban field workers. Dr Barbara Thompson provided much valuable information about the women in Keneba. Mr Ken Day assisted with data preparation.

1 Silas JH, Barker AT, Ramsay LE. Clinical evaluation of Dinamap 845 automated blood pressure recorder. *Br Heart J* 1980;**43**:202–5.
2 Cole TJ. The LMS method for constructing normalized growth standards. *Eur J Clin Nutr* 1990;**44**:45–60.
3 Akinkughe OO. *High blood pressure in the African.* Edinburgh: Churchill Livingstone. 1972.
4 Shaper AG, Saxton GA. Blood pressure and body build in a rural community in Uganda. *East Africa Med J* 1969;**46**:228–45.
5 Horan MJ, Sinaiko AR. Synopsis of the report of the Second Task Force on blood pressure control in children. *Hypertension* 1987;**10**:115–21.
6 Whincup PH, Cook DG, Shaper AG. Early influences on blood pressure: a study of children aged 5 to 7 years. *BMJ* 1989;**299**:587–91.
7 Van Dongen PWJ, Herned Y, Van T Hof MA. Reference values for blood pressures in non-pregnant women over the age of 14 years in two rural Tanzanian Communities. *East Africa Med J* 1983;**60**:739–47.

PART VI
HAEMOSTATIC FACTORS

20: Relation of fetal and infant growth to plasma fibrinogen and factor VII concentrations in adult life

D J P BARKER, T W MEADE, C H D FALL, A LEE,
C OSMOND, K PHIPPS, Y STIRLING

Two groups of men were followed up to investigate whether reduced early growth is associated with higher plasma fibrinogen and factor VII concentrations in adult life. The first group was 597 men who were born in east Hertfordshire during 1920–30 and still lived there. Their weights at birth and at 1 year had been recorded by health visitors. The second group was 142 men who were born in Preston during 1935–43 and still lived in or near the city. Their size at birth had been recorded in detail. Plasma fibrinogen and factor VII concentrations in both groups of men were measured.

Among men in Hertfordshire mean plasma fibrinogen and factor VII concentrations fell with increasing weight at 1 year (from 3.21 g/l in men whose weight had been 18 lb or less to 2.93 g/l in men who had weighed 27 lb or more and from 122% of standard to 103%; $p < 0.001$, $p < 0.005$ respectively). The trends were independent of cigarette smoking, alcohol consumption, body mass index, and social class. Neither plasma fibrinogen nor factor VII concentration was related to birth weight. In men in Preston, however, fibrinogen concentrations fell progressively as the ratio of placental weight to birth weight decreased ($p = 0.01$).

It was concluded that reduced growth in fetal life and

infancy is strongly related to high plasma concentrations of the haemostatic factors, fibrinogen and factor VII. This may be a persisting response to impaired liver development during a critical early period.

Introduction

Retarded growth in utero and during infancy is associated with the development of cardiovascular disease in adult life. Among men born 70 years ago, whose early growth was recorded, those who had had lower birth weights and weights at 1 year had higher death rates from ischaemic heart disease (chapter 13). There were threefold differences in death rates between men with the lowest and highest early weights.

These findings pose the question of which processes associated with retarded early growth lead to ischaemic heart disease. High plasma concentrations of two haemostatic factors, fibrinogen and factor VII, are independently associated with increased rates of the disease.[1] They may predispose to thrombosis and contribute to the development and progression of atheroma.[2] Their association with ischaemic heart disease is at least as strong as that of high plasma cholesterol concentration.[1] We therefore examined whether retarded early growth is associated with higher plasma concentrations of fibrinogen and factor VII.

We measured plasma concentrations of these haemostatic factors in two groups, one group comprising men aged around 64 years whose weight gain in infancy had been recorded, and the other men aged around 50 years whose size at birth had been measured in detail.

Subjects and methods

In Hertfordshire, from 1911 onwards, each birth was notified by the attending midwife. A health visitor saw the child at home periodically throughout its infancy. The data recorded are described in chapter 13.

We traced 1157 singleton boys born in east Hertfordshire during 1920–30; 845 of the men agreed to be interviewed at home. After the interview men were asked to attend a local clinic to have a blood sample taken; from 606 blood was taken with minimum haemostasis and analysed for fibrinogen and factor VII concentrations. Thrombin clottable fibrinogen concentration was measured by the Clauss method, with an electrical impedance end point.[3] Factor VII concentration was measured by a one stage assay with bovine adsorbed deficient plasma and rabbit brain thromboplastin.[4]

In Preston a standardised record form had been kept for each woman admitted to the labour ward at Sharoe Green Hospital during 1935–43.

The data recorded are described in chapter 16. The babies were not followed up after discharge from hospital.

Two hundred and fifty two of the men who had been singleton boys born during 1935–43 still lived in Lancashire; 236 agreed to be interviewed at home and were visited by one of four fieldworkers. Blood pressure, weight, height, waist circumference, and hip girth were recorded as for the Hertfordshire men. Social class was defined as in the Hertfordshire men. Of 204 men living in or close to Preston who were asked to attend Sharoe Green Hospital to have a blood sample taken, 148 did so. Blood was taken with minimum haemostasis and analysed for fibrinogen and factor VII concentrations by the same methods as used for the samples from Hertfordshire men.

As plasma fibrinogen and factor VII concentrations have skewed distributions we transformed them in the analysis by using logarithms. We used multiple regression to analyse the data.

Results

HERTFORDSHIRE MEN

Satisfactory measurements of fibrinogen and factor VII concentrations were obtained for 591 and 582 men respectively; 597 men had one or both measurements performed. Plasma fibrinogen concentration increased by 0·03 g/l with each year of age from 59 to 70 years, and we therefore adjusted the concentrations for age. Plasma factor VII concentration was not related to age.

Both mean plasma fibrinogen and factor VII concentrations fell with increasing weight at 1 year (table I). These trends were strongly significant ($p < 0.001$, $p < 0.005$ respectively). Neither factor showed a significant trend with birth weight ($p = 0.10$, $p = 0.84$ respectively), though the highest concentration of each was found in men with birth weights of 5·5 lb or less.

When the men were grouped into current smokers, ex-smokers, and those who had never smoked (histories for three men were unclassifiable) mean plasma fibrinogen concentration was highest in smokers and higher in ex-smokers than in men who had never smoked (table II). Adjustment for smoking did not change the trend in mean plasma fibrinogen concentration with weight at 1 year. Regression analysis showed that the concentration fell with increasing weight at 1 year in each smoking group (table II). Plasma fibrinogen concentration was lower in men who drank alcohol, the mean value being 2·94 g/l in men who drank more than two units of alcohol a day compared with 3·06 g/l in the remainder. Adjustment for alcohol consumption did not change the trends with weight at 1 year. Mean fibrinogen concentration was not related to body mass index (weight/height^2). It was, however, higher in men with larger waist to hip ratios,

TABLE I—*Mean plasma fibrinogen and factor VII concentrations and systolic blood pressure in Hertfordshire men aged 59–70, according to weight at 1 year and birth weight*

	No of men	Fibrinogen (g/l) (adjusted for age)	Factor VII (% of standard)	Systolic pressure (mm Hg) (adjusted for age and room temperature)
Weight at 1 year (lb):				
≤18	38	3·21	122	167
−20	93	3·10	111	167
−22	178	3·13	108	166
−24	173	2·97	106	162
−26	82	2·93	106	164
>26	33	2·93	103	162
Birth weight (lb):				
≤5·5	21	3·18	118	174
−6·5	70	3·06	104	165
−7·5	187	3·10	108	166
−8·5	183	2·98	107	164
−9·5	96	3·00	112	161
>9·5	40	3·05	109	164
All	597	3·04	108	164
Standard deviation		0·59	27	23

rising by 0·11 g/l with each increase in waist to hip ratio of 0·1. Adjustment for waist to hip ratio did not change the trends with weight at 1 year.

Fibrinogen concentration was lower in taller men. Simultaneous regression of concentration on current height, birth weight, and weight at 1 year showed a significant trend with only weight at 1 year. Fibrinogen concentration fell by 0·03 g/l (95% confidence interval 0·005 to 0·047) with each pound increase in weight at 1 year. In contrast, it fell by only 0·003 g/l with

TABLE II—*Mean plasma fibrinogen concentration (g/l) in Hertfordshire men, according to weight at 1 year and smoking habit. Numbers of men in parentheses*

	History of smoking		
Weight at 1 year (lb)	Never smoked	Ex smoker	Current smoker
≤18	2·87 (6)	3·25 (19)	3·33 (12)
−20	3·25 (11)	2·94 (48)	3·28 (31)
−22	2·98 (31)	3·10 (96)	3·29 (50)
−24	2·81 (32)	2·95 (97)	3·14 (42)
−26	2·78 (16)	2·93 (46)	3·05 (18)
>26	2·62 (4)	3·00 (22)	2·87 (7)
All	2·90 (100)	3·01 (328)	3·20 (160)

each centimetre increase in height (-0.004 to 0.012) and by 0.003 g/l with each pound increase in birth weight (-0.039 to 0.046).

Plasma factor VII concentration was not related to smoking or alcohol consumption. It rose, however, by 0.7% of the standard with each unit increase in body mass index (kg/m^2) and by 0.6% of the standard with each 0.1 increase in waist to hip ratio. Adjustment for body mass index and waist to hip ratio did not change the trends with weight at 1 year (table I). Similarly to fibrinogen, the concentration of factor VII was lower in taller men, but in a simultaneous regression of factor VII concentration with height, birth weight, and weight at 1 year there was a significant trend with only weight at 1 year.

Neither fibrinogen nor factor VII concentration was related to current social class or social class at birth, after adjustment for age, smoking, alcohol intake, body mass index, and waist to hip ratio.

Details of infant feeding were recorded for 588 men: 417 were exclusively breast fed, of whom 306 were weaned by 1 year; 143 were breast and bottle fed; and 28 were exclusively bottle fed. Mean plasma fibrinogen and factor VII concentrations did not differ according to the method of feeding. In all, 411 of the men were recorded as having had one illness or more during infancy. Their mean fibrinogen and factor VII concentrations did not differ from the remainder. Neither did those of men who had had specific illnesses including bronchitis, bronchopneumonia, measles, whooping cough, and diarrhoea.

Systolic blood pressure rose by 0.7 mm Hg with each year of age, fell by 1.2 mm Hg with every degree centigrade of room temperature, and rose by 1.1 mm Hg with each unit of body mass index. In contrast to mean fibrinogen and factor VII concentrations, mean systolic pressure fell with increasing birth weight ($p=0.003$) but showed no significant trend with weight at 1 year (table I) or with height. Table III shows variations in mean

TABLE III—*Mean plasma fibrinogen and factor VII concentration in Hertfordshire men, according to systolic blood pressure*

Systolic pressure (mm Hg) (adjusted for age, room temperature, and body mass)	No of men	Fibrinogen (g/l) (adjusted for age, smoking, alcohol, and waist to hip ratio)	Factor VII (% of standard) (adjusted for waist to hip ratio and body mass)
≤140	83	2·98	107
−150	81	2·94	106
−160	111	2·96	108
−170	120	3·10	109
−190	115	3·12	107
>190	87	3·14	112
All	597	3·04	108

plasma fibrinogen and factor VII concentrations in relation to systolic pressure, after the other variables had been adjusted for. Plasma fibrinogen concentration was strongly related to systolic pressure, rising progressively with increasing pressure (p = 0·005); plasma factor VII concentration was only weakly positively related to blood pressure (p = 0·12) and to fibrinogen concentration (p = 0·12).

PRESTON MEN

Satisfactory measurements of fibrinogen and factor VII concentrations were obtained for 142 of the 148 men. Plasma fibrinogen concentration increased with age, cigarette smoking, and larger waist to hip ratio, but was not related to alcohol intake or social class. As in the Hertfordshire men, fibrinogen concentration was not significantly related to birth weight. Simultaneous analysis of birth weight and placental weight, however, showed that it fell with increasing birth weight (p = 0·06) and rose with increasing placental weight (p = 0·03). The lowest mean plasma fibrinogen concentration (2·82 g/l) was in men who had weighed more than 7·5 lb at birth, with a placental weight of 1·25 lb or less (table IV). The highest value (3·11 g/l) was in men who had weighed 6·5 lb or less, with a placental weight greater than 1·25 lb. Mean plasma fibrinogen concentration rose progressively as the ratio of placental weight to birth weight increased (p = 0·01, table V). These trends were independent of duration of gestation, which was known for 108 of the men.

We examined the separate associations of plasma fibrinogen concentration with head circumference, length, and ponderal index (birth weight/length³) at birth. Simultaneous analysis with placental weight showed that fibrinogen concentration tended to rise as length decreased (p = 0·08), from 2·83 g/l in men who had been 21 inches or longer at birth to 3·06 g/l in men who had been less than 20 inches. Concentration was not associated with head circumference or ponderal index.

TABLE IV—*Mean plasma fibrinogen concentration (g/l), adjusted for age, according to birth and placental weights in Preston men aged 46–54. Numbers of men in parentheses*

Birth weight (lb)	Placental weight (lb)		All
	≤ 1·25	> 1·25	
≤ 6·5	3·00 (31)	3·11 (15)	3·04 (46)
− 7·5	2·95 (28)	2·93 (22)	2·94 (50)
> 7·5	2·82 (11)	2·87 (35)	2·85 (46)
All	2·95 (70)	2·94 (72)	2·94 (142)

TABLE V—*Mean plasma fibrinogen concentration, adjusted for age, and mean factor VII concentration in Preston men, according to ratio of placental to birth weight*

Ratio of placental to birth weight	No of men	Fibrinogen (g/l)	Factor VII (% of standard)
≤0·162	28	2·87	113
−0·182	30	2·89	113
−0·200	27	2·92	110
−0·229	28	2·90	111
>0·229	29	3·15	107
All	142	2·94	111
Standard deviation		0·50	30

Factor VII concentration in the men in Preston was not associated with body mass index or waist to hip ratio. As in Hertfordshire men it was not related to birth weight, nor was it related to the ratio of placental weight to birth weight (table V). Factor VII concentration tended to fall with increasing gestation (p = 0·08, table VI).

Discussion

We have shown that plasma concentrations of fibrinogen and factor VII in adult men are strongly linked with growth in infancy. Both fell progressively with increasing weight at 1 year (table I). The difference in concentrations between men who had weighed 27 lb or more at 1 year and those who had weighed 18 lb or less was statistically equivalent to an increase in cardiovascular death rate of around 40%.[1] This is likely to underestimate the strength of the associations, as the weights of the babies were imprecise. Babies were weighed at home with simple scales, and their weights were often rounded to the nearest half pound.

The study samples comprised men who were born in east Hertfordshire during 1920–30, who were still living there, and men born in Sharoe Green Hospital, Preston, and still living in or close to the town. As our analysis was based on internal comparisons, the selection of the sample would

TABLE VI—*Mean plasma factor VII concentration in Preston men, according to weeks of completed gestation*

	Weeks of gestation			
	≤38	−40	>40	All
Mean plasma factor VII (% of standard)	119	118	103	113
No of men	30	41	37	108

introduce bias only if the relations between early growth and plasma fibrinogen and factor VII concentrations were different in those selected and not selected. This is unlikely. The same relations were found in each social class.

High fibrinogen concentration increases blood viscosity and enhances platelet aggregability and, in rabbits, determines the amount of fibrin deposited when coagulation is initiated.[5] It is suspected to contribute to the development and progression of atheroma. Fibrinogen is an acute phase protein and rises in response to several stimuli.[6] Factor VII, which does not respond to such stimuli, is a key component of the extrinsic coagulation system and thus in the production of thrombin. Both fibrinogen and factor VII may thus have a causal role in ischaemic heart disease.

Consistent with previous findings, a higher plasma fibrinogen concentration was associated with age, smoking, low alcohol intake, and waist to hip ratio.[7 8] A higher plasma factor VII concentration was associated with higher body mass index and waist to hip ratio. The trends with weight at 1 year were not changed by adjustment for these variables. The simultaneous relation of fibrinogen concentration with smoking and weight at 1 year (table II) indicates that effects of the adult environment add to those associated with failure of infant growth.

INFLUENCE OF CONFOUNDING VARIABLES

It may be argued that people born into an adverse environment tend to remain there. Therefore the association between lower weight at 1 year and higher adult concentrations of haemostatic factors could reflect the cumulative effects of adverse influences acting throughout a person's life. After smoking and other known confounding variables had been allowed for, however, average concentrations of fibrinogen and factor VII were not higher in men of lower social class, as would be expected from this argument. Furthermore, they were not independently related to adult height or to birth weight, but only to weight at 1 year. An association with short adult stature would be expected if they were determined by adverse influences acting throughout the period of growth. The argument that higher fibrinogen concentration reflects influences in only the current environment which trigger the acute phase response is not consistent with the absence of a social class gradient in fibrinogen concentration in our study. Nor could it apply to factor VII concentration, as factor VII does not rise as part of the acute phase response.

It could also be argued that the link between early growth and adult plasma fibrinogen and factor VII concentrations reflects genetic influences. Studies using restriction fragment length polymorphisms of the fibrinogen genes showed that genetic variation could account for at least 15% of the total variance in plasma concentration.[9] Fetal and infant growth are, however, strongly influenced by maternal physique, health, and nutrition, and we therefore favour an environmental explanation for our findings.

INFLUENCE OF RESTRICTED GROWTH IN EARLY LIFE

Our results suggest that there may be a critical period in early life when growth is linked with the setting of plasma concentrations of haemostatic factors. Research in animals has shown that influences which restrain growth during critical periods of early life may permanently affect organ size and function.[10 11] For example, in rats weaned on to a low protein diet for only three weeks the insulin response to glucose was permanently impaired.[12] This phenomenon, known as "programming," has been shown in a wide range of tissues. Circulating fibrinogen and factor VII concentrations are largely regulated by the liver. The high adult concentrations associated with reduced infant growth may be a persisting response to impaired liver development during a critical early phase. Plasma concentrations of fibrinogen and factor VII reach values within the adult range by the age of 1 year.[13]

Growth failure in infancy may result from either postnatal or prenatal influences. Postnatal influences include feeding and illness. Concentrations of the haemostatic factors in the Hertfordshire men did not vary in relation to differences in infant feeding and weaning, although these differences were related to adult cholesterol concentrations (chapter 25). Neither were they related to illness during infancy, although the occurrence of bronchitis or bronchopneumonia was associated with impaired adult lung function in these men (chapter 14).

The findings in Preston suggest that prenatal influences may underlie the reduction in infant growth which is associated with high plasma concentrations of fibrinogen. Although fibrinogen concentration was not related to birth weight, simultaneous analysis of birth weight and placental weight disclosed that it fell with increasing birth weight and rose with increasing placental weight (table IV). The highest concentration was in men with the highest ratio of placental weight to birth weight (table V). These trends were independent of gestation.

Low birth weight for placental weight may be interpreted as a sign of fetal growth failure (chapter 17). Previous analyses of the Preston data showed that high blood pressure is also related to low birth weight for placental weight (chapter 16). Failure of a fetus to achieve the size expected from its placental weight occurs in babies within the normal range of birth weight (table IV). It is not confined to low birth weight babies, as defined by conventional criteria for intrauterine growth retardation. Some low birth weight babies, conventionally defined, have disproportionate retardation of growth of the abdominal viscera, especially the liver, as growth of some other organs, notably the brain, tends to be protected.[14] Whether reduced liver size is also a characteristic of babies with low birth weight for placental weight is not known. Reduced liver growth in utero could lead to long term changes in fibrinogen metabolism.

The pattern of infant growth which follows retarded intrauterine growth differs according to whether the babies are short at birth or thin, as measured by low ponderal index.[15][16] Thin babies tend to "catch up" in weight whereas short babies do not. In our data fibrinogen concentration was associated with shortness but not thinness. High adult fibrinogen concentration and infant growth failure may therefore be associated through a common origin in fetal growth failure.

In the Preston data high blood pressure was found in babies who were short and also in those who were thin (chapter 17). The tendency for thin babies to have below average birth weights but to catch up in infancy may explain why high blood pressure in Hertfordshire men was associated with low birth weight but not with weight at 1 year (table I). Association of both fibrinogen concentration and blood pressure with low birth weight for placental weight is consistent with the close relation between fibrinogen concentration and blood pressure in adults, as shown in our data (table III) and in previous studies.[17][18]

Similarly to the Northwick Park study,[1] we found that factor VII concentration was only weakly associated with either fibrinogen concentration or blood pressure level (table III). This is consistent with it having no association with birth weight or placental weight (table V). We found that factor VII concentration tended to be higher in men born before 40 weeks' gestation (table VI). The association was based on only 108 men whose gestation period was known and was not significant; it is interesting, however, as in the neonate factor VII concentration is linked with duration of gestation.[13] Our data gave no other indication that prenatal influences contribute to the association between reduced infant growth and high plasma factor VII concentration.

We conclude that the control of haemostasis in adults is partly programmed by the intrauterine and infant environments. Added to recent findings that fetal and infant growth is linked with adult blood pressure (chapter 16) and glucose tolerance (chapter 22), this is further evidence of the importance of fetal and infant development in the genesis of cardiovascular disease.

We thank all the men who gave us their time; also Hertfordshire county archives and the medical records department at Sharoe Green Hospital, Preston, which preserved the records and allowed us to use them. We thank Dr I Clarke, east Hertfordshire district community physician, for much local help. B E Newland, Princess Alexandra Hospital, Harlow, and the laboratory staff at the Royal Preston Hospital stored the blood samples.

1 Meade TW, Mellows S, Brozovic M, Miller GJ, Chakrabarti RR, North WRS, *et al.* Haemostatic function and ischaemic heart disease: principal results of the Northwick Park heart study. *Lancet* 1986;ii:533–7.

2 Meade TW. The epidemiology of haemostatic and other variables in coronary artery disease. In: Verstraete M, Vermiylen J, Lijnen R, Arnout J, eds. *Thrombosis and haemostasis*. Leuven, Netherlands: University Press. 1987;37–66.

3 Clauss A. Gerinnungsphysiologische Schnellmethode zur Bestimmung des Fibrinogens. *Acta Haematol (Basel)* 1957;**17**:237–46.

4 Brozovic M, Stirling Y, Harricks C, North WRS, Meade TW. Factor VII in an industrial population. *Br J Haematol* 1974;**28**:381–91.

5 Gureweich V, Lipinski B, Hyde E. The effect of the fibrinogen concentration and the leucocyte count on intravascular fibrin deposition from soluble fibrin monomer complexes. *Thromb Haemost* 1976;**36**:605–14.

6 Brozovic M. Physiological mechanisms in coagulation and fibrinolysis. *Br Med Bull* 1977;**33**:231–8.

7 Meade TW, Chakrabarti R, Haines AP, North WRS, Stirling Y. Characteristics affecting fibrinolytic activity and plasma fibrinogen concentration. *BMJ* 1979;i:153–8.

8 Lee AJ, Smith WCS, Lowe GDO, Tunstall-Pedoe H. Plasma fibrinogen and coronary risk factors: the Scottish heart health study. *J Clin Epidemiol* 1990;**43**:913–9.

9 Humphries SE, Cook M, Dubowitz M, Stirling Y, Meade TW. Role of genetic variation at the fibrinogen locus in determination of plasma fibrinogen concentrations. *Lancet* 1987;ii:1452–6.

10 Dubos R, Savage D, Schaedler R. Biological Freudianism: lasting effects of early environmental influences. *Pediatrics* 1966;**38**:789–800.

11 Winick M, Noble A. Cellular response in rats during malnutrition at various ages. *J Nutr* 1966;**89**:300–6.

12 Swenne I, Crace CJ, Milner RDG. Persistent impairment of insulin secretory response to glucose in adult rats after limited period of protein-calorie malnutrition early in life. *Diabetes* 1987;**36**:454–8.

13 Andrew M, Paes B, Johnston M. Development of the hemostatic system in the neonate and young infant. *Am J Pediatr Hematol Oncol* 1990;**12**:95–104.

14 Gruenwald P. Chronic fetal distress and placental insufficiency. *Biol Neonat* 1963;**5**:215–65.

15 Holmes GE, Miller HC, Hassanein K, Lansky SB, Goggin JE. Postnatal somatic growth in infants with atypical fetal growth patterns. *Am J Dis Child* 1977;**3**:1078–83.

16 Villar J, Smeriglio V, Martorell R, Brown CH, Klein RE. Heterogeneous growth and mental development of intrauterine growth retarded infants during the first 3 years of life. *Pediatrics* 1984;**74**:783–91.

17 Kannel WB, Philip AW, Castelli WP, D'Agostino RB. Fibrinogen and risk of cardiovascular disease. The Framingham study. *JAMA* 1987;**258**:1183–6.

18 Wilhelmsen L, Svardsudd K, Korsan-Bengtsen K, Larsson B, Welin L, Tibblin G. Fibrinogen as a risk factor for stroke and myocardial infarction. *N Engl J Med* 1984;**311**:501–5.

PART VII
REVIEW

21: Intrauterine origins of cardiovascular and obstructive lung disease in adult life

The Marc Daniels Lecture 1990, Royal College of Physicians of London

D J P BARKER

The aim of this chapter is to present evidence that retardation of growth during critical periods of development in fetal life and infancy is associated with cardiovascular and obstructive lung disease.

Geographical studies

The large geographical differences in death rates from cardiovascular and obstructive lung disease in England and Wales remain unexplained. Variations in adult diet and cigarette smoking do not explain why the highest cardiovascular death rates are in industrial areas in the north and west of the country, and in some of the less affluent rural areas such as North Wales. Rates are low throughout the south and east, including London. It is a paradox that, although the steep increase in ischaemic heart disease during this century has been associated with rising prosperity, the disease is now more common in poorer areas, and in lower income groups. The highest death rates from obstructive lung disease occur in cities and large towns, and again differences in cigarette smoking may contribute to this distribution but cannot explain it.

One possibility is that these differences in mortality derive not from the current environment but from the environment to which people were exposed during childhood. The existence of detailed records of infant mortality from the beginning of the century allows us to compare current death rates in any area of England and Wales with infant mortality rates 60 or more years ago. This comparison can be made by dividing the country into 212 local authority groupings. The correlations between past infant mortality and current mortality from both cardiovascular and obstructive lung disease are remarkably strong, the correlation coefficients being 0·73 and 0·82 respectively (chapters 1 and 3). Infant mortality is a general indicator of an adverse environment, and the conclusion drawn from these correlations is that poor living conditions in childhood are a risk factor for cardiovascular disease—a conclusion first put forward in 1977 by Forsdahl, who found a similar geographical relation between infant and cardiovascular mortality in the counties of Norway.[1]

The detailed infant mortality records in England and Wales make it possible to distinguish neonatal mortality (deaths before 1 month of age) from postneonatal mortality (deaths from 1 month to 1 year). They give the new and surprising clue that cardiovascular mortality in adults is closely linked to neonatal mortality (chapter 4). In the past, neonatal mortality was high in places where many babies had a low birth weight. High neonatal mortality was generally associated with high maternal mortality rates, which were found in places where women had poor physique and health. There is, therefore, a geographical association between poor maternal physique and health, poor fetal growth, and high death rates from cardiovascular disease.

In contrast, the geographical distribution of chronic obstructive lung disease closely resembles the pattern of postneonatal mortality, and in particular infant deaths from bronchitis and pneumonia (chapter 3). High infant death rates from lower respiratory tract infection occurred in places where overcrowding resulted both from a high density of housing and from overcrowding within houses.

The recent fall in stroke mortality in Britain and many other Western countries is consistent with improvement in maternal health during the past century (chapter 11). The fall in mortality from chronic obstructive lung disease is consistent with the reduction in overcrowding, a consequence of the falling birth rate and improvements in housing. To explain the rise in ischaemic heart disease it seems necessary to postulate two groups of causes: one associated with poor living standards and acting in infancy, and the other associated with prosperity and linked, presumably, to the Western diet.

Follow up studies

Further epidemiological exploration of the relation of early growth and infection to adult disease requires studies of adults in middle and old age for whom records of their early development are available. In Hertford-shire, from 1911 onwards every baby born in the county was weighed at birth, visited periodically by health visitors throughout the first year, and weighed again at one year. From 1923 onwards all illnesses in children aged up to 5 years were recorded. The records for the whole county have been preserved, and it is therefore possible to trace men and women born around 60 years ago, and to relate their early development to the later occurrence of illness and death and the presence of known risk factors (chapters 13 and 14).

Obstructive lung disease

In an early study we followed up 6500 men who had been born in eight districts of east and west Hertfordshire in 1911–30, all of whom had been breast fed at birth. Fifty two had died from obstructive lung disease. In table I death rates are expressed in relation to a national average of 100 allowing for the age distribution of the men. The standardised mortality ratios fell sharply with increasing weight at 1 year of age.

We also measured the lung function of 825 men who still live in the districts where they were born (chapter 14). The forced expiratory volumes in one second (FEV_1) adjusted for the men's current heights are shown in table II. They rise progressively with increasing birth weight. It has been argued that such findings only show that an adverse early environment, indicated by lower birth weight, results in lower adult FEV_1 in conse-quence of the cumulative effects of several influences acting during childhood and adolescence. We reject this. In these men birth weight was not associated with social class, and the same relation between birth weight and FEV_1 was found within each social class. We interpret this relation as evidence of the long term effects of an adverse environment during a critical period of rapid lung growth in utero, an example of so called

TABLE I—*Standardised mortality ratios for obstructive lung disease, according to weight at 1 year, in 6500 men born during 1911–30. Numbers of deaths in parentheses*

Weight at 1 year (lb)	Chronic obstructive lung disease
≤18	103 (5)
−20	98 (14)
−22	52 (13)
−24	70 (14)
−26	48 (5)
≥27	26 (1)
All	66 (52)

1 lb = 0·45 kg

TABLE II—*Forced expiratory volume in one second (FEV₁) adjusted for height in men aged 64, according to birth weight*

Birth weight (lb)	No of men	FEV₁ (litres)
⩽5·5	33	2·28
−6·5	103	2·41
−7·5	258	2·44
−8·5	242	2·52
−9·5	132	2·55
>9·5	57	2·57
All	825	2·48*

* Standard deviation = 0·59

"programming". The adverse environment retards the weight gain of the fetus and constrains irrecoverably the growth of the airways. This interpretation is consistent with findings in rats in whom a period of malnutrition around the time of birth permanently reduces lung size and DNA content.[2]

Another finding which we interpret as an effect of programming is that the mean FEV_1 of 59 men whose records show that they had had an attack of bronchitis or pneumonia during infancy was lower at each birth weight (chapter 14). The FEV_1 was not reduced when the attack of bronchitis or pneumonia had occurred between the ages of 1 and 5 years. This is consistent with infection causing permanent damage to the airways during infancy but not at older ages, when rates of lung growth decline though lung expansion continues. Evidence of a permanent effect of early infection on adult respiratory function has come from other studies, notably those on the 1946 birth cohort.[3]

The reduction in FEV_1 associated with lower birth weight interacts with the effects of smoking, so that the highest FEV_1 (2·79 litres) was in men in the upper third of the birth weight distribution who had never smoked, and the lowest (2·21 litres) was in men in the lower third of the birth weight distribution who were current smokers.

Ischaemic heart disease

Table III shows standardised mortality ratios for ischaemic heart disease in the 6500 men, of whom 469 had died from the disease. The ratios fall steeply with increasing weight at 1 year, a trend not shown by deaths from non-circulatory causes. Ischaemic heart disease mortality also falls with increasing birth weight, though the relation is not as strong as with weight at 1 year. Stroke mortality shows similar trends. An interpretation of this is that programming of cardiovascular disease occurs partly during fetal life and partly in infancy. This interpretation is consistent with the findings on cardiovascular risk factors.

TABLE III—*Standardised mortality ratios for ischaemic heart disease, according to weight at 1 year, in 6500 men born during 1911–30. Numbers of deaths in parentheses*

Weight at 1 year (lb)	Ischaemic heart disease	All non-circulatory disease
⩽18	100 (36)	74 (39)
−20	84 (90)	99 (157)
−22	92 (180)	74 (215)
−24	70 (109)	67 (155)
−26	55 (44)	84 (99)
⩾27	34 (10)	72 (31)
All	78 (469)	78 (696)

Dr T W Meade and his colleagues at Northwick Park Hospital have measured the plasma fibrinogen levels in 597 of the men in Hertfordshire (chapter 20). High plasma fibrinogen concentration is a strong predictor of both ischaemic heart disease and stroke.[45] Levels fall with increasing weight at 1 year (table IV). They do not, however, fall with birth weight. This contrasts with systolic blood pressure, which falls with birth weight (table V) but is unrelated to weight at 1 year. This specificity of the relation

TABLE IV—*Mean plasma fibrinogen concentrations in men aged 64, according to weight at 1 year*

Weight at 1 year (lb)	No of men	Fibrinogen (g/litre)
⩽18	38	3·21
−20	93	3·10
−22	178	3·13
−24	173	2·97
−26	82	2·93
>26	33	2·93
All	597	3·04

TABLE V—*Mean systolic blood pressure in men aged 64, according to birth weight*

Birth weight (lb)	No of men	Systolic pressure (mm Hg)
⩽5·5	21	174
−6·5	70	165
−7·5	187	166
−8·5	183	164
−9·5	96	161
>9·5	40	164
All	597	164

of the two risk factors to weight either at birth or at 1 year is a further argument in favour of long term effects being determined during critical, often brief, periods of early development.

Blood pressure

In table VI the men have been divided roughly into thirds according to birth weight and current body mass index (weight/height^2). Systolic pressure falls with increasing birth weight and rises with body mass index. The highest mean pressures (174 mm Hg) were in men in the lowest third of birth weight and the highest third of body mass index; the lowest pressures (158 mm Hg) were in men in the highest third of birth weight and the lowest third of body mass index.

Birth weight is a summary measure of fetal growth which includes head size, length, and fatness. We now know that it greatly underestimates the relation between fetal growth and blood pressure. To explore the association between measurements at birth and adult blood pressure we examined 449 men and women aged around 50 years who were born in one hospital in Preston (chapter 16). At that hospital, Sharoe Green, unusually detailed observations were made at birth. Table VII shows the mean

TABLE VI—*Mean systolic blood pressure (mm Hg) in men aged 64, according to current body mass index and birth weight. Numbers of men in parentheses*

Body mass index (kg/m^2)	Birth weight (lb)			
	−7·25	−8·25	8·25 +	All
<25·2	162	159	158	159 (192)
25·2–27·9	167	169	161	166 (201)
>27·9	174	165	166	168 (204)
All	168 (177)	164 (203)	162 (217)	164 (597)

TABLE VII—*Mean systolic blood pressures (mm Hg) of men and women aged 46 to 54, according to birth weight and placental weight. Numbers of people in parentheses*

Birth weight (lb)	Placental weight (lb)				
	−1·0	−1·25	−1·5	>1·5	All
−5·5	152 (26)	154 (13)	153 (5)	206 (1)	154 (45)
−6·5	147 (16)	151 (54)	150 (28)	166 (8)	151 (106)
−7·5	144 (20)	148 (77)	145 (45)	160 (27)	149 (169)
>7·5	133 (6)	148 (27)	147 (42)	154 (54)	149 (129)
All	147 (68)	149 (171)	147 (120)	157 (90)	150 (449)

systolic pressures according to birth weight and placental weight. There are opposing trends, such that systolic pressure falls by around 10 mm Hg with increasing birth weight and rises by around 12 mm Hg with increasing placental weight. Adjustment for gestation did not affect these trends.

An important aspect of the findings is that most people with high systolic pressure were not unusually small at birth. Rather, their birth weights were within the normal range but did not match the weight of the placenta. A feature of babies born with the heaviest placentas, weighing more than 1·5 lb, among whom adult blood pressures were highest, was that they were disproportionate at birth, being relatively short in relation to their head circumference. This suggests that one process linking fetal growth with adult blood pressure may be diversion of fetal cardiac output away from the trunk to favour the brain.

Large placental weight is associated with clinical hypertension in later life as well as higher mean blood pressure. Among the 449 men and women the risk of needing treatment for hypertension was 3·7 times greater among those with placentas weighing more than 1·5 lb than among those whose placentas weighed 1·0 lb or less. The causes of large placental size are largely unknown. In Preston, however, only 4/56 (7%) babies born at term to mothers in social classes I and II had placentas heavier than 1·5 lb. This compared with 62/254 (24%) for mothers in the lower social classes. We suggest that the influence that links low social class with large placental weight is poor nutrition. A recent study of 8684 births in Oxford has shown that iron deficiency anaemia is associated with heavier placental weight (chapter 27).

Conclusion

Retarded fetal and infant growth are strongly related to death from obstructive lung disease and cardiovascular disease and to risk factors for these diseases. These long term associations of retarded growth may reflect restraint of tissue growth by an adverse environment during a critical, sometimes brief, period of fetal or infant development. Which tissues are affected depends on the nature of the adverse influence and its timing. The phenomenon of "programming" has been shown on a range of structures and functions in experimental animals.[6-8] It probably occurs widely in human development and has an important effect on the development of degenerative disease. Long term human studies now in progress will extend our knowledge of its occurrence and may give insight into the timing of critical periods.

The relation of early growth with risk factors and disease rates is continuous. FEV_1 rises progressively up to the highest values of birth weight (table II) while systolic blood pressure falls (table V). It follows, therefore, that though an average birth weight is usual it may not be optimum. If the criterion of successful fetal growth is adult health and longevity, assessment of the newborn must at the least include placental weight and the proportions of the baby.

The effects of programming interact with influences in the adult environment, including cigarette smoking and body weight (table VI). The existence of programming does not imply that adult influences should be discounted—though in the past we have probably overestimated their importance.

Our findings are open to the interpretation that genetic influences that are immediately manifest as growth failure in early life show themselves in adult life through the occurrence of degenerative disease. However, studies of the birth weights of the firstborn children of mothers and daughters suggest that genetic factors play only a small part in determining birth weight.[9] Experiments in which newborn mice were randomly assigned to foster mothers show that individual variations in growth rates after weaning are more related to the nutritional status of the foster mother than to the origins of the offspring.[8]

We favour an environmental explanation of our findings and suspect that maternal nutrition is important. Research is needed into the maternal influences that regulate fetal and infant growth. We need to know why the children of women living in rural southern England in the early years of this century have had such low death rates from cardiovascular and obstructive lung disease. We can reasonably suspect that the seeds of ill health in the next century are being sown today wherever girls and mothers have nutritional deficiencies whose nature we do not yet know.

1 Forsdahl A. Are poor living conditions in childhood and adolescence an important risk factor for arteriosclerotic heart disease? *British Journal of Preventive Social Medicine* 1977;**31**:91–5.

2 Winick M, Noble A. Cellular response in rats during malnutrition at various ages. *J Nutr* 1966;**89**:300–6.

3 Colley JRT, Douglas JWB, Reid DD. Respiratory disease in young adults: influence of early childhood lower respiratory tract illness, social class, air pollution, and smoking. *BMJ* 1973;iii:195–8.

4 Meade TW, North WRS. Population-based distributions of haemostatic variables. *Br Med Bull* 1977;**33**:283–8.

5 Meade TW, Mellows S, Brozovic M, *et al.* Haemostatic function and ischaemic heart disease: principal results of the Northwick Park heart study. *Lancet* 1986;ii:533–7.

6 Mott GE, Lewis DS, McGill HC. Programming of cholesterol metabolism by breast or formula feeding. In: *The childhood environment and adult disease*. Chichester: Wiley, 1991. (Ciba Symposium 156).

7 Kahn AJ. Embryogenic effect on post-natal changes in haemoglobin with time. *Growth* 1968;**32**:13–22.

8 Dubos R, Savage D, Schaedler R. Biological Freudianism: lasting effects of early environmental influences *Pediatrics* 1966;**38**:789–800.

9 Carr-Hill R, Campbell DM, Hall MH, Meredith A. Is birthweight determined genetically? *BMJ* 1987;**295**:687–9.

PART VIII
GLUCOSE TOLERANCE

22: Fetal and infant growth and impaired glucose tolerance at age 64

C N HALES, D J P BARKER, P M S CLARK, L J COX, C FALL, C OSMOND, P D WINTER

Men born in east Hertfordshire during 1920–30 were followed up to ascertain whether reduced fetal and infant growth is associated with non-insulin dependent diabetes and impaired glucose tolerance in adult life.

Four hundred and sixty eight of the men who still lived in Hertfordshire had fasting blood samples taken; 370 had glucose tolerance tests. Ninety three of the 370 men had impaired glucose tolerance or hitherto undiagnosed diabetes. They had had a lower mean birth weight and a lower weight at 1 year. The proportion of men with impaired glucose tolerance fell progressively from 26% (6/23) among those who had weighed 18 lb (8·16 kg) or less at 1 year to 13% (3/24) among those who had weighed 27 lb (12·25 kg) or more. Corresponding figures for diabetes were 17% (4/23) and nil (0/24). Plasma glucose concentrations at 30 and 120 minutes fell with increasing birth weight and weight at 1 year. Plasma 32–33 split proinsulin concentration fell with increasing weight at 1 year. All these trends were significant and independent of current body mass. Blood pressure was inversely related to birth weight and strongly related to plasma glucose and 32–33 split proinsulin concentrations.

It was concluded that reduced growth in early life is strongly linked with impaired glucose tolerance and non-insulin dependent diabetes. Reduced early growth is also related to a raised plasma concentration of 32–33 split proinsulin, which is interpreted as a sign of β cell dysfunction. Reduced intrauterine growth is linked with high blood pressure, which may explain the association between hypertension and impaired glucose tolerance.

Introduction

Recent findings suggest that retardation of growth during fetal life and infancy is associated with increased death rates from cardiovascular disease in adult life (chapter 13). They pose the question of what processes link retarded early growth with cardiovascular disease. Blood pressure may be one such link. In a study of men and women aged 50 higher blood pressure was strongly related to lower birth weight and higher placental weight (chapter 16). Impaired glucose tolerance may be another link as it is a known risk factor for ischaemic heart disease,[1] and non-insulin dependent diabetes is associated with hypertension.[2] We therefore examined a sample of the men born in Hertfordshire and measured their glucose tolerance.

There is controversy about the relative importance of insulin deficiency due to pancreatic β cell dysfunction and insulin resistance in the genesis of impaired glucose tolerance and non-insulin dependent diabetes. Recent advances in assay methodology make it possible to measure specifically plasma concentrations of insulin and its precursors, intact and 32–33 split proinsulin.[3] People with non-insulin dependent diabetes have raised plasma concentrations of these precursors, which has been interpreted as evidence of β cell dysfunction.[4] We therefore measured insulin and its precursors in the Hertfordshire men to discover whether retarded early growth is linked to β cell dysfunction.

Subjects and methods

As described in chapter 14, we traced 1157 singleton boys who had been born in east Hertfordshire during 1920–30 and still lived there; 845 of the men agreed to be interviewed at home. After the interview each was asked if he would be willing to attend a local clinic one morning after an overnight fast to have a standard 75 g oral glucose tolerance test. Men known to have diabetes were excluded. A total of 468 men agreed to attend the clinic and have a fasting blood sample taken; 408 had a full glucose tolerance test. Measurements on the blood samples included plasma glucose and insulin concentrations at zero, 30, and 120 minutes and proinsulin and 32–33 split proinsulin concentrations at zero time only. Ethical approval was obtained from the east Hertfordshire ethics committee.

Plasma glucose was measured by a hexokinase method.[5] Plasma insulin, proinsulin, and 32–33 split proinsulin concentrations were determined by two site immunometric assays with either iodine-125 or alkaline phosphatase as labels.[36] The insulin assay was standardised against the first international reference preparation coded 66/304 and the intact and split proinsulin assays against standards obtained from Lilly Research Laboratories (Indianapolis, USA).

Because plasma measurements of glucose, insulin, proinsulin, and 32–33 split proinsulin have skewed distributions we transformed them to normality in the analysis by using logarithms. Values below the lower limit of detection were assigned the value of the lower limit. We analysed the data using linear regression, two sample t tests, and logistic regression for calculating odds ratios.

Results

The 468 men who attended the clinic fasting were aged 59–70 (mean 64) years. Of the 408 who had a glucose tolerance test, 370 had complete measurements on all blood samples. Our analysis is based on the 468 fasting blood samples and the 370 samples from complete glucose tolerance tests. Of the 370 men who had complete measurements on all samples, 66 had impaired tolerance, defined as a two hour plasma glucose concentration of 7·8–11·0 mmol/l, and 27 had diabetes, defined as a two hour plasma glucose concentration of 11·1 mmol/l or over. Compared with the 277 other subjects these men had been on average 0·5 lb (227 g) lighter at birth and 1·0 lb (450 g) lighter at 1 year (table I). They were currently heavier and had higher body mass indices (weight (kg)/height (m)²) and waist to hip ratios. They had higher systolic and diastolic blood pressures. Their fasting glucose concentrations were 1·0 mmol/l higher (6·8 mmol/l compared with 5·8 mmol/l).

Men with impaired glucose tolerance or diabetes had higher mean insulin concentrations two hours after oral glucose (284 pmol/l compared with 124 pmol/l). They had higher mean fasting proinsulin concentrations (4·06 pmol/l compared with 2·66 pmol/l) and higher 32–33 split proinsulin concentrations (4·67 pmol/l compared with 2·72 pmol/l). All these differences were significant at the 5% level.

Tables II and III show that the proportions of men with impaired glucose tolerance or diabetes fell progressively with increasing birth weight and weight at 1 year.

Tables IV and V show the trends with birth weight and weight at 1 year in glucose, insulin, and proinsulin concentrations and blood pressure. Each of these measurements varied with body mass index, which tended to increase with birth weight and weight at 1 year, though the trends were weak. We therefore allowed for body mass index when calculating the significance of trends with early weight. Plasma glucose concentration at

243

TABLE I—*Mean weight, height, body mass index, waist to hip ratio, and systolic and diastolic blood pressures in men with and without impaired glucose tolerance or newly diagnosed diabetes as defined by plasma glucose concentrations two hours after 75 g oral load*

		Two hour glucose concentration (mmol/l)			
		<7·8 (n=277)	≥7·8 (n=93)	Difference (95% confidence interval)	p Value
Birth weight* { lb		8·0	7·5	−0·5 (−0·8 to −0·2) }	0·004
{ g		3621	3411	−210 (−351 to −69) }	
Weight at 1 year* { lb		22·8	21·8	−1·0 (−1·6 to −0·3) }	0·002
{ kg		10·3	9·9	−0·4 (−0·7 to −0·2) }	
Height (m)		1·72	1·71	−0·01 (−0·02 to 0·01)	0·21
Weight (kg)		78·5	81·7	3·2 (0·4 to 5·9)	0·02
Body mass index (kg/m²)		26·6	27·9	1·4 (0·6 to 2·2)	0·001
Waist to hip ratio		0·93	0·95	0·02 (0·01 to 0·03)	0·001
Systolic blood pressure (mm Hg)		163	174	11 (6 to 17)	<0·001
Diastolic blood pressure (mm Hg)		89	92	3 (0 to 6)	0·02

* Original measurements were expressed in pounds (lb) and were rounded.

two hours fell with increasing birth weight and weight at 1 year (tables IV and V). Plasma glucose concentration at 30 minutes showed similar trends. Fasting plasma glucose values showed no trends. Table VI shows the plasma glucose concentrations at two hours with the men divided into approximate thirds according to weight at 1 year and adult body mass

TABLE II—*Proportions of men aged 64 with impaired glucose tolerance or diabetes, according to birth weight*

Birth weight*		No of men	No (%) of men with two hour glucose (mmol/l) of:			Odds ratio (95% confidence interval)†
lb	g		7·8–11·0	≥11·1	≥7·8	
≤5·5	≤2495	20	6 (30)	2 (10)	8 (40)	6·6 (1·5 to 28)
−6·5	−2948	47	10 (21)	6 (13)	16 (34)	4·8 (1·3 to 17)
−7·5	−3402	104	26 (25)	6 (6)	32 (31)	4·6 (1·4 to 16)
−8·5	−3856	117	18 (15)	8 (7)	26 (22)	2·6 (0·8 to 8·9)
−9·5	−4309	54	2 (4)	5 (9)	7 (13)	1·4 (0·3 to 5·6)
>9·5	>4309	28	4 (14)	0	4 (14)	1·0 —
Total		370	66 (18)	27 (7)	93 (25)	

* Original measurements were expressed in lb and were rounded.
† Odds ratio for two hour glucose concentration of ≥7·8 mmol/l adjusted for body mass index (χ^2 for trend = 15·4; p < 0·001).

TABLE III—*Proportions of men aged 64 with impaired glucose tolerance or diabetes, according to weight at 1 year*

Weight at 1 year*		No of men	No (%) of men with two hour glucose (mmol/l) of:			Odds ratio (95% confidence interval)†
lb	kg		7·8–11·0	≥11·1	≥7·8	
≤18	≤8·16	23	6 (26)	4 (17)	10 (43)	8·2 (1·8 to 38)
−20	−9·07	63	13 (21)	7 (11)	20 (32)	4·8 (1·2 to 19)
−22	−9·98	107	24 (22)	8 (7)	32 (30)	4·2 (1·1 to 16)
−24	−10·89	105	14 (13)	5 (5)	19 (18)	2·1 (0·5 to 7·9)
−26	−11·79	48	6 (13)	3 (6)	9 (19)	2·1 (0·5 to 9·0)
≥27	≥12·25	24	3 (13)	0	3 (13)	1·0 —
Total		370	66 (18)	27 (7)	93 (25)	

* Original measurements were expressed in lb and were rounded.
† Odds ratio for two hour glucose of ≥7·8 mmol/l adjusted for body mass index (χ^2 for trend = 14·9; $p < 0.001$).

index. The values rose from 5·8 mmol/l in men with the highest weights at 1 year and lowest body mass indices to 7·7 mmol/l in men with the lowest weights at 1 year and highest body mass indices.

Similarly to plasma glucose, plasma insulin concentrations at two hours fell with increasing birth weight and weight at 1 year (tables IV and V). Thirty minute and fasting plasma insulin values showed no trends with early weights.

Plasma proinsulin concentrations showed no trend with either birth weight or weight at 1 year. Plasma 32–33 split proinsulin concentrations fell slightly with increasing birth weight but showed a strong downward trend with increasing weight at 1 year (tables IV and V). Table VII shows the plasma 32–33 split proinsulin concentrations with the men divided into approximate thirds according to weight at 1 year and adult body mass index. The values rose from 2·1 pmol/l in men with the highest weights at 1 year and lowest body mass indices to 4·8 pmol/l in men with the lowest weights at 1 year and highest body mass indices.

Systolic blood pressure fell with increasing birth weight and weight at 1 year (tables IV and V). The trend with weight at 1 year was abolished by adjustment for birth weight. Systolic pressure rose with increasing plasma glucose concentration at two hours ($p = 0.02$) independently of body mass index. The trend with plasma glucose concentration at 30 minutes was stronger ($p = 0.0006$). Systolic pressure also rose with increasing plasma 32–33 split proinsulin concentration ($p = 0.005$), again independently of body mass index. Diastolic pressure varied with plasma glucose and proinsulin concentrations in the same way as systolic pressure, but the trends were weaker.

TABLE IV—Mean body mass index; geometric mean plasma glucose, insulin, and proinsulin concentrations; and mean systolic blood pressure, according to birth weight

	Birth weight in lb (g)*							Trend test†
	≤5·5 (≤2495)	-6·5 (-2948)	-7·5 (-3402)	-8·5 (-3856)	-9·5 (-4309)	>9·5 (>4309)	All	
Fasting blood samples:								
No of men	21	61	144	141	68	33	468	
Body mass index (kg/m²)	26·7	26·8	26·4	26·9	26·8	29·1	26·9	0·17
Glucose (mmol/l)	6·2	6·0	6·1	6·1	6·0	5·8	6·1	0·15
Insulin (pmol/l)	45	44	41	41	40	46	42	0·24
Proinsulin (pmol/l)	3·5	2·8	3·0	3·0	2·9	2·9	3·0	0·06
32-33 Split proinsulin (pmol/l)	3·6	3·4	3·0	3·1	3·0	3·1	3·1	0·001
Systolic blood pressure (mm Hg)	173	165	166	164	161	161	164	0·001
Glucose tolerance tests:								
No of men	20	47	104	117	54	28	370	
Glucose (mmol/l) { 30 min	10·1	9·9	9·7	9·3	9·2	8·9	9·5	0·001
{ 2 hours	7·5	6·9	6·8	6·5	6·3	5·9	6·6	0·002
Insulin (pmol/l) { 30 min	315	293	254	282	248	296	273	0·22
{ 2 hours	224	192	161	139	124	143	153	0·0005

* Original measurements were expressed in lb and were rounded.
† p Value adjusted for body mass index.

TABLE V—Mean body mass index; geometric mean plasma glucose, insulin, and proinsulin concentrations; and mean systolic blood pressure, according to weight at 1 year

	Weight at 1 year in lb (kg)*							Trend test†
	≤18 (≤8·16)	−20 (−9·07)	−22 (−9·98)	−24 (−10·89)	−26 (−11·79)	≥27 (≥12·25)	All	
Fasting blood samples:								
No of men	28	75	143	132	63	27	468	
Body mass index (kg/m²)	26·2	26·4	26·9	26·9	26·9	28·3	26·9	0·2
Glucose (mmol/l)	6·0	6·1	6·1	6·1	6·0	5·8	6·1	0·11
Insulin (pmol/l)	34	49	43	38	42	43	42	0·11
Proinsulin (pmol/l)	3·1	2·9	3·1	2·8	3·3	2·7	3·0	0·008
32-33 Split proinsulin (pmol/l)	3·4	3·3	3·2	2·8	3·4	2·5	3·1	0·007
Systolic blood pressure (mm Hg)	168	169	165	162	162	161	164	
Glucose tolerance tests:								
No of men	23	63	107	105	48	24	370	
Glucose (mmol/l) { 30 min	9·7	9·7	9·8	9·4	9·0	8·7	9·5	0·004
Glucose (mmol/l) { 2 hours	7·9	7·0	6·7	6·5	6·3	6·0	6·6	0·0006
Insulin (pmol/l) { 30 min	220	286	290	279	253	238	273	0·16
Insulin (pmol/l) { 2 hours	153	201	156	138	129	144	153	0·002

* Original measurements were expressed in lb and were rounded.
† p Value adjusted for body mass index.

TABLE VI—*Geometric mean plasma glucose concentration (mmol/l) two hours after 75 g oral glucose load, according to weight at 1 year and adult body mass index. (Numbers of men given in square brackets)*

Adult body mass index (kg/m²)	Weight at 1 year in lb (kg)*			
	≤21·5 (≤9·75)	−23·5 (−10·66)	>23·5 (>10·66)	Total
≤25·4	6·6 [45]	6·1 [39]	5·8 [36]	6·2 [120]
−28	6·7 [47]	6·9 [44]	5·9 [36]	6·5 [127]
>28	7·7 [39]	7·4 [43]	6·6 [41]	7·2 [123]
Total	7·0 [131]	6·8 [126]	6·1 [113]	6·6 [370]

* Original measurements were expressed in lb and were rounded.
Geometric standard deviation of plasma glucose = 1·4.

TABLE VII—*Geometric mean plasma 32–33 split proinsulin concentration (pmol/l) according to weight at 1 year and adult body mass index. (Numbers of men given in square brackets)*

Adult body mass index (kg/m²)	Weight at 1 year in lb (kg)*			
	≤21·5 (≤9·75)	−23·5 (−10·66)	>23·5 (>10·66)	Total
≤25·4	2·5 [57]	2·2 [56]	2·1 [49]	2·2 [162]
−28	3·2 [57]	3·6 [49]	3·1 [41]	3·3 [147]
>28	4·8 [48]	3·8 [59]	3·9 [52]	4·1 [159]
Total	3·3 [162]	3·1 [164]	2·9 [142]	3·1 [468]

* Original measurements were expressed in lb and were rounded.
Geometric standard deviation of plasma 32–33 split proinsulin = 2·1.

The men's social class either at birth or currently was not related to plasma glucose, insulin, or proinsulin concentration. Adjustment for social class did not change the associations with birth weight and weight at 1 year.

Discussion

In this study of men aged 59–70, 18% (66/370) were found to have impaired glucose tolerance and 7% (27/370) were newly discovered diabetics. These figures are consistent with other surveys.[7] Our study shows that adults with impaired glucose tolerance and non-insulin dependent diabetes have lower weight gain prenatally and during infancy. The proportion of men with impaired glucose tolerance and diabetes fell progressively up to the highest values of birth weight and weight at 1 year (tables II and III). There were threefold differences in the prevalence of impaired tolerance and diabetes between men with the lowest and highest early weights. These trends paralleled the fall in death rates from ischaemic heart disease with increasing birth weight and weight at 1 year described in chapter 13. They suggest that impaired glucose tolerance and ischaemic heart disease may both be determined by influences which reduce fetal and infant growth.

Tables VI and VII illustrate how fetal and infant growth protect against the deleterious effect of higher body mass in adult life and, conversely, how lower body mass protects against the deleterious effect of reduced early growth. Twenty six per cent of men (14/53) whose birth weights and weights at 1 year were below the median and whose body mass indices were above the median had impaired glucose tolerance. Only 5% of the men (3/64) who were above the median for early weights and below the median for body mass index had impaired tolerance. The corresponding figures for diabetes were 15% and 2% (8/53 and 1/64). The study sample comprised 40% of men who were born in east Hertfordshire and still living there. As our analysis was based on internal comparisons, the selection of the sample would introduce bias only if the relations between early growth and plasma glucose, insulin, and proinsulin concentrations were different in those selected and not selected. This is unlikely. The same relations were found in each social class and each body mass group (tables VI and VII).

The correlation of birth weight and weight at 1 year with glucose intolerance might result from a single influence acting prenatally which reduces fetal growth and continues to affect infant growth. The mechanisms which link low fetal and infant growth rates with adult glucose intolerance are still a matter for speculation. We know, however, that much of the development of the islets of Langerhans occurs in utero.[8] The exact timing of islet formation differs among species. In rats the numbers of islets increase rapidly in the last four to six days of intrauterine life. In humans β cell mass increases more than 130-fold between the 12th intrauterine week and the fifth postnatal month.

Overnutrition during intrauterine life is known to influence β cell development, in that diabetes during pregnancy—which has been likened to overnutrition—leads to β cell hyperplasia in the fetus.[9] There are few studies of the effects on β cell development of undernutrition during early life. In rats weaned on to a low protein diet for only three weeks the insulin response to glucose was permanently impaired. This led to the suggestion "that early malnutrition may predispose to diabetes."[10] Infants who are small for dates have fewer β cells.[11] There are conflicting reports on whether the β cell mass is reduced in patients with non-insulin dependent diabetes.[8] In one study, however, in which diabetic patients were compared with people of the same weight, their β cell mass was found to be lower.[12]

249

A WORKING HYPOTHESIS

As a working hypothesis it seems reasonable to propose that nutritional and other factors determining fetal and infant growth influence the size and function of the adult pancreatic β cell complement. Plasma concentrations of 32–33 split proinsulin were higher in men with lower weight at 1 year (table V). A raised plasma 32–33 split proinsulin concentration may indicate production of insulin by a comparatively small complement of β cells. Whether and when non-insulin dependent diabetes supervenes will be determined by the rate of attrition of β cells with aging and by the development of insulin resistance, of which the most important known determinant is obesity. An alternative explanation of the raised 32–33 split proinsulin concentration is that it reflects increased insulin production secondary to insulin resistance. Futher experiments are planned to invest-igate these possibilities or indeed whether processes leading to poor fetal and infant growth might lead to a combination of insulin deficiency and resistance.

An attractive feature of this explanation is that it provides an alternative to the "thrifty genotype" hypothesis.[13] This hypothesis suggests that the high incidence of diabetes in Western or recently affluent societies results from the existence of diabetogenic genes which confer a survival advantage in conditions of subsistence living. We suggest that diabetes is a conse-quence of poor nutrition during critical periods of fetal life and infancy with consequent impaired development of β cell function. If poor nutrition continues the reduced ability to produce insulin is not a disadvantage. It becomes so only if nutrition becomes abundant, when increased demand for insulin outstrips the capacity for production. Ethiopian Jews who migrated to Israel experienced a change from poor to abundant nutrition and had a subsequent high incidence of diabetes.[14] The long term effects of poor nutrition during early life may depend on the nature, timing, and intensity of deprivation, which will determine the specific tissues in which development is impaired. This phenomenon may underlie several Western diseases other than diabetes, most importantly ischaemic heart disease (chapter 13).

Consistent with other studies,[15] we have found that plasma glucose concentrations are strongly related to blood pressure levels independently of body mass index. Blood pressure was inversely related to birth weight, as has also been found before (chapter 16). The association between blood pressure and 32–33 split proinsulin concentrations indicates that similar influences may impair vascular and pancreatic islet cell development in utero. The association of hypertension, non-insulin dependent diabetes, and hyperlipidaemia has been called syndrome X.[16] Insulin resistance has been proposed as the link between these abnormalities. Our study, how-ever, raises the possibility that retarded intrauterine growth may be the link.

Our findings are open to the interpretation that a genetically determined deficiency of insulin production is manifested by growth failure in early life long before the onset of adult glucose intolerance. The high concordance of non-insulin dependent diabetes in monozygotic twins is often cited as strong evidence that the disorder is genetically controlled.[17] Because maternal physique and nutrition have such a strong influence on fetal and infant growth we favour an environmental explanation of our findings. This would necessarily put in question the genetic interpretation of concordance in monozygotic twins. The strong associations which we report suggest that research directed towards the causes of non-insulin dependent diabetes should examine the development of the pancreas in fetal life and infancy and the nutritional and other influences which regulate it.

We are grateful to all the men who gave us their time; to Hertfordshire County Archives, which preserved the records, and to Dr I Clarke for much local help. B Alpha, M Brown, N J Crowther, A E Schneider-Darlinson, and D Wong gave technical assistance. We thank staff of the NHS section of the department of clinical biochemistry, Addenbrooke's Hospital, for glucose analyses, and B Newland, of Princess Alexandra Hospital, Harlow, for storing specimens.

1 Fuller JH, Shipley MJ, Rose G, Jarrett RJ, Keen H. Coronary heart disease risk and impaired glucose tolerance. *Lancet* 1980;i:1373–6.
2 Modan M, Halkin H, Almog S, Lusky A, Eshkol A, Shefi M, *et al.* Hyperinsulinemia: a link between hypertension, obesity and glucose intolerance. *J Clin Invest* 1985;75:809–17.
3 Sobey WJ, Beer SF, Carrington CA, Clark PMS, Frank BH, Gray IP, *et al.* Sensitive and specific two-site immunoradiometric assays for human insulin, proinsulin, 65–66 split and 32–33 split proinsulins. *Biochem J* 1989;260:535–41.
4 Temple RC, Carrington CA, Luzio SD, Owens DR, Schneider AE, Sobey WJ, *et al.* Insulin deficiency in non-insulin dependent diabetes. *Lancet* 1989;i:293–5.
5 Kunst A, Draeger B, Ziegenhorn J. UV-methods with hexokinase and glucose-6-phosphate dehydrogenase. In: Bergmeyer HU, ed. *Methods of enzymatic analysis*. Vol VI. Weinheim: Verlag Chemie Deerfield FL, 1983:163–72.
6 Johannsson A, Stanley CJ, Self CH. A fast highly sensitive colorimetric enzyme immunoassay system demonstrating benefits of enzyme amplifications in clinical chemistry. *Clin Chim Acta* 1985;148:119–24.
7 Harris MI, Hadden WC, Knowler WC, Bennett PH. Prevalence of diabetes and impaired glucose tolerance and plasma glucose levels in US population aged 20–74 years. *Diabetes* 1987;36:523–34.
8 Hellerström C, Swenne I, Andersson A. Islet cell replication and diabetes. In: Lefebvre PJ, Pipeleers DG, eds. *The pathology of the endocrine pancreas in diabetes*. Heidelberg: Springer Verlag, 1988:141–70.
9 Freinkel N. Of pregnancy and progeny. *Diabetes* 1980;29:1023–39.
10 Swenne I, Crace CJ, Milner RDG. Persistent impairment of insulin secretory response to glucose in adult rats after limited period of protein–calorie malnutrition early in life. *Diabetes* 1987;36:454–8.
11 Van Assche FA, Aerts L. The fetal endocrine pancreas. *Contrib Gynecol Obstet* 1979; 5:44–57.
12 Klöppel G, Löhr M, Habich K, Oberholzer M, Heitz PU. Islet pathology and pathogenesis of type 1 and type 2 diabetes revisited. *Survey and Synthesis of Pathology Research* 1985;4:110–25.

13 Thrifty genotype rendered detrimental by progress? [Editorial]. *Lancet* 1989;ii:839–40.
14 Cohen MP, Stern E, Rusecki Y, Zeidler A. High prevalence of diabetes in young adult Ethiopian immigrants to Israel. *Diabetes* 1988;**37**:824–8.
15 Stamler J, Rhomberg P, Schoenberger JA, Shekelle RB, Dyer A, Shekelle S, *et al.* Multivariate analysis of the relationship of seven variables to blood pressure: findings of the Chicago Heart Association detection project in industry, 1967–1972. *J Chronic Dis* 1975;**28**:527–48.
16 Reaven GM. Role of insulin resistance in human disease. *Diabetes* 1988;**37**:1595–607.
17 Newman B, Selby JV, King M-C, Slemenda C, Fabsitz R, Friedman GD. Concordance for type 2 (non-insulin-dependent) diabetes mellitus in male twins. *Diabetologia* 1987;**30**:763–8.

23: Relation of fetal growth to plasma glucose concentrations in young men

S M ROBINSON, R J WALTON, P M S CLARK,
D J P BARKER, C N HALES, C OSMOND

In a study of men aged 59 to 70 plasma glucose concentrations 30 and 120 minutes after a 75 g glucose drink were inversely related to birth weight. To assess whether there are similar relations at a younger age, the 30 minute plasma glucose concentrations of 40 men aged 18 to 25, who had been born in one hospital in the United Kingdom, were measured. Lower birth weight was associated with higher 30 minute plasma glucose concentrations. This trend was independent of gestational age and current body mass, height, and social class.

Introduction

Retarded growth during fetal life and infancy is associated with increased death rates from cardiovascular disease in adult life (chapter 13). This long term association of retarded early growth is thought to result from programming, by which adverse influences at critical periods of fetal or infant development irrecoverably constrain the growth of organs and tissues and permanently change their metabolism or structure, or both (chapter 21). The phenomenon of "programming" has been shown in brain development and in a range of structures and functions in experimental animals.

There is evidence that non-insulin dependent (type II) diabetes mellitus, which is associated with ischaemic heart disease, is programmed in fetal life and infancy. A study of 370 Hertfordshire men aged 59 to 70 showed that plasma glucose concentrations 30 and 120 minutes after a 75 g glucose drink were inversely related to birth weight and to weight at 1 year (chapter 22).

It could be argued that lower birth and infant weights merely indicate an adverse early environment, and that people born into an adverse environment tend to remain in one. Associations with early growth could therefore reflect influences acting later in life, though the associations described in chapter 22 are strong and graded, which makes this unlikely. It is also possible that the associations depend on influences which affected fetal growth in the past but are no longer present in the environment today. We have therefore studied glucose tolerance in a group of young men aged 18 to 25.

Subjects and methods

Sixty seven men aged 18–25, who were on the general practice list of one of the authors (RJW) and had been born in Southampton Hospital maternity unit, were asked to take part in the study; 42 (63%) agreed to do so. Obstetric data were obtained from their mothers' antenatal and delivery records. These data included birth weight, placental weight, and head circumference. Gestational age derived from the date of the mother's last menstrual period had been recorded for each of the men except two. The final sample size represented all men in the age range who were on the practice list and who had complete obstetric records.

All 42 men were seen at the health centre having fasted overnight. Using a structured questionnaire we asked them about their medical history, smoking habits, and alcohol intake. Their waist and hip circumferences were measured. We measured height using a portable stadiometer and weight with a portable Seca scale. Blood pressure was measured with an automated recorder (Dinamap; Critikon, Tampa, USA) while the subject was sitting down. Readings were taken on the left arm using the cuff size recommended for the arm circumference. Two readings were taken and the average used in the analysis.

The men were given a standard 75 g glucose drink. A blood sample was taken after 30 minutes and tested for glucose, insulin, and proinsulin concentrations. Plasma glucose concentration was measured by a hexokinase method. Plasma insulin and proinsulin concentrations were measured using two site immunoradiometric assays.[1] The insulin assay was standardised against the first international reference preparation coded 66/304 and the proinsulin assay against a standard obtained from Lilly Research Laboratories (Indianapolis, USA).

Ethical permission for the study was given by the Southampton ethics committee.

STATISTICAL ANALYSIS

Statistical analysis was by multiple linear regression and tabulation of means. Because the plasma measurements of insulin and proinsulin have skewed distributions we transformed them in the analysis by using logarithms. Social class was defined according to father's occupation.[2] The social class of three fathers was unknown.

Results

The age of the 42 men ranged from 18 to 25 with a mean (SD) of 21·1 (2·0) years. Their mean (SD) birth weight was 3413 (373) g. The mean (SD) age of the 25 men who declined to take part in the study was 21·2 (2·0) years. Their mean (SD) birth weight was 3282 (372) g. The 42 men taking part had a mean plasma glucose concentration at 30 minutes of 8·2 mmol/l. Two men had values of 11·2 and 11·5 mmol/l, which exceed the level defining diabetes.[3] Those two men, who are likely to have insulin dependent (type I) rather than non-insulin dependent (type II) diabetes, were excluded from the analyses. Their birth weights were 3402 g and 3983 g.

The table shows the 40 men divided into three groups according to birth weights. Thirty minute plasma glucose concentrations were highest in those with the lowest, and lowest in those with the highest, birth weights. The inverse association between birth weight and plasma glucose concentration was such that an increase of 1000 g in birth weight corresponded to a decrease of 1·5 mmol/l in 30 minute glucose (95% confidence interval 0·4 to 2·6, p = 0·01). The trend was independent of gestational age. Thirty minute plasma glucose concentration was not related to head circumference at birth or placental weight, or to current body mass index (weight (kg)/ height (m)^2), waist to hip ratio, height, alcohol intake, or smoking.

Neither 30 minute plasma insulin nor proinsulin concentrations were related to birth weight, head circumference, or placental weight. Both 30 minute plasma insulin and proinsulin concentrations were related to 30

Mean plasma glucose, insulin, and proinsulin concentrations, body mass index, and systolic blood pressure according to birth weight

Birth weight (g)	n	Plasma glucose (mmol/l)	Plasma insulin* (pmol/l)	Plasma proinsulin* (pmol/l)	Body mass index (kg/m^2)	Systolic blood pressure (mm Hg)
− 3204	14	8·8	244	4·3	22·5	145
− 3572	13	8·2	314	5·3	24·6	149
> 3572	13	7·3	241	4·7	23·3	144
All	40	8·1	264	4·7	23·4	146
Standard deviation		1·4	1·7	1·8	2·6	14

* Geometric means and standard deviations.

minute plasma glucose concentration. An increase of 1 mmol/l in 30 minute glucose concentration was associated with an increase of 0·19 (95% confidence interval 0·10 to 0·29, p = 0·0004) in log 30 minute insulin and an increase of 0·17 (95% confidence interval 0·05 to 0·30, p = 0·01) in log 30 minute proinsulin concentrations. They were also weakly related to body mass index. The corresponding figures resulting from a 1 kg/m^2 increase in body mass index were an increase of 0·06 (95% confidence interval 0·00 to 0·12; p = 0·05) in log 30 minute insulin and an increase of 0·06 (− 0·01 to 0·13; p = 0·09) in log 30 minute proinsulin concentrations. In a multiple regression with plasma glucose and body mass index both plasma insulin and proinsulin levels rose with birth weight. An increase of 1000 g in birth weight corresponded to an increase of 0·36 (95% confidence interval 0·00 to 0·72, p = 0·05) in log 30 minute insulin and an increase of 0·46 (95% confidence interval − 0·02 to 0·94, p = 0·07) in log proinsulin concentrations. These trends were independent of gestational age.

Systolic blood pressure increased with body mass index. An increase in body mass index of 1 kg/m^2 was associated with an increase of 2·6 mm Hg (95% confidence interval 1·2 to 4·0, p = 0·001). After allowing for body mass index, systolic blood pressure increased with plasma glucose concentration. An increase of 1 mmol/l in 30 minute plasma glucose was associated with a 2·9 mm Hg increase in systolic blood pressure (95% confidence interval 0·4 to 5·4, p = 0·03). There was no association of systolic blood pressure with birth weight, placental weight, head circumference, or plasma insulin or proinsulin concentrations.

Mean plasma glucose concentrations according to subject's social class at birth were 8·0 mmol/l in classes I, II, and III non-manual (n = 8), 8·0 mmol/l in social class III manual (n = 22), and 8·4 mmol/l in classes IV and V (n = 7). The corresponding mean (SD) birth weights were 3558 (423) g, 3353 (376) g, and 3450 (301) g.

Discussion

We have shown that among men aged 21, 30 minute plasma glucose concentrations are higher in those who had lower birth weights whereas, after allowance for glucose and body mass, 30 minute plasma insulin and proinsulin concentrations are lower. Our sample was selected from male subjects born in the maternity unit in Southampton. Though the sample is unlikely to be representative of all young men in Southampton, their mean birth weight, 3413 g, is around the national average. Our analysis was based on internal comparisons, and bias would be introduced only if the relation between fetal growth and plasma glucose in the sample was unusual. This seems unlikely.

Our findings are consistent with those in the study of men aged 64 in whom 30 minute and two hour plasma glucose concentrations, and the risk of impaired glucose tolerance and diabetes, fell progressively with increasingly birth weight independently of waist to hip ratio and body mass index (chapter 22). The strength of the association in men aged 21 is such that 30 minute plasma glucose decreased by 0·70 mmol/l per lb (454 g) of birth weight. The corresponding figure for men aged 64 was 0·22 mmol/l, which just exceeds the lower confidence limit for the figure for men aged 21.

The association between 30 minute plasma glucose concentration and birth weight in the present study was independent of social class at birth and adult height. This suggests that the association is not the result of confounding environmental influences, which are associated both with retarded fetal growth and with the later development of impaired glucose tolerance.

Blood pressure was related to 30 minute plasma glucose concentration in keeping with previous observations on children and adults.[45] The association was independent of body mass index. The unexpectedly high mean systolic pressure of 146 mm Hg may be a consequence of recording blood pressure on the same occasion as glucose tolerance testing. Unlike plasma glucose concentration, blood pressure was not associated with lower birth weight, though this association has been found in larger studies (chapters 15, 16, and 18).

The trends of association of 30 minute plasma glucose, insulin, and proinsulin concentrations with birth weight were independent of gestational age. They may therefore reflect retarded fetal growth. The relation between retarded fetal growth and higher 30 minute plasma glucose but lower 30 minute plasma insulin and proinsulin concentrations (allowing for plasma glucose concentration and body mass index) suggests deficient insulin production by men who had lower birth weights. Our findings are consistent with the hypothesis that impaired glucose tolerance and diabetes in adult life may result from nutritional and other influences, which retard growth of the pancreas and reduce the number or size, or both, of the pancreatic β cell complement.

We thank the men who took part in the study and the staff at Shirley Health Centre for their cooperation.

1 Sobey WJ, Beer SF, Carrington CA, Clark PMS, Frank BH, Gray IP, et al. Sensitive and specific two site immunoradiometric assays for human insulin, proinsulin, 65–66 split and 32–33 split proinsulins. Biochem J 1989;260:535–41.
2 Office of Population Censuses and Surveys. Classification of occupations 1980. London: HMSO, 1980.
3 National Diabetes Data Group. Classification and diagnosis of diabetes mellitus and other categories of glucose intolerance. Diabetes 1979; 28:1039–57.
4 Florey C du V, Uppal S, Lowy C. Relation between blood pressure, weight, and plasma sugar and serum insulin levels in school children aged 9–12 years in Westland Holland. BMJ 1976;i:1368–71.
5 Cambien F, Warnet JM, Eschweg E, Jacqueson A, Richard JL, Rosselin G. Body mass, blood pressure, glucose and lipids. Does plasma insulin explain their relationships? Arteriosclerosis 1987;7:197–202.

24: Non-insulin dependent (type II) diabetes mellitus: thrifty phenotype hypothesis

C N HALES, D J P BARKER

In this contribution we put forward a new hypothesis concerning the aetiology of non-insulin dependent (type II) diabetes. The concept underlying our hypothesis is that poor fetal and early postnatal nutrition imposes mechanisms of nutritional thrift on the growing individual. We propose that one of the major long term consequences of inadequate early nutrition is impaired development of the endocrine pancreas and a greatly increased susceptibility to the development of non-insulin dependent diabetes. In the first section we outline our research which has led to this hypothesis. We then review the relevant publications. Finally, we show that the hypothesis suggests a reinterpretation of some findings and an explanation of others which are at present not easy to understand.

Insulin deficiency in non-insulin dependent diabetes

The controversy concerning the relative roles of insulin deficiency and insulin resistance in non-insulin dependent (type II) diabetes continues unresolved. Despite the early demonstration that obese people have raised plasma insulin concentrations,[1] many studies over the years have failed to control adequately for the influence of obesity. Another difficulty with the interpretation of plasma insulin concentrations is that sustained hyperglycaemia could have detrimental effects on insulin secretion.

In the 1960s one of us (CNH) attempted to assess whether people with a normal fasting glucose concentration but a delayed return to the fasting concentration after being given oral glucose (a condition similar to but not identical with that now defined as "impaired glucose tolerance") had poor

258

insulin secretion early in a glucose tolerance test.[2] People thus identified were studied again five years later to assess their tendency to deteriorate to diabetes. Obese people in this group showed the greatest deterioration in glucose tolerance.[3] It was concluded that obese people with defective initial rises in plasma insulin concentration were those most likely to develop diabetes. Unfortunately the relatively small numbers of people who could be studied in those days meant that this finding could only be taken as suggestive rather than definitive.

While that work was in progress the discovery of proinsulin,[4] the later demonstration of its presence in plasma,[5 6] and its high concentrations in the plasma of people with non-insulin dependent diabetes[7-9] raised a question concerning the specificity of insulin measurements in plasma. It was apparent from early days that proinsulin cross reacted strongly in many insulin radioimmunoassays. A potential solution to the assay problem lay in the exploitation of immunoassay techniques using labelled antibodies, which are termed "immunoradiometric" assays. These were developed in various configurations in one of our laboratories over the years,[10-14] which led to what was termed an "indirect two site immunoradiometric assay" of human proinsulin.[15] It was something of a surprise to discover subsequently, with the advent of bioengineered human proinsulin,[16] that this assay did not detect intact human proinsulin but rather the sum of the partially proteolysed derivatives on the pathway of conversion to insulin.[17] This finding led to the inevitable conclusion that an appreciable amount of the proinsulin-like material in plasma was partially split rather than intact. Further work, this time exploiting the monoclonal antibody technique,[18] was required to devise assays with adequate specificity to resolve the complex mixture of insulin-like molecules present in plasma.[19]

The new assays were used to reinvestigate plasma insulin concentrations in people with established non-insulin dependent diabetes.[20 21] The main conclusions to emerge from these studies were as follows. (1) The major proinsulin-like molecule in the plasma of many people with non-insulin dependent diabetes was the 32–33 split form. (The assays developed do not discriminate between des 31, 32, des 32, and 32–33 split proinsulin or between des 64, 65, des 65, or 65–66 split proinsulin. As Sobey et al pointed out, des 31, 32 or des 64, 65 are probably the main products in plasma,[19] but for simplicity the term 32–33 split is used here.) (2) The total concentration of proinsulin-like molecules in plasma from people with non-insulin dependent diabetes was one third to two thirds of the total concentration of insulin-like molecules in plasma. (3) Measuring the relatively biologically inactive proinsulin-like molecules as "insulin" could lead to the erroneous conclusion that a patient with diabetes was insulin resistant rather than insulin deficient. (4) Specific measurement of insulin showed that there was a clear separation between the 30 minute insulin responses of controls compared with the lower response of people with non-insulin dependent diabetes. (5) Insulin radioimmunoassays often measured the sum of all the insulin and proinsulin-like molecules present in plasma.

Another possibility that arose from this work was that 32–33 split proinsulin might have a pathogenic importance.[22] Risk factors for ischaemic heart disease, such as high plasma cholesterol, triglyceride, high density lipoprotein cholesterol, plasminogen activator inhibitor concentrations and high blood pressure, were more strongly correlated with 32–33 split proinsulin than was insulin itself. We return to the interpretation of this finding below.

Although the finding of a uniformly reduced early insulin response to oral glucose in people with non-insulin dependent diabetes seemed to be received as something of a shock a couple of years ago, review of reports of studies controlled for obesity published over the years show this to be an almost universal finding.[23-32] Disagreement over the insulin status of people with non-insulin dependent diabetes has often resulted from the use of different aspects of the plasma insulin response to oral glucose to assess status. Emphasis has been placed variously on the early insulin response, the two hour insulin concentration, or the area under the insulin curve or a combination of these. It is now clear that the early insulin response is of critical importance in determining glucose tolerance.[33] Thus in the absence of a normal early insulin response, high two hour insulin concentrations or a large area under the two hour insulin concentration curve cannot be accepted as evidence of insulin resistance. Studies of people with impaired glucose tolerance give less clear cut findings than in non-insulin dependent diabetes, but provide little evidence of universally raised early insulin responses as might be expected of a condition that has been suggested as being largely determined by insulin resistance.[25-28 32 34-37]

Studies such as those listed above, however, cannot assess whether insulin deficiency, insulin resistance, or a combination of the two leads to non-insulin dependent diabetes. A large prospective study of adult men and women living in Ely, Cambridgeshire has been initiated to address this issue. An early and surprising finding to emerge from this work is that there is in this population a continuous relation between height and glucose tolerance and that both men and women subjects with impaired glucose tolerance are significantly shorter than matched controls.[38]

Fetal and infant growth and non-insulin dependent diabetes

Previous work has led to the conclusion that cardiovascular disease in adult life results from restraint of growth during fetal life and infancy (chapter 21). Cardiovascular disease is viewed as a "programmed" effect of interference with early growth and development. (Programming may be defined as a permanent or long term change in the structure or function of an organism resulting from a stimulus or insult acting at a critical period of early life.[39]) The first evidence for this came from geographical studies which showed that differences in death rates from cardiovascular disease in different areas of England and Wales were closely related to differences in neonatal mortality (deaths before 1 month of age) 70 and more years ago (chapters 1 and 4). As most neonatal deaths were associated with low birth weights these findings suggest that cardiovascular disease is linked to impaired fetal growth.

This link was subsequently shown in studies of individual men and women whose fetal and infant growth was recorded at the time. The first study was carried out in the county of Hertfordshire where, since 1911, all babies born have been weighed at birth and at one year. Among 5654 men, those who had the lowest weight at birth and at 1 year had the highest death rates from ischaemic heart disease as adults (chapter 13). The differences in death rates were large, around threefold. This posed the question of what processes link lower rates of fetal and infant growth with cardiovascular disease. Subsequent studies in Hertfordshire and in the city of Preston, Lancashire, showed that lower birth weight, especially if associated with disproportionately high placental weight, is linked with raised blood pressure in adult life and to high plasma concentrations of fibrinogen (chapters 16 and 20). We concluded that these long term associations reflect restraint of growth of certain tissues, including blood vessels and the liver, by an adverse environment during a critical period of fetal or infant development. Poor maternal nutrition was suggested as an important environmental influence.

The known associations of non-insulin dependent diabetes and impaired glucose tolerance with ischaemic heart disease and hypertension,[40][41] plus awareness of the rapid growth of β cells during fetal life,[42] suggested to us that reduced glucose tolerance may be another outcome of early growth restraint.

Of the Hertfordshire men who still live in the county, 468 attended for venous blood sampling in the fasting state, and 370 of them agreed to have a full 75 g oral glucose tolerance test. From this study some strong relations have emerged (chapter 22). The percentage of men with impaired glucose tolerance or non-insulin dependent diabetes fell progressively with increasing birth weight and weight at 1 year. Two hour plasma glucose concentrations of 7·8 mmol/l or over were found in 40% (8/20) of men with birth weights of 5·5 lb (250 g) or less compared with 14% (4/28) of men with birth weights over 9·5 lb (4300 g), and in 43% (10/23) of men with weights at 1 year of 18 lb (8·18 kg) or less compared with 13% (3/24) of men with weights at 1 year of 27 lb (12·27 kg) or more. Some infants with heavier birth weights were possibly the outcome of pregnancies complicated by gestational diabetes. Such babies would have been few, however, and their survival 60 or more years ago would probably have been poor. Though there is evidence that gestational diabetes predisposes to diabetes in the offspring,[43] this could not explain our finding that the largest babies are those least likely to develop diabetes.

Analysis of the effects of obesity, measured as body mass index (weight (kg)/height $(m)^2$), showed that its diabetogenic effect adds to that of poor early growth. The mean two hour glucose concentration ranged from 5·8 mmol/l in men who had been above the highest tertile of weight at 1 year but were at or below the lowest tertile of current body mass index ($\leqslant 25\cdot4$) to 7·7 mmol/l in men below the lowest tertile of weight at 1 and above the highest tertile of current body mass index (> 28). Interestingly, there was a similar addition of the effects of obesity and low weight at 1 year on current fasting 32–33 split proinsulin concentration. The extremes of the range, defined as above, were 2·1 and 4·8 pmol/l respectively. When the men were divided into fifths according to the fasting 32–33 split proinsulin concentration, this measurement was highly correlated with systolic blood pressure (table). This association is consistent with earlier findings linking 32–33 split proinsulin and risk factors for ischaemic heart disease[22] and requires an explanation.

The concentrations of 32–33 split proinsulin measured in the Hertfordshire study are in the low pmolar range. Any biological activity of this derivative at these low concentrations has yet to be described. It seems to us that a more likely explanation of its association with blood pressure is that the pathogenic mechanisms leading to changes in both measurements are linked. This is reminiscent of the proposal by Reaven in relation to what he termed syndrome X, which includes glucose intolerance, hypertension, and some types of hyperlipidaemia.[44] He suggested that insulin resistance is the underlying factor linking these phenomena.

Our data suggest a different interpretation. Consistent with previous findings (chapter 16), blood pressure in the Hertfordshire men was inversely related to birth weight, though unlike two hour plasma glucose

---

Mean systolic blood pressure (adjusted for body mass index, age, and room temperature) in men aged 59–70 related to 32–33 split proinsulin plasma concentration after overnight fast

32–33 Split proinsulin (pmol/l)	Mean (SD) systolic pressure (mm Hg)	No. of men
− 1·5	161	96
− 2·5	164	90
− 3·6	163	93
− 5·8	165	96
> 5·8	170	93
Total	164 (23)	468

p Value for trend $= 0\cdot003$

concentration it was not related to weight at 1 year. Factors affecting early growth may therefore lead to either high blood pressure or impaired glucose tolerance (or non-insulin dependent diabetes), or to a mixture of hypertension and glucose intolerance, depending on the exact timing of the growth impairment during fetal or infant life. Our working hypothesis is that the varying components and combinations of syndrome X, possibly including insulin resistance, are late outcomes of abnormal growth and development processes occurring in fetal and early infant life.

At first sight it may seem improbable that events occurring in the first two years of existence could produce changes 50–70 years later. However, looked at in another way it is perhaps less surprising. It has been calculated that the fertilised ovum goes through some 42 rounds of cell division in developing into a full term infant.[45] After birth there need be only a further five cycles of division. The number of these divisions and their timing in development varies widely between different tissues. For example at birth a virtually full complement of brain neurons and of renal glomeruli are present, and available data suggest that at the age of 1 year at least half the adult complement of β cells is present.[46 47] Adverse influences, in particular poor nutrition, acting at this early time could permanently impair the size and structure of organs and tissues. Poor intrauterine nutrition may lead either to generalised growth retardation, or growth of the brain may be protected at the expense of the viscera. Evidence for selective growth retardation comes from the studies of blood pressure in Preston where one group of people with high blood pressure as adults was characterised at birth by their shortness in relation to their head circumference (chapter 17). There is good reason to believe that development of β cells, which proceeds rapidly during fetal life and early infancy,[42] would be vulnerable to poor nutrition. Poor fetal nutrition may be caused by poor maternal nutrition. A link with poor maternal nutrition would explain the high rates of impaired glucose tolerance and diabetes in parts of the third world and is also consistent with the occurrence of non-insulin dependent diabetes in more affluent countries. A recent survey in Oxford, for example, found evidence of iron deficiency in 47% of all pregnant women (chapter 27).

Thus we propose that poor nutrition of the fetus and infant leads to permanent changes in the structure and function of certain organs and tissues. The timing and precise nature of the deficiencies determine the pattern of metabolic and functional abnormalities seen in later life, including diabetes and hypertension and possibly also including some hyperlipidaemias and even insulin resistance. We suggest that poor early development of islets of Langerhans and β cells is a major factor in the aetiology of non-insulin dependent diabetes.

In referring to poor early development we do not at this stage consider this necessarily to be a solely quantitative deficiency of β cells but include the possibility that the cells themselves may be altered, or that the more complex aspects of islet structure and function, such as vasculature[48] and innervation, may be abnormally developed. There is a disproportionally large flow of blood to the islets (10–20%) compared to that of the pancreas as a whole.[47] Therefore major changes in islet vasculature such as have been described[48] could make a large contribution to changes in islet and particularly β cell function.

Brief review of evidence

We briefly review six key questions central to the hypothesis.

(1) IS THERE A DEFICIENCY OF β CELLS IN NON-INSULIN DEPENDENT DIABETES?

Many of the histological studies which have been carried out thus far have failed to control for the effects of obesity on β cells. However, as reviewed by Klöppel and colleagues,[49] there is now a general consensus that the number and total area of islets are reduced, mainly due to a decrease in the volume of β cells. But is a 50% reduction really enough to cause diabetes? Dogma has it that an 80–90% loss is needed.

(2) WHAT DEGREE OF DEFICIENCY OF β CELLS IS REQUIRED TO REDUCE GLUCOSE TOLERANCE?

A recent paper from the University of Minnesota pancreas transplant programme showed that even hemipancreatectomy in humans leads to a considerable deterioration of insulin secretion and glucose tolerance. The early insulin response was virtually arithmetically halved in these people, and 7/28 developed severely abnormal glucose tolerance.[50]

In parallel with this data, work from Weir's laboratory has shown that careful measurement of the degree of deficiency produced by pancreatic ablation in animals is needed. Both after neonatal streptozotocin and pancreatectomy considerable regeneration of β cells occurs in rats. These workers have been able to produce good models of non-insulin dependent diabetes in rats which retain 46% of normal β cell mass after neonatal streptozotocin and 42% after pancreatectomy.[51]

Our assertion that poor fetal growth is associated with non-insulin dependent diabetes in later life begs the question:

(3) WHAT ARE THE MAJOR NUTRITIONAL DETERMINANTS OF FETAL GROWTH?

Many studies have shown the key role of amino acids in fetal growth. Not only are they essential for laying down the protein required by the growing fetus but interestingly they are also a major source of substrate for energy production.[52] Looking at it teleologically this is not too surprising as the fetus clearly has to gear its growth to the availability of amino acids.

The availability of amino acids may be monitored by the β cell, just as the β cell senses the availability of nutrients in the adult. Thus it is important to understand what effect amino acids have on the development and growth of β cells in the fetus and also whether they control fetal insulin secretion. Evidence available to date strongly suggests that amino acids are the major factors controlling β cell growth and development and insulin secretion until late fetal life. Glucose has little effect until late gestation.[53][54] Insulin in turn appears to be a key regulator of fetal growth.[55][56]

If the key sequence of events is the supply of amino acids leading to insulin secretion leading to fetal growth, then we should ask:

(4) IS THE AMINO ACID SUPPLY ABNORMAL IN GROWTH RETARDED BABIES?

A recent collaborative study between Milan and Denver has shown that this is indeed the case and that the deficiency is large.[57] Furthermore, whether as a cause or an effect, there is deficient amino acid transport in placentas of small babies.[58]

If a major cause of defective intrauterine and early postnatal growth is linked to insulin deficiency, and this in turn leads to adult diabetes, then we should be able to show that there is defective production and performance of β cells in this situation and that such defects are irreversible.

(5) DOES DEFECTIVE β CELL GROWTH AND FUNCTION RESULT FROM MALNUTRITION? IF SO IS IT IRREVERSIBLE?

There is in fact quite a considerable body of evidence both in man and experimental animals that the answer to both these questions is yes.

James and Coore studied treated malnourished children and suggested that they showed a permanent reduction of insulin response to glucose.[59] Milner studied malnourished children before and after treatment and found the same. He even questioned whether this might predispose to adult diabetes.[60] These two studies were of postnatally malnourished children, although it is possible of course that the children might also have been malnourished in the uterus. Certainly there is evidence of a major effect of intrauterine malnutrition. Growth retarded newborn infants have reduced numbers of β cells and reduced insulin secretion.[61] Studies in experimental animals show clearly that these changes can be reproduced by subjecting either fetal or early postnatal animals to general protein energy malnutrition[62] or, interestingly, to protein deficiency alone.[48] It is notable that the degree of loss of insulin secretion in protein energy malnutrition is much more severe than would have been expected from the degree of reduction of islet volume.[62] This of course is reminiscent of the situation in human non-insulin dependent diabetes. An explanation of the discrepancy between the deficit of β cells and the severe loss of insulin secretion may lie in the finding that protein deficiency not only reduced β cell mass but produced an even larger effect on islet vascularisation.[48] Thus poor insulin secretion may be due not only to fewer β cells but also to abnormal islet structure and vascularisation. Indeed one cannot help wondering whether poor vascularisation might lead to poor clearance of insoluble peptides. Or in other words could amyloid deposition be secondary to vascular changes? This would of course have an accelerating effect on the underlying pathology.

In addition, underfeeding young rats lowers adult plasma insulin. This is not restored by refeeding normally.[63] Indeed the finding of irreversible loss from an early growth failure applies generally to tissue growth. Work in the 'sixties and early 'seventies showed clearly that a failure of early cell multiplication leads to an irrecoverable deficit in cell numbers.[64][65]

In reviewing the effects of poor fetal and early postnatal nutrition on β cell growth and function we have placed great emphasis on the role of protein and amino acids. We have done this because there is considerable evidence that, as far as insulin production is concerned, protein and amino acid supply are critically important. However, optimum nutrition in pregnancy and early life depends on a complex interaction of many nutrients concerning which we are still largely ignorant. It is probable that other nutrients play a part in non-insulin dependent diabetes and other components of syndrome X.

Relation of hypothesis to current concepts of the aetiology of non-insulin dependent diabetes

How do we reconcile the views that we are putting forward with the widely accepted theory that non-insulin dependent diabetes is totally genetically determined? In the first place the mechanisms we propose by no means exclude genetically based changes. We do suggest, however, that in thinking of candidate genes in non-insulin dependent diabetes we should widen our horizons considerably and consider genes that affect fetal growth and development.

The evidence that we have presented raises a question about the interpretation of concordance in identical twin data. A genetic interpretation of concordance rates of non-insulin dependent diabetes in identical twins may not be justifiable as identical twins share a common early nutritional environment. The familial pattern of non-insulin dependent diabetes may have a similar explanation. Family members share a similar socioeconomic environment, which is known to be linked to the incidence and prevalence of non-insulin dependent diabetes.[66] Poor maternal nutrition may be the key influence associated with low socioeconomic status. The stronger maternal than paternal influence on the development of non-insulin dependent diabetes[67] is consistent with our hypothesis. So too is the result of a large genetic study of non-insulin dependent diabetes.[68] This study of families with non-insulin dependent diabetes looked for evidence of genetic inheritance of poor insulin secretion. Instead it was discovered that the strongest influence was the common environment shared by the siblings.

We should also reconsider the Neal "thrifty genotype" hypothesis—that the diabetogenic gene or genes persist at a high level in the population because they somehow confer a survival advantage in times of nutritional deprivation, though detrimental at times of adequate or overnutrition.[69 70] For reasons outlined above we are suggesting a thrifty phenotype hypothesis. We propose that non-insulin dependent diabetes is the outcome of the fetus and early infant having to be nutritionally thrifty. This thrift results in impaired growth of the β cells of the islets of Langerhans. As long as the individual persists in the undernourished state there is no need to produce much insulin. A sudden move to good or overnutrition, however, exposes the reduced state of β cell function, and diabetes results. This situation was shown recently in the Ethiopian Jews transported to Israel, among whom a high prevalence of diabetes was observed.[71] The effect of a rapid transition from subsistence to good or overnutrition was also seen in the Nauruan islanders, who suffered severe nutritional deficiency before and during the last world war. After the war, they became affluent from phosphate mining. Diabetes on the island became epidemic. An interesting consequence of what we are suggesting is that the advent of good nutrition should start to result in better infant and fetal growth which in turn will reduce the incidence of diabetes, provided always of course that the population does not become fatter and less active. It was therefore interesting to see the outcome of the most recent survey of the islanders.[72] Though obesity, exercise, and other risk factors had not decreased since 1975/76, when the first survey was carried out, there had nevertheless been a dramatic reduction in impaired glucose tolerance and non-insulin dependent diabetes. The authors attributed this to a eugenic affect of lower reproduction in people with diabetes. The size and speed of the improvement, however, makes this explanation unlikely. We suggest that it was due to a great improvement of fetal and infant nutrition consequent on postwar affluence. Thus infants born after 1945 are now aged up to 46. It was among them that the reduction in diabetes was seen.

Conclusions

We propose a "thrifty phenotype" hypothesis of the aetiology of non-insulin dependent diabetes. The essence of the hypothesis is that poor nutrition in fetal and early infant life are detrimental to the development and function of the β cells of the islets of Langerhans. Such defects of structure and function, which may include more complex features of islet anatomy such as the vasculature and innervation, predispose to the later

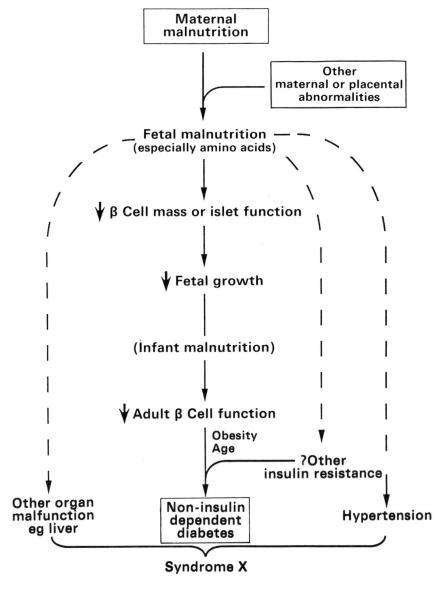

Diagramatic representation of key features of the "thrifty phenotype" hypothesis of the aetiology of non-insulin dependent (type II) diabetes. Also outlined is the suggestion that the features of syndrome X[49] may have closely related origins in failures of early growth and development. Not shown for the sake of simplicity and clarity are the additional possibilities that (i) an early reduction of insulin production could have secondary consequences for the growth and development of other organs affected in syndrome X; (ii) infant malnutrition may be involved in processes contributing to components of syndrome X.

development of non-insulin dependent diabetes. Existing evidence points to a key role for protein and amino acids in this process, but other nutritional defects are not excluded. Indeed the complex interactions of the type and timing of nutritional defects in early life are suggested as underlying the pathogenesis of the variable abnormalities sometimes described as syndrome X. Though these early changes powerfully determine susceptibility, additional factors such as obesity, ageing, physical inactivity, and possibly other processes leading to insulin resistance must also play a part in deciding the time of onset and severity of non-insulin dependent diabetes (figure).

1 Karam JH, Grodsky GM, Forsham PH. Excessive insulin response to glucose in obese subjects as measured by immunochemical assay. *Diabetes* 1963;**12**:197–204.

2 Hales CN, Greenwood FC, Mitchell FL, Strauss WT. Blood-glucose, plasma-insulin and growth hormone concentrations of individuals with minor abnormalities of glucose tolerance. *Diabetologia* 1968;**4**:73–82.

3 Strauss WT, Hales CN. Plasma insulin in minor abnormalities of glucose tolerance: a 5 year follow-up. *Diabetologia* 1974:**10**:237–43.

4 Steiner DF, Oyer PE. The biosynthesis of insulin and a probable precursor of insulin by a human islet cell adenoma. *Proc Natl Acad Sci USA* 1967;**57**:473–80.

5 Roth J, Gorden P, Postan I. "Big insulin": a new component of plasma insulin detected by immunoassay. *Proc Natl Acad Sci USA* 1968;**61**:138–45.

6 Rubenstein AH, Cho S, Steiner DF. Evidence for proinsulin in human urine and serum. *Lancet* 1968;i:1353–5

7 Duckworth WC, Kitabchi AE, Heinemann M. Direct measurement of plasma proinsulin in normal and diabetic subjects. *Am J Med* 1972; **53**:418–27.

8 Gorden P, Hendricks CM, Roth J. Circulating proinsulin-like component in man: increased proportion in hypoinsulinaemic states. *Diabetologia* 1974;**10**:469–74.

9 Mako ME, Starr JI, Rubenstein AH. Circulating proinsulin in patients with maturity onset diabetes. *Am J Med* 1977; **63**:865–9.

10 Miles LEM, Hales CN. Labelled antibodies and immunological assay systems. *Nature* 1968;**219**: 186–9.

11 Miles LEM, Hales CN. The preparation and properties of purified ^{125}I-labelled antibodies to insulin. *Biochem J* 1968;**108**:611–8.

12 Addison GM, Hales CN. The immunoradiometric assay. In: Kirkham KE, Hunter WM, (eds.) *Radioimmunoassay methods*. Edinburgh: Churchill Livingstone, 1971:481–7.

13 Addison GM, Hales CN. Two site assay of human growth hormone. *Horm Metab Res* 1971;**3**:59–60.

14 Beck P, Hales CN. Immunoassay of serum polypeptide hormones by using ^{125}I-labelled anti-(immunoglobulin G) antibodies. *Biochem J* 1975;**145**:607–16.

15 Rainbow SJ, Woodhead JS, Yue DK, Luzio SD, Hales CN. Measurement of human proinsulin by an indirect two-site immunoradiometric assay. *Diabetologia* 1979;**17**:229–34.

16 Frank BH, Pettee JM, Zimmerman RE, Burck PH. The production of human proinsulin and its transformation to human insulin and C-peptide. In: Rich DH, Gross E, eds. *Peptides: synthesis-structure-function. Proceedings of the 7th American Peptide Symposium.* Pierce Chemical Company, 1981:729–38.

17 Gray IP, Siddle K, Docherty K, Frank BH, Hales CN. (1984) Proinsulin in human serum: problems in measurement and interpretation. *Clin Endocrinol (Oxf)* 1984;**21**:43–7.

18 Kohler G, Milstein C. Continuous cultures of fused cells secreting antibody of predefined specificity. *Nature* 1975;**256**:495–7.

19 Sobey WJ, Beer SF, Carrington CA, Clark PMS, Frank BH, Gray IP, et al. Sensitive and specific two-site immunoradiometric assays for human insulin proinsulin 65–66 split and 32–33 split proinsulins. Biochem J 1989;260:535–41.

20 Temple RC, Carrington CA, Luzio SD, Owens DR, Schneider AE, Sobey WJ, et al. Insulin deficiency in non-insulin dependent diabetes. Lancet 1989;i:293–5.

21 Temple RC, Clark PMS, Nagi DK, Schneider AE, Yudkin JS, Hales CN. Radio-immunoassay may overestimate insulin in non-insulin dependent diabetics. Clin Endocrinol 1989;32:689–93.

22 Nagi DK, Hendra TJ, Ryle AJ, Cooper TM, Temple RC, Clark PMS, et al. The relationship of concentrations of insulin, intact proinsulin and 32–33 split proinsulin with cardiovascular risk factors in Type 2 (non-insulin-dependent) diabetic subjects. Diabetologia 1990;33:532–7.

23 Perley MJ, Kipnis DM. Plasma insulin responses to oral and intravenous glucose: studies in normal and diabetic subjects. J Clin Invest 1967;46:1954–62.

24 Chiles R, Tzagounis M. Excessive serum insulin response to oral glucose in obesity and mild diabetes. Diabetes 1970; 19:458–64.

25 Jackson WPU, Van Mieghem W, Keller P. Insulin excess as the initial lesion in diabetes. Lancet 1972;i:1040–4.

26 Savage PJ, Dippe SE, Bennett PH, Gordon P, Roth J, Rushforth NB, et al. Hyperinsulinemia and hypoinsulinemia. Insulin responses to oral carbohydrate over a wide spectrum of glucose tolerance. Diabetes 1975;24:362–8.

27 Reaven GM, Bernstein R, Davis B, Olefsky JM. Nonketotic diabetes mellitus: insulin deficiency or insulin resistance? Am J Med 1976;60:80–8.

28 Kosaka K, Hagura R, Kuzuya T. Insulin responses in equivocal and definite diabetes, with special reference to subjects who had mild glucose intolerance but later developed definite diabetes. Diabetes 1977;26:944–52.

29 Savage PJ, Bennion LJ, Flock EV, Nagulesparan M, Mott D, Roth J, et al. Diet-induced improvement of abnormalities in insulin and glucagon secretion and in insulin receptor binding in diabetes mellitus. J Clin Endocrinol Metab 1979;48:999–1007.

30 Mohan V, Sharp PS, Cloke HR, Burrin JM, Schumer B, Kohner EM. Serum immuno-reactive insulin responses to a glucose load in Asian Indian and European Type 2 (non-insulin-dependent) diabetic patients and control subjects. Diabetologia 1986;29:235–7.

31 Deacon CF, Schleser-Mohr S, Ballmann M, Willims B, Conlon JM, Creutzfeldt W. Preferential release of proinsulin relative to insulin in non-insulin-dependent diabetes mellitus. Acta Endocrinol (Copenh) 1988;119:549–54.

32 Yoshioka N, Kuzuya T, Matsuda A, Taniguchi M, Iwamoto Y. Serum proinsulin levels at fasting and after oral glucose load in patients with Type 2 (non-insulin-dependent) diabetes. Diabetologia 1988;31:355–60.

33 Bruce DG, Chisholm DJ, Storlein LH, Kraegen EW. Physiological importance of deficiency in early prandial insulin secretion in non-insulin-dependent diabetes. Diabetes 1988;317:736–44.

34 Johansen K. Normal initial plasma insulin response in mild diabetes. Metabolism 1972; 21:1177–80.

35 Danowski TS, Khurana RC, Nolan S, Stephan T, Gegick CG, Chae S, et al. Insulin patterns in equivocal glucose tolerance test (chemical diabetes). Diabetes 1973;22:808–12.

36 Reaven GM, Olefsky JM. Relationship between heterogeneity of insulin responses and insulin resistance in normal subjects and patients with chemical diabetes. Diabetologia 1977;13:201–6.

37 Berntorp K, Eriksson KF, Lindgärde F. The importance of diabetes heredity in lean subjects on insulin secretion, blood lipids and oxygen uptake in the pathogenesis of glucose intolerance. Diabetes Res 1986;3:231–6.

38 Brown DC, Byrne CD, Clark PMS, Cox BD, Day NE, Hales CN, et al. Height and glucose tolerance in adults. Diabetologia 1991;34:531–3.

39 Lucas A. Programming by early nutrition in man. In: Bock GR, Whelan J, eds. The childhood environment and adult disease. Chichester: Wiley, 1991:38–50. (Ciba Foundation Symposium No.156).

40 Fuller JH, Shipley MJ, Rose G, Jarrett RJ, Keen H. Coronary heart disease risk and impaired glucose tolerance. *Lancet* 1980;i:1373–6.

41 Modan M, Halkin H, Almog S, Lusky A, Eshol A, Shefi M, *et al.* Hyperinsulinaemia: a link between hypertension, obesity and glucose tolerance. *J Clin Invest* 1985;75:809–17.

42 Hellerström C, Swenne I, Andersson A. Islet cell replication and diabetes. In: Lefebvre PJ, Pipeleers DG, eds. *The pathology of the endocrine pancreas in diabetes.* Heidelberg: Springer 1988:141–70.

43 Pettitt DJ, Aleck KA, Baird HR, Carraker MJ, Bennett PH, Knowler WC. Congenital susceptibility to NIDDM. Role of intrauterine environment. *Diabetes* 1988;37:622–8.

44 Reaven GM. Role of insulin resistance in human disease. *Diabetes* 1988;37:1595–607.

45 Milner RDG. Mechanisms of overgrowth. In: Sharp F, Fraser RB, Milner RDG, eds. *Fetal growth. Proceedings of the 20th study group of the Royal College of Obstetricians and Gynaecologists.* London: Royal College of Obstetricians and Gynaecologists, 1989:139–48.

46 Rahier J, Wallon J, Henquin J-C. Cell populations in the endocrine pancreas of human neonates and infants. *Diabetologia* 1981;20:540–6.

47 Bonner-Weir S. Anatomy of the islet of Langerhans. In: Samols E, ed. *The endocrine pancreas.* New York: Raven Press, 1991,15–27.

48 Snoeck A, Remacle C, Reusens B, Hoet JJ. Effect of a low protein diet during pregnancy on the fetal rat endocrine pancreas. *Biol Neonate* 1990;57:107–18.

49 Klöppel G, Löhr M, Habich K, Oberholzer M, Heitz PU. Islet pathology and the pathogenesis of Type 1 and Type 2 diabetes mellitus revisited. *Survey and Synthesis of Pathology Research* 1985;4:110–25.

50 Kendall DM, Sutherland DER, Najarian JS, Goetz FC, Robertson RP. Effects of hemipancreatectomy on insulin secretion and glucose tolerance in healthy humans. *N Eng J Med* 1990;322:898–903.

51 Weir GC, Leahy JL, Bonner-Weir S. Experimental reduction of B-cell mass: implications for the pathogenesis of diabetes. *Diabetes Metab Rev* 1986;2:125–61.

52 Battaglia FC, Meschia G. Principle substrates of fetal metabolism. *Physiol Rev* 1978;58:499–527.

53 De Gasparo M, Milner GR, Norris PD, Milner RDG. Effect of glucose and amino acids on foetal rat pancreatic growth and insulin secretion *in vitro. J Endocrinol* 1978;77:241–8.

54 Swenne I. Pancreatic B-cell growth and diabetes mellitus. *Diabetologia* (in press).

55 Fowden AL. The role of insulin in prenatal growth. *J Dev Physiol* 1989;12:173–82.

56 Philipps AF, Rosenkrantz TS, Clark RM, Knox I, Chaffin DG, Raye JR. Effects of fetal insulin deficiency on growth in fetal lambs. *Diabetes* 1991;40:20–7.

57 Cetin I, Marconi AM, Bozzetti P, Sereni LP, Corbetta C, Pardi G, *et al.* Umbilical amino acid concentrations in appropriate and small for gestational age infants: a biochemical difference present *in utero. Am J Obstet Gynecol* 1988;158:120–6.

58 Dicke JM, Henderson GI. Placental amino acid uptake in normal and complicated pregnancies. *Am J Med Sci* 1988;295:223–7.

59 James WPT, Coore HG. Persistent impairment of insulin secretion and glucose tolerance after malnutrition. *Am J Clin Nutr* 1970; 23:386–9.

60 Milner RDG. Metabolic and hormonal responses to glucose and glucagon in patients with infantile malnutrition. *Pediat Res* 1971;5:33–9.

61 Van Assche FA, Aerts L. The fetal endocrine pancreas. *Contrib Gynecol Obstet* 1979;5:44–57.

62 Weinkove C, Weinkove EA, Pimstone BL. Insulin release and pancreatic islet volume in malnourished rats. *S Afr Med J* 1974;48:1888.

63 Swenne I, Crace CJ, Milner RDG. Persistent impairment of insulin secretory response to glucose in adult rats after limited period of protein-calorie malnutrition early in life. *Diabetes* 1987;36:454–8.

64 Winick M, Noble A. Cellular response in rats during malnutrition at various ages. *J Nutr* 1966;89:300–6.

65 Widdowson EM, Crabb DE, Milner RDG. Cellular development of some human organs before birth. *Arch Dis Child* 1972;47:652–5.

66 Barker DJP, Gardner MJ, Power C. Incidence of diabetes amongst people aged 18–50 years in nine British towns: a collaborative study. *Diabetologia* 1982;**22**:421–5.
67 Alcolado JC, Alcolado R. Importance of maternal history of non-insulin dependent diabetic patients. *BMJ* 1991;**302**:1178–80.
68 Iselius L, Lindsten J, Morton NE, Efendic S, Cerasi E, Haegermark A, *et al.* Evidence for an autosomal recessive gene regulating the persistence of the insulin response to glucose in man. *Clin Genet* 1982;**22**:180–94.
69 Neel JV. Diabetes mellitus: a thrifty genotype rendered detrimental by "progress"? *Am J Hum Genet* 1962;**14**:353–62.
70 Anonymous. Thrifty genotype rendered detrimental by progress? [Editorial] *Lancet* 1989;ii:839–40.
71 Cohen MP, Stern E, Rusecki Y, Zeidler A. High prevalence of diabetes in young adult Ethiopian immigrants to Israel. *Diabetes* 1988;**37**:824–8.
72 Dowse GK, Zimmet PZ, Finch CF, Collins VR. Decline in incidence of epidemic glucose intolerance in Nauruans: implications for the "thrifty genotype". *Am J Epidemiol* 1991;**133**:1093–104.

PART IX
CHOLESTEROL

25: Relation of infant feeding to adult serum cholesterol concentration and death from ischaemic heart disease

C H D FALL, D J P BARKER, C OSMOND,
P D WINTER, P M S CLARK, C N HALES

A total of 5718 men born in Hertfordshire, England during 1911–30 was followed up. Their birth weights, weights at 1 year, and method of feeding as infants had been recorded at the time by health visitors.

Four hundred and seventy four of the men had died from ischaemic heart disease. Standardised mortality ratios were 97 (confidence interval 81 to 115) in men who had been breast fed and not weaned at 1 year, compared with 79 in men who had been breast fed and weaned at one year, and 73 in men who had been breast and bottle fed. In a subgroup of 495 men born in the county during 1920–30 and still living there, those who had been breast fed and not weaned at 1 year had higher mean serum concentrations of total and low density lipoprotein cholesterols and apolipoprotein B. The highest concentrations were found in men who had been heavy at birth and light at 1 year. Men who had been exclusively bottle fed also had a high standardised mortality ratio (95) for ischaemic heart disease and high mean serum concentrations of total and low density lipoprotein cholesterols and apolipoprotein B.

Therefore, in a group of men born 60–70 years ago, those who had not been weaned off breast milk within 1 year had higher serum low density lipoprotein cholesterol concentrations and higher death rates from ischaemic heart disease. Similar results were seen in men who had been exclusively bottle fed (bottle feeds available 70 years ago differed from modern formulas). One interpretation of these findings is that delayed weaning and different methods of infant feeding may programme lipid metabolism throughout life.

Introduction

There has been speculation that the high cholesterol and saturated fat content of milk received by infants may influence lipid metabolism throughout life.[1] In humans there is little evidence to support this, as comparisons of serum cholesterol concentrations in people who were breast fed or bottle fed after birth have given conflicting results.[2-7] Nevertheless, some observations give credibility to the speculation. An infant's serum cholesterol concentration, unlike that of an older child or an adult, is strongly related to its intake of cholesterol and saturated fat.[4 8-10] Follow up studies of children have shown that serum cholesterol concentrations tend to track, so that children maintain their rank order by serum cholesterol concentration over several years.[11 12] Tracking has been observed from the age of 6 months. Experiments in animals have clearly shown that different early feeding regimens can lead to permanent changes in serum lipid concentrations and the metabolic activity of enzymes controlling cholesterol synthesis and excretion.[13-15]

We measured serum lipids in a group of men born in Hertfordshire, England, where the method of feeding of all babies was routinely recorded from 1911 onwards (chapter 13). The recorded information included whether infants were breast or bottle fed and whether they were weaned at 1 year of age. We have also examined death rates from ischaemic heart disease in relation to method of infant feeding.

Subjects and methods

As described in chapter 13, from 1911 onwards all births in Hertfordshire were notified by the attending midwife and the birth weight recorded. A health visitor saw the babies at home periodically through infancy (the first year of life) and recorded how each baby was fed, using one of three categories: breast feeding, bottle feeding, or a combination of breast and bottle feeding. When children were 1 year old their weight, whether or not they were weaned, and how many teeth had erupted were recorded. Weights were measured in pounds (1 lb = 0·45 kg) and were often rounded to the nearest half pound. We have therefore used the original units.

We traced 5718 (74%) of the singleton boys born in six districts of east Hertfordshire during 1911–30 (see chapter 14). For 5471 of them the method of infant feeding was recorded. We analysed death rates for ischaemic heart disease and all non-circulatory disease (all causes of death excluding ICD 390–459) in relation to birth weight, weight at 1 year, and method of infant feeding.

There were 1157 men who were born during 1920–30 and still lived in the six districts. As described in chapter 14, 845 of them (73%) agreed to be interviewed at home and were visited by one of four fieldworkers. The fieldworkers had not seen the infant data recorded for the men. Blood pressure, height, weight, and waist and hip circumferences were measured. After the interview the men were asked if they would be willing to attend a local clinic to have blood samples taken. They were asked to attend twice: once after fasting overnight for 12 hours, and once for a non-fasting sample. Men known to have diabetes were excluded. In all, 485 (57%) men provided fasting blood samples, of whom 431 also provided non-fasting samples.

The fasting blood samples were analysed for serum total cholesterol, high density lipoprotein cholesterol, triglyceride, apolipoproteins A1 and B, and Lp(a) lipoprotein concentrations. The non-fasting samples were analysed for only total cholesterol. Serum total cholesterol, high density lipoprotein cholesterol, and triglyceride concentrations were measured using standard enzymatic methods.[16–19] Interassay coefficients of variation for these assays were in the range 1·7% to 2·7%. Low density lipoprotein cholesterol concentration was derived by the Friedwalk-Fredrickson formula.[20] Apolipoprotein A1 and B concentrations were measured by immunoturbimetric assays with interassay coefficients of variation of less than 5%.[21] Lp(a) lipoprotein concentration was measured by immunoenzymometric assay (Enzyquick, Immuno, Sevenoaks) with an interassay coefficient of variation of 11%.[22]

Serum concentrations of triglyceride, apolipoprotein A1 and B, and Lp(a) lipoprotein had skewed distributions and we transformed them using logarithms. The geometric standard deviation is the antilog of the standard deviation measured on the log scale. We analysed the data using tabulation of means, multiple linear regression, and two sample t tests. Standardised mortality ratios were calculated by the method of person years.[23]

Results

Of the 5471 men, 1381 had been both breast and bottle fed, 3733 had been exclusively breast fed, and 357 had been exclusively bottle fed. Only 2592 (69%) of the men who had been exclusively breast fed had been weaned at 1 year, compared with 1244 (90%) of those who had been breast and bottle fed and 336 (94%) of those who had been exclusively bottle fed.

A total of 1314 men had died, of whom 474 had died from ischaemic heart disease. The death rate from this disease was below the national average, the overall standardised mortality ratio being 83. Analysis according to method of infant feeding showed that the standardised mortality ratio was 73 in the men who had been breast and bottle fed, 85 in the men who had been exclusively breast fed, and 95 in the men who had been exclusively bottle fed. We divided the exclusively breast fed men according to whether or not they were weaned at 1 year. The standardised mortality ratio in those who had been weaned was 79 compared with 97 in those who were not weaned (table I). In contrast with these differences in mortality from ischaemic heart disease there were no significant differences in mortality from non-circulatory disease (table I).

As we have shown previously (chapter 13), standardised mortality ratios fell with increasing weight at 1 year (table I). This trend was seen in each feeding group. In each weight group, however, standardised mortality ratios tended to be higher in men who had been breast fed and had not been weaned at 1 year and in those who had been exclusively bottle fed. In all feeding groups combined standardised mortality ratios fell with increasing birth weight (from 105 in those who weighed 5·5 lb or less at birth to 81 in those who weighed more than 9·5 lb) though the fall was not so great as with weight at 1 year. In men who had been breast fed and not weaned at 1 year, however, standardised mortality ratios rose with increasing birth weight.

The ages of the 485 men who still lived in the six districts of east Hertfordshire ranged from 59 to 70 (mean 64) years; 116 had been breast

TABLE I—*Standardised mortality ratios for ischaemic heart disease in 5471 men born in east Hertfordshire 1911–30, according to method of feeding and infants. (Numbers of deaths are in parentheses)*

Weight at 1 year (lb)	Breast and bottle fed	Breast fed		Bottle fed	All
		Weaned at 1 year	Not weaned at 1 year		
≤18	87 (8)	93 (14)	140 (10)	126 (4)	104 (36)
−20	88 (21)	93 (39)	95 (26)	97 (6)	93 (92)
−22	90 (37)	92 (77)	121 (55)	75 (9)	97 (178)
−24	66 (22)	69 (51)	65 (21)	109 (13)	71 (107)
−26	42 (8)	67 (24)	87 (13)	104 (6)	68 (51)
>26	26 (2)	23 (3)	73 (4)	50 (1)	36 (10)
All weights	73 (98)	79 (208)	97 (129)	95 (39)	83 (474)
95% Confidence interval	59 to 89	69 to 90	81 to 115	68 to 130	75 to 90
Ratio for non-circulatory disease	74 (147)	84 (329)	85 (166)	69 (42)	81 (684)
95% Confidence interval	62 to 87	75 to 94	73 to 99	50 to 94	75 to 87

and bottle fed, 344 exclusively breast fed, and 25 exclusively bottle fed. Only 253 (74%) of the men who had been exclusively breast fed had been weaned at 1 year compared with 102 (88%) of those who had been breast and bottle fed and 25 (100%) of those who had been exclusively bottle fed.

Men who had been breast fed and had not been weaned at 1 year and those who were exclusively bottle fed had higher serum concentrations of total cholesterol in fasting and non-fasting samples, and of low density lipoprotein cholesterol, and higher ratios of low density lipoprotein to high density lipoprotein cholesterol than men in the other two feeding groups (table II). Differences in apolipoprotein B concentration showed the same pattern as those in total and low density lipoprotein cholesterol, though they were not significant.

There were no differences between feeding groups in mean serum concentrations of high density cholesterol, triglycerides, apolipoprotein A1 and Lp(a) lipoprotein or in mean height and body mass index (table II). The percentages of men who were current smokers or who were in social class IV or V were similar in all infant feeding groups. Despite the

TABLE II—*Mean serum lipid concentrations, height, body mass index, percentage of smokers and men of low social class in 485 men aged 59–70, according to method of feeding as infants*

| | Breast and bottle fed (n = 116) | Breast fed | | Bottle fed (n = 25) | All groups (No of men) (n = 485) | SD |
		Weaned at 1 year (n = 253)	Not weaned at 1 year (n = 91)			
Cholesterol (mmol/l)	6·6	6·6	6·9*	7·0*	6·7 (485)	1·2
Non-fasting cholesterol (mmol/l)	6·4	6·4	6·9**	7·1**	6·5 (431)	1·2
Low density lipoprotein cholesterol (mmol/l)	4·6	4·6	5·0**	5·1*	4·7 (470)	1·1
High density lipoprotein cholesterol (mmol/l)	1·2	1·2	1·2	1·2	1·2 (470)	0·3
Low density lipoprotein/ high density lipoprotein ratio	3·8	3·8	4·2**	4·2	3·9 (470)	1·5
Triglyceride (mmol/l)†	1·4	1·5	1·4	1·4	1·4 (485)	1·6
Apolipoprotein A1 (g/l)†	1·31	1·30	1·29	1.35	1·30 (466)	1·2
Apolipoprotein B (g/l)†	1·08	1·08	1·14	1.14	1·09 (464)	1·3
Lp(a) lipoprotein (mg/l)†	92	100	96	83	97 (469)	3·6
Height (m)	1·71	1·72	1·72	1·72	1·72 (485)	0·07
Body mass index (kg/m²)	26·5	27·0	27·1	27·1	26·9 (485)	3·5
% Current smokers	23	28	27	28	27 (482)	44
% Current social class IV or V	25	24	29	24	25 (480)	43
% Social class IV or V at birth	46	48	64**	50	51 (458)	50

SD = standard deviation.

* p < 0·05, ** p < 0·01, comparison with breast and bottle fed group combined with breast fed and weaned group.

† Logarithms were used in the analysis, therefore means and standard deviations are geometric.

similarity in current social class, a higher percentage of men who had been breast fed and had not been weaned at 1 year were born into families of social class IV or V. Table III shows, however, that the higher concentrations of low density lipoprotein cholesterol in the men in this feeding group were found for all social classes at birth. Findings for total cholesterol and apolipoprotein B were similar.

Men who had been breast and bottle fed and men who had been breast fed and weaned at 1 year had similar mortality from ischaemic heart disease (table I) and mean values of all variables in table II. Only 14 of the breast and bottle fed men had not been weaned at 1 year. We excluded these 14 and combined the remaining 102 with the 253 breast fed men who had been weaned at 1 year. This defined a "weaned" group, which we contrast with the 91 men who were breast fed and not weaned at 1 year, the "not weaned" group. Because of the small numbers of men who had been exclusively bottle fed we excluded them from further analysis.

Table IV shows mean fasting serum cholesterol concentrations according to weight at 1 year and birth weight. In the weaned group there were no trends with weight at 1 year or with birth weight. The mean fasting serum cholesterol concentrations in the not weaned group rose with increasing birth weight. In the weaned group a simultaneous regression analysis with weight at 1 year and birth weight showed that serum cholesterol concentration fell by 0·15 mmol/l for every pound increase in weight at 1 year and rose by 0·43 mmol/l for every pound increase in birth weight (table V). Mean fasting cholesterol concentrations were higher in men with higher body mass indices (p = 0·02) and waist to hip ratios (p = 0·005). They did not vary in relation to age, smoking, alcohol consumption, or social class, either currently or at birth. Adjustment for body mass index and waist to hip ratio did not change the trends in mean cholesterol concentration shown in table IV.

In the not weaned group the trends in non-fasting serum cholesterol, low density lipoprotein cholesterol, and in apolipoprotein B concentrations

TABLE III—*Mean serum low density lipoprotein cholesterol concentration (mmol/l) in men aged 59–70 according to method of feeding as infants and social class at birth*

Social class at birth	Breast and bottle	Breast fed Weaned at 1 year	Not weaned at 1 year	Bottle fed	All groups (No of men)	Standard deviation
I, II, III (Non-manual)	4·8	4·6	5·1	4·9	4·7 (62)	1·0
III (Manual)	4·5	4·7	5·0	5·6	4·7 (157)	1·1
IV, V	4·6	4·6	5·0	5·0	4·7 (225)	1·2
All classes	4·6	4·6	5·0	5·2	4·7 (444)	1·1

TABLE IV—*Mean fasting serum cholesterol concentration (mmol/litre) in men aged 59–70, according to weight at 1 year, birth weight, and whether weaned at 1 year. (Numbers of men are in parentheses)*

	Weaned	Not weaned
Weight at 1 year (lb):		
≤ 18	6·7 (20)	7·5 (5)
− 20	6·7 (53)	7·2 (17)
− 22	6·7 (103)	6·8 (35)
− 24	6·5 (107)	6·6 (19)
− 26	6·2 (52)	6·9 (9)
> 26	6·9 (20)	7·1 (7)
Birth weight (lb):		
≤ 5·5	6·5 (18)	6·1 (1)
− 6·5	6·9 (41)	6·4 (15)
− 7·5	6·6 (109)	6·6 (28)
− 8·5	6·5 (106)	7·3 (27)
− 9·5	6·7 (54)	7·0 (14)
> 9·5	6·2 (27)	7·2 (6)
All weights	6·6 (355)	6·9 (91)
Standard deviation:	1·2	1·3

were similar to those in fasting cholesterol concentrations (table V). In table VI the men are divided into three roughly equal groups according to weight at 1 year, and three equal groups according to birth weight. Among men in the not weaned group the highest low density lipoprotein cholesterol value was 5·7 mmol/l in men who weighed more than 8·25 lb at birth but 21 lb or less at 1 year. In the weaned group the mean low density lipoprotein cholesterol concentrations were more evenly distributed

TABLE V—*Regression of serum lipid concentrations on birth weight and weight at 1 year simultaneously in men aged 59–70 who had not been weaned at 1 year*

Dependent variable	Birth weight (lb)		Weight at 1 year (lb)	
	Regression coefficient (95% CI)	p Value	Regression coefficient (95% CI)	p Value
Fasting cholesterol (mmol/l)	0·43 (0·19 to 0·68)	< 0·001	− 0·15 (− 0·27 to − 0·04)	0·01
Non-fasting cholesterol (mmol/l)	0·34 (0·04 to 0·64)	0·03	− 0·22 (− 0·35 to − 0·09)	0·001
Low density lipoprotein cholesterol (mmol/l)	0·39 (0·16 to 0·62)	0·001	− 0·12 (− 0·22 to − 0·01)	0·04
Apolipoprotein B (log g/l)	0·06 (0·01 to 0·11)	0·03	− 0·04 (− 0·06 to − 0·01)	0·007

CI = confidence interval

TABLE VI—*Mean serum low density lipoprotein cholesterol concentration (mmol/l) in men aged 59–70, according to weight at 1 year, birth weight, and whether weaned at 1 year. (Numbers of men are in parentheses)*

Birth weight (lb)	Weight at 1 year (lb)			
	≤21	−23	>23	All
Weaned:				
≤7	4.8 (45)	4·8 (29)	4·6 (10)	4·8 (84)
−8·25	4.8 (41)	4·5 (47)	4·5 (39)	4·6 (127)
>8·25	4.8 (22)	4·6 (45)	4·5 (64)	4·6 (131)
All*	4.8 (108)	4·6 (121)	4·5 (113)	4·6 (342)
Not weaned:				
≤7	4.8 (18)	4·1 (7)	3·9 (1)	4·6 (26)
−8·25	4.9 (13)	4·9 (12)	5·1 (10)	4·9 (35)
>8·25	5.7 (8)	5·3 (9)	5·2 (12)	5·4 (29)
All†	5.0 (39)	4·8 (28)	5·1 (23)	5·0 (90)

* Overall standard deviation = 1·1.

† Overall standard deviation = 1·2.

according to birth weight and weight at 1 year. In contrast to findings for total cholesterol and low density cholesterol, mean apolipoprotein B concentrations in the weaned group fell with increasing weight at 1 year and birth weight (table VII).

TABLE VII—*Mean fasting serum apolipoprotein B concentration (g/l) in men aged 59–70, according to weight at 1 year, birth weight, and whether weaned at 1 year. (Numbers of men are in parentheses).*

	Weaned	Not weaned	All men
Weight at 1 year (lb):			
≤18	1·08 (19)	1·30 (5)	1·12 (24)
−20	1·18 (52)	1·24 (15)	1·19 (67)
−22	1·09 (99)	1·14 (33)	1·10 (132)
−24	1·06 (104)	1·08 (18)	1·06 (122)
−26	1·01 (47)	1·11 (8)	1·03 (55)
>26	1·05 (20)	1·05 (6)	1·05 (26)
Birth weight (lb):			
≤5·5	1·13 (18)	1·12 (1)	1·13 (19)
−6·5	1·20 (39)	1·09 (15)	1·17 (54)
−7·5	1·08 (104)	1·12 (25)	1·08 (129)
−8·5	1·06 (102)	1·21 (26)	1·09 (128)
−9·5	1·05 (51)	1·15 (13)	1·07 (64)
>9·5	1·01 (27)	1·08 (5)	1·02 (32)
All weights	1·08 (341)	1·14 (85)	1·09 (426)
Geometric standard deviation	1·31	1·29	1·31

Mean systolic blood pressure in the weaned and not weaned groups were similar: 164 mm Hg and 167 mm Hg respectively. Mean diastolic blood pressure was 90 mm Hg in both groups. We have previously analysed plasma concentrations of fibrinogen, factor VII, and glucose in this sample of men (chapters 20 and 22), though without separate analysis by feeding group. Mean concentrations were similar in the weaned and not weaned groups: fibrinogen 3·03 g/l (weaned) and 3·05 g/l (not weaned); factor VII 108% of standard and 108% of standard; glucose two hours after a 75 g oral glucose load 6·6 mmol/l and 6·5 mmol/l. The percentages of men with impaired glucose tolerance or newly diagnosed diabetes mellitus were 24% in the weaned group and 25% in the not weaned group.

We examined the early weights and numbers of teeth at 1 year in the weaned and not weaned group. Mean birth weights were identical (7·9 pounds) but mean weight at 1 year was lower in the not weaned group (22·6 lb weaned v 22·3 lb not weaned). This difference was not significant. Mean numbers of teeth were, however, significantly lower in the not weaned group (6·9 weaned v 6·2 not weaned). The difference between the two groups in numbers of teeth was greatest for babies who had been heaviest at birth. In the three birth weight groups: ⩽7 lb, −8·25 lb, and >8·25 lb, the mean numbers of teeth at 1 year in the weaned group were 6·3, 6·6, and 7·6 respectively compared with 5·8, 6·3, and 6·2 in the not weaned group.

Discussion

We have shown that serum lipid concentrations among adult men and death rates from ischaemic heart disease are related to the method of infant feeding. Among 5471 men born in part of one county in England around 70 years ago those who had been breast fed and had not been weaned at 1 year and those who were exclusively bottle fed from birth had higher death rates from ischaemic heart disease (table I). Examination of those still living in the county showed that these two groups of men also had higher serum total cholesterol, low density lipoprotein cholesterol, and apolipoprotein B concentrations (table II). Each of these is known to be associated with increased risk of ischaemic heart disease. Serum cholesterol concentrations in these two groups of men were raised in fasting and non-fasting blood samples.

The subsample of men whose serum cholesterol concentrations were measured comprised men who were born in east Hertfordshire during 1920–30 and still lived there. As our analysis was based on internal comparisons the selection of the sample would introduce bias only if the relations between infant feeding and serum cholesterol were different in those selected and not selected. This is unlikely. There were no differences in mean birth weight, weight at 1 year, or percentages of men in each infant feeding group between the 485 men examined and the total group of 5471 men who were traced.

The health visitors in Hertfordshire recorded that each baby either was or was not weaned at 1 year. The term weaned can imply either that breast feeding has stopped or that solid food has been introduced. The evidence from the Hertfordshire chief health visitor's annual reports, anecdotal evidence from health visitors who worked in Hertforshire around this period, and contemporary records in Derbyshire (unpublished) suggest that weaned usually meant stopping of breast feeding. In her annual reports the chief health visitor for Hertfordshire quoted percentages of breast fed babies weaned at 12 months but gave no comparable information for bottle fed babies, presumably because the word did not usually apply.[24]

In our analysis the not weaned group comprised babies who were exclusively breast fed. It did not include the few babies who were bottle fed, or breast and bottle fed, who had not been weaned at 1 year. Babies in the not weaned group were therefore still receiving some breast milk at 1 year, but we do not know how much or whether they were receiving solid food as well.

In England at the beginning of the century breast feeding was continued for longer than is usual now but commonly stopped at around 9 months and usually before 1 year.[25 26] More of the men in Hertfordshire who were not weaned at 1 year were born into low social class families. Anecdotal evidence from Hertfordshire suggests that women in lower social classes prolonged breast feeding beyond 1 year as a form of contraception. It could be argued that the raised low density lipoprotein cholesterol concentrations in these men were a consequence of different diet in later life rather than of infant feeding. However, they had raised low density lipoprotein cholesterol concentrations regardless of which social class they had been born into (table III) or of their social class at the time of the survey. Furthermore, these men were similar to those in the other infant feeding groups in respect of all other cardiovascular risk factors, including body mass index and factor VII concentration, which are known to be influenced by adult diet.[27]

EFFECT OF PROLONGED BREAST FEEDING

Our findings suggest that, in babies born 70 years ago who were breast fed and weaned relatively late, a process was established which led to raised serum concentrations of low density lipoprotein cholesterol and increased death rates from ischaemic heart disease in adult life. This process was not linked to high density lipoprotein cholesterol, triglyceride, apolipoprotein A1, or Lp(a) lipoprotein concentrations. Findings from previous studies in Hertfordshire and Preston suggest that adult blood pressure and concentrations of fibrinogen, factor VII, and glucose are partly determined or programmed during critical periods in fetal life and infancy. The critical period may differ for each variable and may be linked to times of rapid growth of the blood vessels, liver, and endocrine pancreas (chapters 16, 20, and 22). The regulation of serum lipid and lipoprotein concentrations involves several tissues, most importantly the liver and gut. Mechanisms by which late weaning of infants may programme lipid metabolism in adults and the tissues which are programmed are a matter of speculation.

Experiments in animals have shown that manipulation of the diets of newborn and weanling animals can produce long term increases in serum lipid, lipoprotein, and apolipoprotein concentrations and changes in the activity of rate limiting hydroxymethyl-glutaryl coenzyme A reductase (cholesterol synthesis) and 7α hydroxylase (bile acid synthesis).[13-15] Though it is not clear which nutrients effect these long term changes, the experiments are clear demonstrations of programming. Experiments with the timing of weaning have shown that premature weaning can raise serum cholesterol in adult animals.[28 29] There have been no studies on the long term effects of late weaning.

INFANT FOODS

Different infant foods are known to have different immediate effects in the human infant. Babies fed on breast milk or cows' milk have higher serum cholesterol concentrations than those fed on modern milk formulas, which have a lower cholesterol content and a higher ratio of polyunsaturated to saturated fatty acid.[9 10] This sensitivity of infants to the fat content of the diet contrasts with the low correlation between dietary fat intake and serum cholesterol concentrations in older children and adults.[4 30 31]

Different infant foods also affect the excretion of bile acids. Breast fed and formula fed infants differ in the quantity of bile acids excreted and in the timing of appearance of secondary bile acids, which depends on the action of gut flora.[32] Breast milk contains several hormones and growth factors that can influence lipid metabolism, including thyroid hormones and steroids.[33 34] Though the effect of these maternal hormones on the infant is unknown, experiments have shown that breast fed baboons have different circulating concentrations of triiodothyronine and cortisol from bottle fed ones (G Mott, personal communication). Babies in Hertfordshire who were not weaned at 1 year would have continued to have a high fat intake from milk and also maternal hormones.

Breast milk provides ideal nourishment for the young infant, but there is evidence that some babies who are exclusively breast fed after 6 months receive inadequate energy.[35] Human breast milk contains low iron concentrations and exclusively breast fed babies commonly develop low iron stores in the latter half of infancy.[36] Breast milk may also be deficient of vitamins, notably vitamin D, if the mother is poorly nourished.[37] In Hertfordshire infants who were not weaned weighed less at 1 year and had fewer teeth than those who were weaned. This may be evidence of poorer

285

nutrition in the not weaned babies, although we cannot say whether these differences were due to late weaning or a cause of it. Among men who had not been weaned it was those who had had higher birth weights but lower weights at 1 year who had the higher death rates from ischaemic heart disease. They also had higher serum total and low density lipoprotein cholesterol concentrations (tables IV, V, and VI). One interpretation of this is that larger babies tended to outgrow an inadequate supply of nutrients.

The men who were exclusively bottle fed, who comprised only 5% of the sample, were similar to the not weaned group in having higher death rates from ischaemic heart disease and higher serum concentrations of low density lipoprotein cholesterol and apolipoprotein B. We do not know what was contained in the bottle feeds because this was not specified in the Hertfordshire records. Bottle foods available 70 years ago included patent preparations of dried cows' milk, unmodified cows' milk, diluted condensed milk, and patent foods made from wheatflour or arrowroot.[38 39] Modern baby-milk formulas differ from these foods: they are fortified with iron and vitamins; the fat content is mainly unsaturated, and the electrolyte content is similar to that of breast milk. It is therefore difficult to assess the relevance of these findings for bottle fed babies today.

We have shown that men who had higher birth weights and weights at 1 year had lower serum concentrations of apolipoprotein B. This was independent of whether or not they had been breast fed beyond 1 year (table VII). A relation between birth weight and apolipoprotein B concentrations has been shown in infants, though in the opposite direction.[40]

CONCLUSIONS

This is the first study of the relation between breast and bottle feeding, age at weaning, and lipids and apolipoprotein concentrations in middle to late life. Previous studies in humans have been limited to children and young adults and related serum cholesterol concentrations to breast or bottle feeding in infancy.[2-7] The results have been inconclusive and largely negative. Our data suggest that age of weaning, and possibly type of milk, may permanently influence serum low density lipoprotein cholesterol concentrations and death rates from ischaemic heart disease.

We thank all the men who gave us their time; and Hertfordshire County archives, which preserved the records. We thank Dr I Clarke for much local help; H Whiteside, C Carr, and staff of the NHS section of the department of clinical biochemistry, Addenbrooke's Hospital, for technical assistance; and B Newland of Princess Alexandra Hospital, Harlow, for storing samples.

1 Chaplin HD. Biology as the basic principle in infant feeding. *Postgraduate (NY)* 1909;24:272–80.
2 Friedman G, Goldberg SJ. Concurrent and subsequent serum cholesterols of breast and formula fed infants. *Am J Clin Nutr* 1975;28:42–5.

3 Hodgson PA, Ellefson RD, Elveback LR, Harris LE, Nelson RA, Weidman WH. Comparison of serum cholesterol in children fed high, moderate or low cholesterol milk diets during neonatal period. *Metabolism* 1976;25:739–46.

4 Anderson GE, Lifschitz C, Früs-Hansen B. Dietary habits and serum lipids during first four years of life. *Acta Paediatr Scand* 1979;68:165–78.

5 Marmot MG, Page CM, Atkins E, Douglas JWB. Effect of breast feeding on plasma cholesterol and weight in young adults. *J Epidemiol Community Health* 1980;34:164–7.

6 Huttunen JK, Saarinen UM, Kostiainen E, Sümes MA. Fat composition of the infant diet does not influence subsequent serum lipid levels in man. *Atherosclerosis* 1983;46:87–94.

7 Fomon SJ, Rogers RR, Ziegler EE, Nelson SE, Thomas LN. Indices of fatness and serum cholesterol at age eight years in relation to feeding and growth during early infancy. *Pediatr Res* 1984;18:1233–8.

8 Fomon SJ, Bartels DJ. Concentrations of cholesterol in serum of infants in relation to diet. *Am Med Assoc J Dis Child* 1960;99:43–6.

9 Darmady JM, Fosbrooke AS, Lloyd JK. Prospective study of serum cholesterol levels during first year of life. *BMJ* 1972;ii:685–8.

10 Van Biervliet JP, Rosseneu M, Caster H. Influence of dietary factors on the plasma lipoprotein composition and content of neonates. *Eur J Pediatr* 1986;144:489–93.

11 Labarthe D, Eissa M, Vara C. Childhood precursors of high blood pressure and elevated cholesterol. *Ann Rev Public Health* 1991;12:519–41.

12 Sporik R, Johnstone JH, Cogswell JJ. Longitudinal study of cholesterol values in 68 children from birth to 11 years of age. *Arch Dis Child* 1991;66:134–7.

13 Mott GE, Jackson EM, McMahan CA, McGill HC. Cholesterol metabolism in adult baboons is influenced by infant diet. *J Nutr* 1990;120:243–51.

14 Hassan AS, Subbiah MTR. Manipulation of cholesterol metabolism in early life: its effect on cholesterol handling and atherosclerosis in adult life. In: Subbiah MTR, ed. *Atherosclerosis: a pediatric perspective*. London: CRC Press, 1989:221–31.

15 Hahn P. Late effects of early nutrition. In: Subbiah MTR, ed. *Atherosclerosis: a pediatric perspective*. London: CRC Press, 1989:155–64.

16 Allain CC, Poon LS, Chan CSG, Richmond W, Fu PC. Enzymatic determination of serum total cholesterol. *Clin Chem* 1974;20:470–5.

17 Lie AF, Schmitz JM, Pierre KJ, Gochman N. Cholesterol oxidase-based determination by continuous flow analysis of total and free cholesterol in serum. *Clin Chem* 1976;22:1627–30.

18 Lopes-Virella MF, Stone P, Ellis S, Colwell JA. Cholesterol determination in high density lipoproteins separated by three different methods. *Clin Chem* 1977;23:882–4.

19 Fossati P, Prencipe L. Serum triglycerides determined colorimetrically with an enzyme that produces hydrogen peroxide. *Clin Chem* 1982;28:2077–80.

20 Friedwalk WT, Levy RI, Fredrickson DS. Estimation of the concentration of low density lipoprotein cholesterol in plasma without use of the preparative ultracentrifuge. *Clin Chem* 1972;18:499–502.

21 Bhatnagar D, Durrington PN. Clinical value of apolipoprotein measurement. *Ann Clin Biochem* 1991;28:427–37.

22 Dagen MM, Packard CJ, Shepherd J. A comparison of commercial kits for the measurement of lipoprotein (a). *Ann Clin Biochem* 1991;28:359–64.

23 Berry G. The analysis of mortality by the subject-years method. *Biometrics* 1983;39:173–84.

24 Burnside EM. Annual report of the Lady Inspector of Midwives. In: *The county medical officer of health's annual report*. Hertfordshire, 1915:41.

25 Whitehead R, Paul A. Changes in infant feeding in Britain during the last century. In: *Infant nutrition and cardiovascular disease*. Southampton: MRC Environmental Epidemiology Unit, 1987:1–10. (Medical Research Council Environmental Epidemiology Unit scientific report No 8.)

26 Breast feeding and weaning. In: *Series II: Baby. Ten minute talks to centre mothers prepared for the use of health visitors*. London: Women Public Health Officers' Association, 1942:1–5.

27 Miller GJ, Martin JC, Webster J, Wilkes H, Miller NE, Wilkinson WH, *et al.* Association between dietary fat intake and plasma factor VII coagulant activity—a predictor of cardiovascular mortality. *Atherosclerosis* 1986;**60**:269–77.

28 Subbiah MTR, Yunker RL, Menkaus A, Poe B. Premature weaning-induced changes of cholesterol metabolism in guinea pigs. *Am J Physiol* 1985;**249**:E251–6.

29 Hahn P, Koldovsky O. Late effect of premature weaning on blood cholesterol levels in adult rats. *Nutrition Reports International* 1976;**13**:87–91.

30 Berenson GS, McMahan CA, Voors AW, Weber LS, Srinivasan SR, Frank GC, *et al.* Dietary studies and the relationship of diet to cardiovascular risk-factor variables in children. In: *Cardiovascular risk factors in children.* New York: Oxford University Press, 1980:289–307.

31 Kannel WB, Gordon T. *The Framingham study: an epidemiological investigation of cardiovascular disease.* Section 24. *The Framingham diet study: diet and the regulation of serum cholesterol.* Washington DC: Department of Health, Education and Welfare, 1978.

32 Hammans JL, Jordan WE, Stewart RL, Jaulbee JD, Berg RW. Age and diet effects on fecal bile acids in infants. *J Ped Gastroenterol Nutr* 1988;**7**:30–8.

33 Koldovsky O, Thornburg W. Hormones in milk: a review. *J Pediatr Gastroenterol Nutr* 1987;**6**:172–96.

34 Salter AM, Fisher SC, Brindley DN. Interactions of triiodothyronine, insulin and dexamethasone on the binding of human LDL to rat hepatocytes in monolayer culture. *Atherosclerosis* 1988;**71**:77–80.

35 Whitehead RG, Paul AA, Ahmed EA. Weaning practices in the UK and variations in anthropometric development. *Acta Paediatr Scand* 1986;Suppl**323**:14–25.

36 Saarinen UM. Need for iron supplementation in infants on prolonged breast feeding. *J Pediatr* 1978;**93**:177–80.

37 Belton NR. Rickets—not only the "English Disease". *Acta Paediatr Scand* 1986;Suppl**323**:68–75.

38 Cheadle WB. *Artificial feeding and food disorders of infants.* 6th ed. London: Smith and Elder, 1906.

39 Paterson D. The next best thing: correct artificial feeding. In: *A chance for every child: a report of lectures given at the 9th winter school for health visitors and school nurses held at Bedford College for Women, University of London, Dec 30th 1929 to Jan 10th 1930.* London: Women Sanitary Inspectors' and Health Visitors' Association, 1930:22–6.

40 Wang XL, Wilken DEL, Dudman NPB. Apolipoproteins A-1 and B and the B/A-1 ratio in the first year of life. *Paediatr Res* 1991;**30**:544–9.

PART X
BODY FAT DISTRIBUTION

26: Early growth and abdominal fatness in adult life

C M LAW, D J P BARKER, C OSMOND, C H D FALL, S J SIMMONDS

Two groups of men were followed up to investigate whether reduced early growth is associated with abdominal fatness in adult life. The first group was 845 men who were born in east Hertfordshire during 1920–30 and still lived there. Their weight at birth and 1 year had been recorded by health visitors. The second group was 239 men who were born in Preston, Lancashire during 1935–42 and still lived in or near the city. Their size at birth had been measured in detail. The ratio of waist circumference to hip girth was measured in both groups of men.

After allowing for body mass index, mean waist to hip ratio fell with increasing birth weight and rose as the ratio of placental weight to birth weight increased. These trends were independent of duration of gestation and therefore reflected retarded fetal growth. Waist to hip ratio also fell with increasing weight at 1 year. All these trends were independent of adult height, alcohol consumption, smoking, social class, and age.

The tendency to store fat abdominally, which is known to increase the risk of cardiovascular disease and diabetes independently of obesity, may be a persisting response to adverse conditions and growth failure in fetal life and infancy.

Introduction

People who are obese, being heavy in relation to their height, have an increased incidence of cardiovascular disease and diabetes.[1] Heavy weight in relation to height, however, which is quantified by a high body mass index (weight/height²), gives no indication of the relative distribution of fat on different parts of the body.[2] Abdominal fatness, as measured by the ratio of waist circumference to hip circumference,[2] increases the risk of cardiovascular disease and diabetes independently of body mass index.[2-7] It is independently associated with high blood pressure,[2-4 6 7] serum concentrations of cholesterol and triglycerides,[2-4 7] and high plasma concentrations of glucose[4-7] and fibrinogen.[2]

Excess intra-abdominal and extra-abdominal fat could have a direct pathogenic effect or it could simply be a marker of other processes. Mechanisms to support both possibilities have been suggested. Lipid mobilisation from the omental and mesenteric fat depots could lead to high concentrations of free fatty acids in the portal blood. This in turn could stimulate synthesis of very low density lipoprotein and low density lipoprotein cholesterol, increase glucose production, and decrease insulin clearance.[8] Alternatively, adrenal overactivity may lead to abdominal fatness and separately to hypertension and impaired glucose tolerance, as occurs in Cushing's disease.[29] These hypotheses are not mutually exclusive,[2] and as yet there is little evidence bearing on either.

Cardiovascular disease and diabetes are associated with retarded growth during fetal life and infancy (chapters 13 and 22). These associations are thought to reflect the long term consequences of growth restraint on the developing vasculature, pancreas, liver, and other tissues. They suggest an explanation for the association between abdominal fatness and disease. A tendency to store fat centrally could be a persisting response to early growth restraint and a marker of it. We have examined the relation between the waist to hip ratio and fetal growth in two samples of adult men.

Subjects and methods

PRESTON

In the city of Preston, England, a standardised record form was kept for each woman admitted to the labour ward at Sharoe Green Hospital during 1935–43. These records are described in chapter 16. Of the singleton boys born during 1935–43, 252 still lived in Lancashire; 239 agreed to be interviewed at home and were visited by one of four fieldworkers. Height was measured with a portable stadiometer, and weight with a portable Seca scale. The waist circumference and hip girth were measured. The man was asked about his social history, smoking, and drinking habits. Alcohol consumption was converted to the total number of units each week (1 unit = 10 ml ethanol). Current social class was derived from the man's occupation.[10] Before starting the study the procedures for the measurements were standardised and the fieldworkers trained.

HERTFORDSHIRE

In the county of Hertfordshire, England, from 1911 onwards, each birth was notified by the attending midwife. A health visitor saw the child at home periodically through infancy and recorded the data described in chapter 13. We traced singleton boys born in east Hertfordshire during 1920–30. Of those who had both birth weight and weight at 1 year recorded, 1157 still live there; 845 agreed to be interviewed at home and were visited by one of four fieldworkers. Height, weight, waist circumference and hip girth, social history, smoking, and alcohol consumption were recorded in the same way as in Preston.

Statistical analysis was by multiple linear regression. For clarity of presentation waist to hip ratio has been expressed as a percentage.

Results

The characteristics of the men in each place are given in table I. Men in Hertfordshire weighed more at birth, were older, drank less alcohol, and smoked less. Placental weight was not available in Hertfordshire and weight at 1 year was not available in Preston.

In both places waist to hip ratio was positively related to weight and body mass index but not to height. In Preston the regression coefficients were

TABLE I—*Characteristics of the men, by place of study*

	Preston (n = 239)			Hertfordshire (n = 845)		
	Mean (standard deviation)			*Mean (standard deviation)*		
Birth weight (lb)	7·0 (1·2)			7·9 (1·3)		
Placental weight (lb)	1·4 (0·3)			Not available		
Weight at 1 year (lb)	Not available			22·6 (2·6)		
Age (years)	51 (2)			64 (3)		
Height (m)	1·72 (0·07)			1·72 (0·07)		
Weight (kg)	79·8 (13·5)			78·9 (12·7)		
Body mass index (kg/m²)	26·9 (4·3)			26·8 (3·8)		
Waist to hip ratio (%)	93·3 (6·2)			93·5 (5·3)		
		Quartiles			*Quartiles*	
	(lower)	*(median)*	*(upper)*	*(lower)*	*(median)*	*(upper)*
Alcohol consumption (units)	2	11	29	0	3	9
		No (%)			*No (%)*	
Never smoker		51 (21)			129 (15)	
Current smoker		94 (39)			243 (29)	
Ex-smoker		94 (39)			468 (56)	

0·22 (standard error 0·026) for weight in kilograms and 0·70 (0·083) for body mass index in kg/metre². In Hertfordshire they were 0·22 (0·012) for weight and 0·82 (0·040) for body mass index. In both places waist to hip ratio was positively related to alcohol consumption but this did not reach significance. Waist to hip ratio was positively related to smoking in Preston and negatively related to smoking in Hertfordshire, but neither of these reached significance.

Waist to hip ratio was not related to birth weight in either place, nor to placental weight in Preston or to weight at 1 year in Hertfordshire. Body weight and mass, however, were related to both birth weight and weight at 1 year. We therefore allowed for body mass index in our analysis of the relations between waist to hip ratio and early weight. Waist to hip ratio was inversely related to birth weight (table II(a)). In contrast, it was positively related to placental weight, though this did not reach significance (table II(b)). In a simultaneous regression with body mass index, waist to hip ratio rose as the ratio of placental weight to birth weight increased (p = 0·05). Although waist to hip ratio was inversely related to weight at 1 year, this relation was not significant in a simultaneous analysis with birth weight (table II(c)).

In Preston and Hertfordshire the association of birth weight and the waist to hip ratio was stronger in men with higher body mass indices. This interaction was significant in Hertfordshire.

Duration of gestation, age, social class, smoking, and alcohol consumption were not related to waist to hip ratio after allowing for body mass index.

TABLE II—*Simultaneous effects of adult body mass index and weights at birth and at 1 year on waist to hip ratio (%)*

	Preston Regression coefficient (95% confidence interval)	Hertfordshire Regression coefficient (95% confidence interval)
(a):		
Adult body mass index (kg/m²)	0·70 (0·54 to 0·86)	0·83 (0·75 to 0·91)
Birth weight (lb)	−0·56 (−1·12 to 0·00)	−0·29 (−0·52 to −0·05)
(b):		
Adult body mass index (kg/m²)	0·70 (0·54 to 0·86)	
Birth weight (lb)	−0·83 (−1·50 to −0·15)	
Placental weight (lb)	1·76 (−0·73 to 4·24)	
(c):		
Adult body mass index (kg/m²)		0·83 (0·75 to 0·91)
Birth weight (lb)		−0·20 (−0·46 to −0·06)
Weight at 1 year (lb)		−0·10 (−0·23 to −0·03)

Discussion

We have shown that in adult men a higher waist to hip ratio, which is an indicator of abdominal fatness,[2] is associated with reduced growth during fetal life and infancy. Waist to hip ratio rose with increasing obesity, as measured by the body mass index, but at any level of obesity there was more abdominal fat in men who weighed less at birth and at 1 year (table II). This relation was most pronounced in those with the highest body mass indices. The associations between early growth and waist to hip ratio were independent of alcohol consumption, cigarette smoking, and social class.

The association between waist to hip ratio and lower birth weight was independent of the duration of gestation, and must therefore reflect an association with reduced fetal growth. At any birth weight waist to hip ratio increased with placental weight (table II(b)) so that the highest waist to hip ratios were in men who had low birth weight in relation to their placental weight. Low birth weight for placental weight may be interpreted as a sign of fetal growth failure (chapter 17). Other analyses of the Preston data have shown that low birth weight for placental weight is also related to high systolic and diastolic blood pressure (chapter 16), high plasma fibrinogen concentrations (chapter 20) and impaired glucose tolerance (unpublished data). The processes which link reduced fetal growth with increased abdominal fat deposition are unknown. Sustained adrenal overactivity,[2] initiated by early growth restraint, is one possible explanation.

Differences in the waist to hip ratio have been shown to correspond with substantial differences in risk of ischaemic heart disease, even after adjustment for body mass index.[2] In a study of men aged 54 who had a similar distribution of waist to hip ratio to that described here, those who were in the highest fifth of waist to hip ratio had a risk 2·5 times higher than those in the lowest fifth.[3]

It could be argued that people who experience an adverse early environment, which restrains fetal and infant growth, tend to remain in adverse environments and that the association between lower early weight and higher adult waist to hip ratio reflects influences acting later in life. In our data, however, the mean waist to hip ratio did not differ with different social classes, as would be expected from this argument.

Our findings are also open to the interpretation that genetic influences determine both reduced early growth and later abdominal fatness. The similarity of fat distribution in siblings, especially identical twins, has led to the suggestion that, unlike body mass, abdominal fat distribution has an important genetic contribution.[11 12] These similarities could, however, reflect similar intrauterine and infant environments rather than genetic resemblance.

1 Jarrett R. Is there an ideal body weight? *BMJ* 1986;**293**:493–5.
2 Bjorntrop P. The associations between obesity, adipose tissue distribution, and disease. *Acta Med Scand* 1988;Suppl723:121–34.
3 Larsson B, Svardsudd K, Welin L, Wilhelmsen J, Bjorntrop P, Tibblin G. Abdominal adipose tissue distribution, obesity, and risk of cardiovascular disease and death: 13 year follow up of participants in the study of men born in 1913. *BMJ* 1984;**288**:1401–4.
4 Lapidus L, Bengtsson C, Larsson B, Pennert K, Rybo E, Sjostrom L. Distribution of adipose tissue and risk of cardiovascular disease and death: a 12 year follow up of participants in the population study of women in Gothenburg, Sweden. *BMJ* 1984;**289**:1257–61.
5 Ohlson L-O, Larsson B, Svardsudd K, *et al.* The influence of body fat distribution on the incidence of diabetes mellitus: 13·5 years of follow-up of the participants in the study of men born in 1913. *Diabetes* 1985;**34**:1055–8.
6 Hartz A, Rupley D, Rimm A. The association of girth measurements with disease in 32,856 women. *Am J Epidemiol* 1984;**119**:71–80.
7 Despres JP, Moorjani S, Lupien PJ, Tremblay A, Nadeau A, Bouchard C. Regional distribution of body fat, plasma lipoproteins and cardiovascular disease. *Arteriosclerosis* 1990;**10**:497–511.
8 Bjorntrop P. "Portal" adipose tissue as a generator of risk factors for cardiovascular disease and diabetes. *Arteriosclerosis* 1990;**10**:493–6.
9 Seidell JC, Cigolini M, Charzewska J, *et al.* Androgenicity in relation to body fat distribution and metabolism in 38 year old women—the European fat distribution study. *J Clin Epidemiol* 1990;**43**:21–34.
10 Office of Population Censuses and Surveys. *Classification of occupations 1980*. London: HMSO, 1980.
11 Bouchard C. Genetic factors in the regulation of adipose tissue distribution. *Acta Med Scand (Suppl)* 1988;(suppl)723:135–41.
12 Selby JV, Newman B, Quesenberry CP, *et al.* Genetic and behavioural influences on body fat distribution. *Int J Obesity* 1990;**14**:593–602.

PART XI
FETAL GROWTH

27: Effect of maternal anaemia and iron deficiency on ratio of fetal weight to placental weight

K M GODFREY, C W G REDMAN, D J P BARKER,
C OSMOND

Large placental weight and a high ratio of placental weight to birth weight are known predictors of adult blood pressure. To examine the maternal influences that determine them, the obstetric and haematology records of 8684 pregnant women were analysed.

Large placental weight was associated with a low maternal haemoglobin and a fall in maternal mean cell volume during pregnancy. The highest ratio of placental weight to birth weight occurred in the most anaemic women with the largest falls in mean cell volume. Large placental weight and a high ratio of placental weight to birth weight were also independently associated with a high maternal body mass index. Maternal smoking reduced placental weight, but increased the ratio of placental weight to birth weight.

It was concluded that anaemia and iron deficiency during pregnancy are associated with large placental weight and a high ratio of placental weight to birth weight. This points to maternal nutritional deficiency as a cause for discordance between placental and fetal growth. This may have important implications for the prevention of adult hypertension, which appears to have its origin in fetal life.

Introduction

High blood pressure in adult life is linked to lower birth weight (chapter 16). In a recent follow up study of 449 men and women aged around 50 years who had been born in Preston, Lancashire the highest systolic and diastolic blood pressures occurred in people who had had heavy placentas and whose birth weight had been lower than might be expected from their placental weight. These relations between measurements at birth and adult blood pressure were independent of current body mass index and alcohol intake.

Birth weight below that expected from placental weight was not limited to babies with low birth weight as currently defined. Most of the babies who failed to match their placental weight were of around the average birth weight but had a larger than average placenta. The maternal influences which lead to this discordance between fetal and placental weight and hence high blood pressure are not known. Impaired nutrition and smoking are two possibilities.

We have therefore analysed antenatal data recorded routinely for 8684 women attending a maternity hospital in Oxford. Maternal dietary intakes are not of course measured during routine antenatal care. Haemoglobin and other red cell indices, however, are established indicators of nutrition.[1] The Oxford record linkage system allows haematology files to be linked direct to birth outcomes.

Subjects and methods

Between January 1987 and January 1989 there were 12 929 deliveries of liveborn singleton babies at the John Radcliffe Hospital, Oxford whose antenatal care had been in Oxford. The Oxford record linkage system enabled the obstetric data for 11 312 of these pregnancies to be linked to the results of full blood counts taken during the pregnancy. Failure to link the remainder largely resulted from a switch during the study period from unit number allocation by the maternity hospital to unit number allocation by the district. We limited our analysis to the 8684 pregnancies with two or more blood counts.

The obstetric data included maternal age, parity, height, weight at booking and at the last antenatal visit before delivery, smoking habits, first and maximum blood pressure, proteinuria, gestational age at delivery (estimated from the last menstrual period and ultrasound scan), infant sex, birth weight, placental weight, and head circumference. Untrimmed placentas were weighed immediately after delivery. Complete data were available for 7903 pregnancies. Data on social class (coded by head of household's occupation) were available for 7423 of them.

Blood counts were determined on Technicon H6000 and Coulter S Plus

4 analysers using standard automated techniques. Changes in mean cell volume during the pregnancy were assessed by comparison with the mean cell volume at booking. Maternal body mass index, calculated as weight/height^2, was estimated only for women whose first recorded weight measurement was before 20 weeks' gestation. Discordance between birth weight and placental weight was assessed by calculating the placental ratio, as placental weight/birth weight, and by adjusting the placental weight for the birth weight.[2] These indices gave similar results, so we present those for the placental ratio. The simultaneous trends in placental weight and in placental ratio with the lowest maternal haemoglobin concentration and fall in mean cell volume were analysed by multiple regression.

Results

Both the lowest maternal haemoglobin concentration during pregnancy and the fall in mean cell volume were independently related to increased placental weight. In table I the divisions of maternal haemoglobin are based on the definition given by the World Health Organisation of pregnancy anaemia as a haemoglobin concentration of $< 11\cdot0$ g/dl,[3] and on a commonly used clinical definition of $10\cdot0$ g/dl.[4] A fall in mean cell volume is probably the most sensitive indicator of iron deficiency assessable from serial routine full blood count measurements.[5] At each level of haemoglobin, mean placental weight increased with falling mean cell volume. The increase in mean placental weight associated with a fall in mean cell volume greater than 6 fl ranged between 31 and 56 g at different haemoglobin levels. Likewise, at each level of fall in mean cell volume, placental weight rose as haemoglobin fell. The highest mean placental weights therefore occurred in women with a low haemoglobin concentration and a large fall

TABLE I—*Mean placental weights (g), according to lowest maternal haemoglobin concentration during pregnancy and fall in mean cell volume. Number of women in parentheses*

Lowest haemoglobin concentration (g/dl)	Fall in mean cell volume (fl)			
	$\leqslant 4$	4–6	> 6	All
$\leqslant 9\cdot9$	634 (485)	673 (95)	672 (270)	650 (850)
$10\cdot0$–$10\cdot9$	622 (1777)	629 (331)	653 (392)	628 (2500)
$11\cdot0$–$11\cdot9$	605 (2841)	617 (312)	639 (222)	608 (3375)
$\geqslant 12\cdot0$	583 (1780)	594 (129)	639 (50)	585 (1959)
All	606 (6883)	624 (867)	654 (934)	613* (8684)

* Standard deviation = 129 g.

in mean cell volume, and the lowest weights occurred in women with a high haemoglobin and little or no fall in mean cell volume. The associations between placental weight and both minimum haemoglobin and fall in mean cell volume were highly significant (p < 0·0001).

As expected, lowest haemoglobin values and the fall in mean cell volume were associated. A fall in mean cell volume of > 4 fl occurred in 43, 29, 16, and 9% of women whose lowest haemoglobin concentrations were < 10·0, 10·0–10·9, 11·0–11·9, and ⩾ 12·0 g/dl respectively.

Birth weight increased with lower maternal haemoglobin and with larger fall in mean cell volume (table II). The differences, however, were proportionally smaller than those with placental weight (table I).

Because placental weights approach term values at an earlier stage of gestation than do birth weights, it follows that the ratio of placental weight to birth weight increases with increasing degree of fetal immaturity. In turn, and consistent with previous findings,[6] low maternal haemoglobin was associated with preterm delivery. In view of this, we analysed the placental ratio only for babies born after 38 completed weeks' (266 days') gestation estimated from the last menstrual period or an ultrasound scan before 20 weeks' gestation (table III). Overall, there were independent significant trends towards increasing placental ratios in association with lower maternal haemoglobin (p < 0·0001) and with larger falls in mean cell volume (p < 0·0001). The highest placental ratios therefore occurred in the most anaemic women with the largest falls in mean cell volume, and the lowest ratios in women with a high haemoglobin concentration and little or no fall in mean cell volume.

Table IV shows the percentage distribution of lowest haemoglobin values for women in each of three social class groupings: 41% of women in social classes IV and V had a haemoglobin below 11·0 g/dl, compared with 33% of women in social classes I and II (difference 8%, 95% confidence intervals 5% to 11%). Likewise, 23% of women in social classes IV and V

TABLE II—*Mean birth weights (g), according to lowest maternal haemoglobin concentration during pregnancy and fall in mean cell volume. Number of women in parentheses*

Lowest haemoglobin concentration (g/dl)	Fall in mean cell volume (fl)			
	⩽4	4–6	>6	All
⩽9·9	3384 (485)	3536 (95)	3483 (270)	3432 (850)
−10·9	3353 (1777)	3404 (331)	3481 (392)	3380 (2500)
−11·9	3333 (2841)	3388 (312)	3454 (222)	3346 (3375)
⩾12·0	3232 (1780)	3252 (129)	3428 (50)	3238 (1959)
All	3315 (6883)	3390 (867)	3472 (934)	3340* (8684)

* Standard deviation = 545 g

TABLE III—*Mean ratio of placental weight to birth weight (placental ratio), according to lowest maternal haemoglobin concentration during pregnancy and fall in mean cell volume for babies born after 265 days' gestation. Number of women in parentheses*

Lowest haemoglobin concentration (g/dl)	Fall in mean cell volume (fl)			
	≤4	4–6	>6	All
≤9·9	0·185 (436)	0·188 (84)	0·192 (254)	0·188 (774)
−10·9	0·184 (1642)	0·184 (311)	0·187 (369)	0·185 (2322)
−11·9	0·180 (2623)	0·181 (291)	0·184 (210)	0·181 (3124)
≥12·0	0·179 (1596)	0·182 (115)	0·186 (47)	0·179 (1758)
All	0·181 (6297)	0·183 (801)	0·187 (880)	0·182* (7978)

* Standard deviation = 0·028.

experienced a fall in mean cell volume of >4 fl, compared with 19% of women in social classes I and II (difference 4%, 95% confidence interval 2% to 7%).

We used multiple regression analysis to analyse the simultaneous relations of maternal haemoglobin, fall in mean cell volume, smoking habits, and physique with the placental ratio for babies born after 38 weeks of gestation (table V). The placental ratio in each group is given as the difference from that of the baseline group. The size of the trends in placental ratio with lowest haemoglobin and fall in mean cell volume shown in table III was only slightly changed by adjustment for the other variables. Inclusion of gestational age at delivery in the regression equation confirmed that these associations were independent of the length of gestation. Maternal smoking was associated with a small reduction in placental weight and a larger reduction in birth weight and therefore with an increase in placental ratio. Women with the highest body mass index had a mean placental ratio 0·0069 higher than those with the lowest body mass index as

TABLE IV—*Percentage distribution of lowest haemoglobin concentration during pregnancy by social class. Number of women in parentheses*

Lowest haemoglobin concentration (g/dl)	Social class			
	I and II	III	IV and V	All
≤9·9	7 (209)	10 (317)	12 (151)	9 (677)
−10·9	26 (757)	30 (964)	29 (372)	28 (2093)
−11·9	42 (1230)	38 (1200)	39 (496)	39 (2926)
≥12·0	26 (754)	22 (704)	21 (269)	23 (1727)
All	100 (2950)	100 (3185)	100 (1288)	100 (7423)

TABLE V—*Multiple regression analysis of the ratio of placental weight to birth weight (placental ratio) (95% confidence interval) associated with maternal lowest haemoglobin concentration, fall in mean cell volume, smoking habits, and body mass index for babies born after 265 days' gestation*

	No of women	Increase in placental ratio relative to baseline group ($\times 10^{-3}$)
Lowest haemoglobin concentration (g/dl)		
≤9·9	706	7·0 (4·4 to 9·5)
−10·9	2130	4·2 (2·3 to 6·0)
−11·9	2833	1·2 (−0·5 to 2·9)
≥12·0	1590	0
Fall in mean cell volume (fl)		
≤4	5717	0
−6	729	0·8 (−1·4 to 2·9)
>6	813	4·4 (2·3 to 6·5)
Cigarettes smoked/day during pregnancy		
0	5725	0
1–10	814	8·8 (6·8 to 10·8)
≥11	720	9·4 (7·2 to 11·5)
Maternal body mass index (kg/m²)*		
≤21·5	1295	0
−23·5	1447	3·2 (1·2 to 5·3)
−26·0	1293	3·5 (1·4 to 5·6)
>26·0	1354	6·9 (4·8 to 9·0)
Not estimated	1870	4·6 (2·6 to 6·5)

Intercept = 0·174.

* Maternal body mass index was not estimated for women who booked after 20 weeks' gestation.

a consequence of an increase in placental weight that was not matched by the smaller increase in birth weight. In contrast to the findings for body mass index, the increase in placental weight associated with tall maternal stature was fully matched by a similar increase in birth weight, such that there was no significant relation between maternal stature and the placental ratio (data not shown).

Further analysis showed no significant associations between the placental ratio and maternal age, parity, blood pressure, and proteinuria.

Discussion

We have shown that large placental weight and a high placental ratio, both known predictors of higher adult blood pressure (chapter 16), are related to low maternal haemoglobin and to a fall in mean cell volume.

This series of pregnant women came from the total population of women who had antenatal and intrapartum care during two years in the maternity hospital in Oxford. They were selected only by their obstetric records being linked with results of two or more full blood counts taken during the pregnancy. The mean placental ratio for pregnancies that were not linked to two or more blood count results was similar to that for pregnancies that were linked, 0·186 compared with 0·185. The mean haemoglobin concentration in the first half of pregnancy was 12·3 g/dl for both the study population and for pregnancies excluded because they had fewer than two blood counts.

Maternal smoking and body mass index were also significantly associated with the placental ratio, but the relations with low maternal haemoglobin and the fall in mean cell volume were independent of these variables. In a study of 4 year old children in Salisbury, blood pressure was related to maternal anaemia and low mean cell volume, but not to maternal smoking and body mass index (chapter 18). The relation of pregnancy anaemia and low mean cell volume with blood pressure at 4 years of age suggests that factors influencing haemoglobin synthesis during pregnancy may be associated not only with discordance between placental weight and birth weight, but also with adult hypertension.

Severe maternal anaemia is known to be associated with large placental weight.[4] The dilutional fall in maternal haemoglobin during pregnancy due to a disproportionate increase in plasma volume may be thought of as reflecting good placental function, and thus likely to be associated with larger placental weight. In a study of normal pregnant women, however, stainable bone marrow stores of iron were absent in all women with haemoglobin values below 10·4 g/dl.[7] In the same study, oral iron treatment from early pregnancy completely prevented the mid trimester fall in haemoglobin that is commonly seen. WHO committees have concluded that pregnancy haemoglobin values below 11·0 g/dl should not be considered physiological,[3] but rather as nutritional in origin.[8] The association of low social class with lower minimum haemoglobin (table IV) and higher falls in mean cell volume during pregnancy strengthens the argument that these variables reflect poor maternal nutrition.

The fall in mean cell volume associated with a high placental ratio contrasts with the usual small rise in mean cell volume in normal pregnancy.[9] It points to iron deficiency.[5] A fall in mean cell volume of > 4 fl occurred in 43% of the pregnancies with lowest haemoglobin levels $< 10·0$ g/dl and in 29% of those with lowest haemoglobin levels between 10·0 and 10·9 g/dl.

There are several possible explanations for the association between iron deficiency and both large placental weight and high placental ratio. It is unlikely that a relatively larger placenta would itself lead to greater consumption of maternal iron stores because the total iron content of the placenta is so much smaller than that of the fetus.[10] Rather, we suggest that the large placental weight and high placental ratio are a consequence of iron deficiency, which induces placental hypertrophy that is disproportionate to fetal size.

As yet we can only speculate on mechanisms linking maternal anaemia and iron deficiency with high blood pressure. One possible explanation is that placental hypertrophy leads to a fast fetal growth path. The most rapidly growing fetuses are then most susceptible to nutrient deficiency, leading to relative failure of somatic growth and abnormal blood vessel growth.

A haemoglobin below the WHO definition of pregnancy anaemia or a fall in mean cell volume greater than 4 fl occurred in 47% of our study population. This suggests that pregnancy associated iron deficiency is still an extremely common condition in this country.

At present our view is that the importance of advice to pregnant women to follow a balanced healthy diet should be reinforced. A recent study showed that supplementation with vitamins and minerals including iron during pregnancy had no effect on birth dimensions when given during the last two trimesters of pregnancy. In contrast, there was a strong relation between birth dimensions and the recorded maternal intake of many nutrients in the first trimester.[11] More specific advice to pregnant women must await further studies.

We thank the coding staff of the Oxford Obstetric Data System, and Dr J McVittae of the Oxford Department of Clinical Biochemistry, for their help in preparing the data.

1 Medical Research Council. *Haemoglobin levels in Great Britain in 1943*. London: HMSO, 1945. Special report series No 252.

2 Heath D, Williams DR. Fetal and placental size and risk of hypertension in adult life. *BMJ* 1990;**301**:441.

3 World Health Organisation. Nutritional anaemias. *WHO Tech Rep Ser* 1968; No 405.

4 Beischer NA, Sivasamboo R, Vohra S, Silpisornkosal S, Reid S. Placental hypertrophy in severe pregnancy anaemia. *Journal of Obstetrics and Gynaecology of the British Commonwealth* 1970;**77**:398–409.

5 Taylor DJ. Prophylaxis and treatment of anaemia during pregnancy. *Clin Obstet Gynecol* 1981;**8**:297–314.

6 Kaltreider DF, Kohl S. Epidemiology of preterm delivery. *Clin Obstet Gynecol* 1980;**23**:17–31.

7 de Leeuw NKM, Lowenstein L, Hsieh Y-S. Iron deficiency and hydremia in normal pregnancy. *Medicine* 1966;**45**:291–315.

8 DeMaeyer EM. *Preventing and controlling iron deficiency anaemia through primary health care*. Geneva: World Health Organisation, 1989.

9 Chanarin I, McFadyen IR, Kyle R. The physiological macrocytosis of pregnancy. *Br J Obstet Gynaecol* 1977;**84**:504–8.

10 Widdowson EM. Demands of the fetal and maternal tissues. In: Dobbing J, ed. *Maternal nutrition in pregnancy—eating for two?* New York and London: Academic Press, 1981:8.

11 Doyle W, Crawford MA, Wynn HA, Wynn SW. The association between maternal diet and birth dimensions. *Journal of Nutrition and Medicine* 1990;**1**:9–17.

28: Fetal heart rate and intrauterine growth

S M ROBINSON, T WHEELER, M C HAYES,
D J P BARKER, C OSMOND

A prospective study of fetal heart rates in 63 primigravid women was carried out to investigate whether fetal heart rate in early and late pregnancy relates to the size of babies at birth.

There were no differences in heart rate between the sexes at 18 weeks gestation, but by 36 weeks the boys had rates which were 4·4 beats per minute lower than those of the girls. Higher fetal heart rate at 18 weeks was associated with lower ponderal index, smaller head circumference, and smaller mid-arm circumference. There were no trends in fetal heart rate at 36 weeks with any birth measurements.

Babies born at term who have a pattern of neonatal measurements which reflect growth retardation have raised heart rates in early pregnancy. Influences which impair fetal growth appear to take effect early in gestation.

Introduction

Recent studies have shown that patterns of fetal growth are strongly associated with blood pressure in adult life. In 449 men and women aged around 50 who had been born in Preston, Lancashire, blood pressure was inversely related to birth weight but was positively associated with placental weight (chapter 16). Men and women who had had relatively low birth weights but high placental weights were at the highest risk of developing hypertension. Further analyses of these data characterised two groups of babies, born at term, who developed high blood pressure as adults. The first were thin, having a below average birth weight, head circumference, and placental weight. The second were short in relation to their head circumference, and had above average birth weight and placental weight (chapter 17).

The processes established prenatally which are associated with thinness at birth, or disproportionate head size and length, and which lead thereafter to high adult blood pressure, are not known. One such process could be the intrauterine "setting" of heart rate, as pulse rate is known to relate positively to blood pressure both in children and in adults (chapter 15).[1]

The aim of the present study was to investigate the changes in fetal heart rate occurring during gestation, and to relate these to birth weight, placental weight, and anthropometric measurements made on the infant at birth.

Subjects and methods

In total, 75 out of a series of 86 primigravid women approached while attending their first antenatal clinic at the Princess Anne Hospital, Southampton agreed to take part in the study. All subjects were normotensive and without any relevant medical history. Their mean (SD) age was 24·7 (4·5) years. Measurements of fetal heart rate were made in early pregnancy (15–21 weeks) and later pregnancy (34–39 weeks). Gestational age was estimated from the date of the last menstrual period, and checked by a routine ultrasound scan made in early pregnancy; for nine women in whom these were discrepant by more than two weeks the scan age was used. Overall 70 women (93%) completed the study. Of the remaining five women, three had fetuses who died before 24 weeks gestation and two were delivered before a second measurement of fetal heart rate was made. Two women were not included in the analysis because their placental weights were not recorded. Five women had preterm deliveries (<37 weeks' gestation) and were also excluded. We present therefore an analysis of 63 babies (31 boys and 32 girls). Complications occurred in five pregnancies (8%); these were mild pregnancy induced hypertension in two, minor antepartum haemorrhage in two, and anaemia in one. The value taken for the mothers' systolic blood pressure was their highest level recorded in the antenatal clinics during pregnancy. The study was approved by the local ethics committee.

MEASUREMENT OF FETAL HEART RATE

Fetal heart rate was measured using wide beamed pulsed Doppler ultrasound (Hewlett Packard 8041A), over a 20–30 minute period while the woman rested in a semirecumbent position. The fetal heart rate record was divided into five-minute epochs, and the average baseline heart rate was calculated for each epoch. The final heart rate was usually derived from the average of at least four epochs. However, problems were encountered in some of the early pregnancy recordings when contact with the fetal heart could be lost for several minutes as a result of fetal activity. In these fetuses the average of at least three five-minute epochs was used to derive the heart rate. From 34 weeks' gestation, heart rate was measured during periods of low heart rate variation.[23] All heart rate recordings were analysed at the end of the study by the same observer (SR) and a sample of 95 traces was assessed independently by a second observer (TW). The mean (SD) difference between observers was 0·1 beats/min (2·9). Analysis of variation in fetal heart rate in early pregnancy, measured in a sample of six babies studied on three occasions during the same week, showed a within subject standard deviation of 1·6 beats/min.

ANTHROPOMETRIC MEASUREMENTS

The measurements made on each infant were head (maximum occipito-frontal) circumference, chest and mid-arm circumferences, crown to heel length, and subscapular skinfold thickness. All measurements were made three times, with the exception of subscapular skinfold thickness, which was measured once. A mean of the three values was calculated. All measurements were made by one person (SR): 72% were made on the second day after delivery, and all were made within three days.

DATA ANALYSIS

Unpaired t tests were used to compare means for the two sexes. Regression was used to examine relations between variables. An assessment of discordance between placental weight and birth weight was made by calculating the placental ratio (placental weight/birth weight). The fetal heart rate data from the 70 women who completed the study, including 36 additional measurements obtained between 28 and 34 weeks, were analysed using the LMS method of Cole.[4] Standard normal scores for fetal heart rates in early (15–21 weeks) or late (34–39 weeks) pregnancy were derived. These scores were transformed to become standardised heart rates at 18·0 or 36·0 weeks, permitting direct comparison between individuals regardless of the exact date of their measurement.

Results

The figure shows the values of fetal heart rate for the 63 babies. Fetal heart rate fell with advancing gestation while the spread in values among the babies increased. The rate of fall in fetal heart rate changed over the course of gestation, being greatest in early pregnancy (15–21 weeks) and slowing in later pregnancy (34–39 weeks).

The mean values of fetal heart rate, standardised as described, are given in table I. At 18 weeks, values for the two sexes were similar, but by 36 weeks a significant difference had emerged, with boys having heart rates 4·4 beats/min lower than those of the girls (95% confidence interval 0·8 to 8·0,

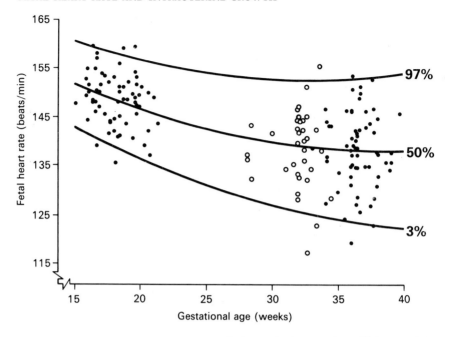

Fetal heart rates recorded from 63 women during early (•; n=63), mid (○; n=35), and late (•; n=63) gestation. Centiles derived from 70 women (see subjects and methods).

p=0·02). The two sexes were of similar size at birth. Using a test at the 5% level, there were no significant differences in average weight, length, head, chest, and mid-arm circumference or in placental weight or placental ratio. The girls were, however, fatter than the boys, having greater mean subscapular skinfold thickness—5·1 mm compared with 4·5 mm (difference 0·7 mm, 95% confidence interval 0·2 to 1·2, p=0·01)—and a higher mean ponderal index—2·79 compared with 2·67 (difference 0·12, 95% confidence interval 0·01 to 0·23, p=0·03).

Mean values of birth measurements and maternal blood pressure are given in table II. Higher heart rate at 18 weeks' gestation was associated

TABLE I—*Mean fetal heart rates (beats/min) in early and late gestation*

Gestation (weeks)	Fetal heart rate (beats/min)	
	Boys (n=31)	Girls (n=32)
18	148·5 (6·1)	148·7 (4·4)
36	135·7* (8·8)	140·1 (5·3)

Figures in parentheses are standard deviations.
* p=0·02 boys *v* girls.

TABLE II—*Regressions of birth measurements and maternal blood pressure with fetal heart rate at 18 and 36 weeks*

Dependent variable	Mean (SD)	18 weeks			36 weeks		
		Slope/beat	95% CI	p	Slope/beat	95% CI	p
Birthweight (g)	3469 (407)	−22·0	−40·9 to −3·1	0·02	−0·65	−15·1 to 13·8	0·93
Head circumference (cm)	35·0 (1·3)	−0·08	−0·14 to −0·02	0·01	−0·03	−0·07 to 0·02	0·27
Length (cm)	50·3 (1·8)	−0·02	−0·11 to 0·07	0·63	0·01	−0·05 to 0·08	0·75
Gestation (weeks)	40·2 (1·3)	−0·05	−0·12 to 0·01	0·09	0·00	−0·05 to 0·05	0·95
Ponderal index (g/cm³ × 100)	2·73 (0·23)	−0·01	−0·02 to 0·00	0·01	0·00	−0·01 to 0·01	0·49
Mid-arm circumference (cm)	10·9 (0·8)	−0·04	−0·08 to 0·00	0·05	0·01	−0·02 to 0·04	0·60
Placental weight (g)	647 (111)	−0·63	−6·05 to 4·80	0·82	−1·29	−5·26 to 2·68	0·52
Maximum maternal systolic blood pressure (mm Hg)	126·5 (9·9)	−0·24	−0·70 to 0·22	0·30	0·16	−0·18 to 0·49	0·36

CI = confidence interval.

with lower birth weight and smaller head circumference, but there was no association with length. Lower fetal heart rates at 18 weeks tended to be associated with a longer gestation, though this was not significant. Allowance for duration of pregnancy reduced, but did not abolish, the associations of heart rate with birth weight and head circumference. Higher fetal heart rate at 18 weeks was associated with a lower ponderal index at birth, an association which was independent of duration of pregnancy. Heart rate was also inversely related to mid-arm circumference. It was not related to placental weight, placental ratio, maximum maternal systolic pressure, subscapular skinfold thickness, or chest circumference. The slope and 95% confidence interval for the association between each birth measurement and fetal heart rate at 36 weeks are also given in table II. Heart rate at 36 weeks was not related to any birth measurement or to the maternal blood pressure.

Table III shows that there were significant associations between ponderal index and head circumference ($p = 0.0003$), mid-arm circumference ($p < 0.0001$), and subscapular skinfold thickness ($p = 0.0004$).

Although maternal systolic pressure was not related to fetal heart rate at 18 or 36 weeks (table II), the magnitude of the fall in heart rate over the period was inversely related to the maternal blood pressure. This relation was not, however, significant ($p = 0.08$). The smallest falls in heart rate were found in babies of mothers whose maximum systolic blood pressure was above 130 mm Hg, the fall being 8·4 beats/min compared with 12·3 beats/min in the babies whose mothers had a maximum blood pressure of ≤ 120 mm Hg. There were no significant differences in heart rate between the babies of mothers who smoked during pregnancy ($n = 15$) and those who did not smoke ($n = 48$).

Discussion

We have examined fetal heart rates at 18 and 36 weeks in 63 primigravid women whose babies were born at term. The fall in basal fetal heart rate

TABLE III—*Head and mid-arm circumferences and subscapular skinfold thickness, in relation to thirds of ponderal index*

Thirds of ponderal index (g/cm³ × 100)	Head circumference (cm)	Mid-arm circumference (cm)	Subscapular skinfold thickness (mm)
−2·62	34·4 (1·3)	10·4 (0·8)	4·2 (0·8)
−2·81	34·9 (1·4)	10·9 (0·8)	4·8 (1·0)
>2·81	35·6 (0·9)	11·3 (0·7)	5·4 (1·2)

Figures in parentheses are standard deviations.

with advancing gestation which we found accords with the findings of other studies.[5 6] Our data confirm those of Wheeler and Murrills who showed a slowing in the rate of fall together with an increasing variability among fetuses in the values in late pregnancy.[2]

To our knowledge a difference in fetal heart rate between the sexes at 36 weeks has not been found in other studies. It is possible that, by calculating a "standardised" 36 week value which takes into account the important effect of gestational age on heart rate, we have been able to show a difference which has been obscured in studies where this has not been done. The difference between the sexes was not explained by size at birth. A higher pulse rate of 3 beats/min in girls over boys at the age of 10 years has been recorded (chapter 15) and similarly was not explained by a difference in height.

We found that babies who had a lower birth weight, had a smaller head circumference at birth, and were thin, having a low ponderal index, had higher heart rates at 18 weeks' gestation. The association with lower birth weight and head circumference partly resulted from earlier birth in babies with higher heart rates. The remainder of the association may therefore be due to retarded growth. The association of heart rate with ponderal index was independent of gestation. We found no associations between birth measurements and fetal heart rate at 36 weeks' gestation. This could be due to the small number of individuals studied at a time of increasing variability among individuals in the values. However, Gagnon et al reported that basal fetal heart rates in a group of fetuses between 30 and 40 weeks' gestation that were small for gestational age were similar to those in a group exhibiting normal growth.[7]

As the association of lower birth weight and head size with faster heart rate at 18 weeks partly depended on retarded fetal growth rather than shorter gestation, it is possible that the faster heart rates resulted from the babies already being small in mid-gestation. Alternatively the faster heart rate could be an early adaptive response to adverse influences which later cause both growth failure and early delivery. Whatever the explanation, our results show that term babies with low ponderal indices, small heads, thin arms, and less subcutaneous fat (table III) already differ from other babies in early gestation. A study of men and women aged 50 years has shown that such babies have high adult blood pressure (chapter 17). A study of 4 year old children similarly showed that they had higher systolic blood pressure (chapter 18). Our findings suggest that these babies would have had raised heart rates in early gestation.

Maternal blood pressure was not related to fetal heart rate at 18 or 36 weeks (table II). We found, however, that when the highest maternal systolic pressure in pregnancy was > 130 mm Hg, the fall in fetal heart rate during gestation was less. This is consistent with the findings of Dawson et al,[5] who showed reduced falls in fetal heart rate in the babies of six women who became hypertensive compared with controls.[5] We found no effect of maternal smoking habits on fetal heart rate.

In conclusion, we have shown that babies born at term with low ponderal indices and small head and mid-arm circumferences have raised heart rates in early pregnancy. This pattern of neonatal measurements, which reflects impaired fetal growth, has been shown to predict high blood pressure in adult life. Intrauterine "setting" of heart rate may be one mechanism linking impaired fetal growth with later high blood pressure. The influences which impair growth appear to take effect early in gestation and are at present not known.

We thank Hewlett-Packard for the loan of the fetal heart rate monitor.

1 Gillum RF. The epidemiology of resting heart rate in a national sample of men and women: associations with hypertension, coronary heart disease, blood pressure and other cardiovascular risk factors. *Am Heart J* 1988;**116**:163–74.
2 Wheeler T, Murrills A. Patterns of fetal heart rate during normal pregnancy. *Br J Obstet Gynaecol* 1978;**85**:18–27.
3 Visser GHA, Dawes GS, Redman CWG. Numerical analysis of the normal antenatal fetal heart rate. *Br J Obstet Gynaecol* 1981;**88**:792–802.
4 Cole TJ. Fitting smoothed centile curves to reference data. *Journal of the Royal Statistical Society (A)* 1988;**151**:385–418.
5 Dawson AJ, Dalton KJ, Newcombe RG. Baseline fetal heart rates from 15 to 38 weeks gestation in normotensive and hypertensive pregnancies. *Br J Obstet Gynaecol* 1985; **92**:60–4.
6 Ibarra-Polo AA, Guiloff E, Gomez-Rogers C. Fetal heart rate throughout pregnancy. *Am J Obstet Gynecol* 1972;**113**:814–8.
7 Gagnon R, Hunse C, Bocking AD. Fetal heart rate patterns in the small-for-gestational-age human fetus. *Am J Obstet Gynecol* 1989;**161**:779–84.

29: Review: maternal and fetal origins of cardiovascular disease

D J P BARKER, C N MARTYN

The limited ability of known risk factors to predict the occurrence of cardiovascular disease in individuals is often forgotten.[1] Rose has pointed out that for a man falling into the lowest risk groups for plasma lipid concentrations, blood pressure, cigarette smoking, and presence of pre-existing symptoms of coronary heart disease, the commonest cause of death is coronary heart disease.[2] Nor is the paradoxical social and geographical distribution of ischaemic heart disease understood. Why is it that a disease that is associated globally with affluence is now commonest in the poorest parts of Britain and among people with the lowest incomes?

Geographical studies

A possible explanation for the geographical differences in mortality from cardiovascular disease in England and Wales is that its causes begin to operate not in adult life but during fetal development and infancy. Records of infant mortality dating from the beginning of the century allow current death rates in the 212 local authority areas of England and Wales to be compared with infant mortality rates in the same places 60 or more years ago. The correlation between past infant mortality and current mortality from cardiovascular disease ($r = 0.73$) is strikingly close (chapter 1). Infant mortality is, of course, no more than a general indicator of adverse environmental conditions. But such a strong relation is, at the very least, suggestive that some aspect of poor living conditions in early childhood determines risk of cardiovascular disease in adult life.

The records of infant mortality in England and Wales are sufficiently detailed to allow neonatal mortality (that is, deaths before 1 month of age) to be distinguished from postneonatal mortality (that is, deaths between the ages of 1 month and 1 year). A further analysis using these separate categories showed that adult cardiovascular mortality is more closely linked to neonatal mortality 60 years earlier than to postneonatal mortality (chapter 4).

Neonatal mortality in the past was high in places where many babies were born with low birth weight. Neonatal mortality is also known to have been associated with high maternal mortality. High rates for both neonatal and maternal mortality were found in places where the physique and health of women were poor. Cardiovascular disease is therefore associated more strongly with poor maternal physique and health and poor fetal growth than with conditions, such as overcrowding, that predispose to high postneonatal death rates.

Animal studies

Ideas about the importance of early life in determining risk of disease in adulthood are reinforced by studies in animals. Transient events in prenatal or early postnatal life have permanent and profound effects on physiology, though such effects may remain latent until the animal is mature. A female rat injected with a few micrograms of testosterone propionate during the first four days of life develops normally until puberty. Only then does it become apparent that the hypothalamic neuronal substrate that mediates the cyclic release of gonadotrophins has been irreversibly altered to a male pattern when, despite adequate ovarian and pituitary function, the animal fails to ovulate or show normal patterns of female sexual behaviour.[3] The same injection of androgen given when the animal is 10 days old has no effect on reproductive function. An example more directly relevant to the theme of this paper is provided by the results of experiments in which the nutrition of pregnant and lactating rats was manipulated. The adult body size of these rats was more powerfully determined by their mothers' nutrition during pregnancy and lactation than by their genetic constitution.[4] Undernutrition during pregnancy stunted the growth of the offspring, and this effect could not be reversed by an optimum diet after birth.[5]

Nutritional deprivation in early life affects the size and DNA content of different organ systems, depending on the precise time at which it occurs. In rats, a brief period of energy restriction immediately after birth caused a profound reduction in the weight of the liver, spleen, and thymus, while brain and skeletal muscle were spared.[6] Energy restriction immediately after weaning reduced only the weight of the thymus.

The metabolic activity of rate limiting enzymes that control cholesterol synthesis seems to be especially sensitive to the content of the diet in infancy. The early nutrition of rats has been shown to determine the response to a dietary fat challenge in adult life[7] and, in baboons, serum concentration and biliary secretion of cholesterol are strongly influenced by the type of diet that they were fed in the neonatal period.[8]

Studies in humans

Whether these ideas about the programming effect of the early environment are applicable to the pathogenesis of cardiovascular disease in humans can be explored by studying adults in middle and old age whose growth and development in infancy was recorded. As described in chapter 13, from 1911 onwards every baby born in the county of Hertfordshire was weighed at birth, visited periodically by a health visitor throughout the first year, and weighed again at 1 year of age. The records of these visits have survived so that it is possible to trace men and women born about 60 years ago and to relate these measurements to the later occurence of illness and death and to the level of known risk factors for cardiovascular disease.

In the first study, 6500 men born in eight districts of the county between 1911 and 1930 were followed up. Table I shows their standardised mortality ratios for ischaemic heart disease according to weight at 1 year; the ratios fall steeply as weight at 1 year increases. There are similar trends with increasing birth weight, though the relation is not as strong as with weight at 1 year.

These findings prompt questions about mechanism. There is now evidence that haemostatic variables, glucose tolerance, blood pressure, and lipid metabolism are all susceptible to the programming effects of the environment in early life (chapters 15–25). In this chapter we have chosen examples that illustrate general points.

High plasma concentration of fibrinogen is a strong predictor of increased risk of both ischaemic heart disease and stroke.[9 10] Fibrinogen

TABLE I—*Standardised mortality ratios for ischaemic heart disease, according to weight at 1 year in 6500 men born during 1911–30. Numbers of deaths in parentheses*

Weight at 1 year (lb)	Ischaemic heart disease	All non-circulatory disease
≤18	100 (36)	74 (39)
−20	84 (90)	99 (157)
−22	92 (180)	74 (215)
−24	70 (109)	67 (155)
−26	55 (44)	84 (99)
≥27	34 (10)	72 (31)
All	78 (469)	78 (696)

TABLE II—*Mean plasma fibrinogen concentrations in men aged 59 to 70, according to weight at 1 year*

Weight at 1 year (lb)	No of men	Fibrinogen (g/litre)*
≤18	38	3·21
−20	93	3·10
−22	178	3·13
−24	173	2·97
−26	82	2·93
≥27	33	2·93
All	597	3·04

* Geometric mean values adjusted for age and cigarette smoking

concentrations have been measured in 597 men aged 59 to 70 still living in Hertfordshire (chapter 20). Table II shows that concentrations are inversely related to weight at 1 year of age. Fibrinogen concentrations are not related to birth weight and only weakly related to adult height. In a simultaneous regression with weight at 1 year, the effect of adult height is no longer apparent. Cigarette smoking, as expected, was also associated with increased plasma levels of fibrinogen but the relation with weight at 1 year was not diminished by adjustment for cigarette smoking.

Glucose tolerance tests have been carried out on 370 of these men (chapter 22). The percentage of men with impaired glucose tolerance or diabetes, defined by a plasma glucose concentration of 7·8 mmol/litre or more at two hours falls progressively with both increasing birth weight and weight at 1 year (table III). There are threefold differences in the prevalence of impaired glucose tolerance and diabetes between men with the highest and lowest early weights. Concentrations of plasma 32–33 split

TABLE III—*Impaired glucose tolerance or diabetes (two hour glucose ≥7·8 mmol/litre) in men aged 59 to 70*

Weights at 1 year (lb)	No of men	Impaired glucose tolerance		Odds ratio adjusted for body mass index (95% confidence interval)
		No	%	
≤18	23	10	43	8·2 (1·8 to 38)
−20	63	20	32	4·8 (1·2 to 19)
−22	107	32	30	4·2 (1·1 to 16)
−24	105	19	18	2·1 (0·5 to 7·9)
−26	48	9	19	2·1 (0·5 to 9·0)
≥27	24	3	13	1·0
Total	370	93	25	χ^2 for trend = 14·9 (p < 0·001)

proinsulin are also inversely related to weight at 1 year. Raised concentrations of this insulin precursor are thought to be an indicator of pancreatic β cell dysfunction. These findings suggest that factors which retard fetal and infant growth impair pancreatic development and limit the eventual size or function of the adult pancreatic β cell complement.

The inverse relation between systolic blood pressure and birth weight present in the Hertfordshire men is shown in table IV (chapter 20). A similar relation has also been found in a national sample of men and women at the age of 36 (chapter 15). In contrast to plasma concentrations of fibrinogen and rates of glucose intolerance, blood pressure in these men is not related to weight at 1 year independently of birth weight, nor is it related to adult height. This may indicate that the critical period when blood pressure is sensitive to programming is during fetal life rather than infancy.

These discoveries have implications both for the pathogenesis of cardiovascular and other diseases, and also for maternal and infant health. The relations between early growth and risk factors and rates of disease are continuous. Plasma concentrations of fibrinogen (table II), the prevalence of impaired glucose tolerance (table III), and levels of systolic blood pressure (table IV) reduce progressively up to the highest values of weight at 1 year or birth weight. If the criterion for successful fetal and infant growth is adult health and longevity, we may no longer be entitled to assume that a baby of average birth weight and weight in infancy has necessarily achieved its optimum weight.

Birth weight is a summary measure of fetal growth; it mixes up head size, body length, and the amount of fat that the baby has stored. To explore the relation between different aspects of fetal growth and adult blood pressure in greater detail, we examined 449 men and women now aged around 50 years who had been born in Sharoe Green hospital in Preston (chapter 16), where unusually detailed observations were made on newborn babies. Table V shows the mean systolic pressures according to placental weight

TABLE IV—*Mean systolic pressure in men aged 59 to 70, according to birth weight*

Birth weight (lb)	No of men	Systolic pressure (mm Hg)
≤5·5	21	174
−6·5	70	165
−7·5	187	166
−8·5	183	164
−9·5	96	161
>9·5	40	164
All	597	164

TABLE V—*Mean systolic pressures (mm Hg) of men and women aged 46 to 54 according to birth weight and placental weight. Numbers of people in parentheses*

Birth weight (lb)	Placental weight (lb)				
	−1·0	−1·25	−1·5	>1·5	All
≤5·5	152 (26)	154 (13)	153 (5)	206 (1)	154 (45)
−6·5	147 (16)	151 (54)	150 (28)	166 (8)	151 (106)
−7·5	144 (20)	148 (77)	145 (45)	160 (27)	149 (169)
>7·5	133 (6)	148 (27)	147 (42)	154 (54)	149 (129)
All	147 (68)	149 (171)	147 (120)	157 (90)	150 (449)

and birth weight. These two variables act in opposite directions; blood pressure falls by around 10 mm Hg from the lowest to the highest groups of birth weight but rises by around 12 mm Hg from the lowest to the highest groups of placental weight. Adjusting for gestational age, current body mass index, and alcohol consumption did not affect these trends. Large placental weight was also associated with clinical hypertension in adult life. Among these 449 men and women the rate of being treated for hypertension was 3·7 times higher in those whose placentas had weighed more than 1·5 lb (680 g) than among those whose placentas had weighed less than 1·0 lb (450 g). A recent survey of the blood pressures of 405 children aged 4 showed the same opposite associations with birth weight and placental weight as were found in the men and women aged 50 (chapter 18).

It is worth emphasising that most of the people in Preston who had high systolic blood pressure were not especially small at birth. Their birth weights were within the normal range, but their placentas were large. An interesting feature of these babies with the heaviest placentas is that their bodies were disproportionately short in relation to their head circumference. In animals it is known that a fetal response to hypoxia results in blood being preferentially diverted to the brain and myocardium at the expense of depriving other tissues of blood flow.[11] It is not too far fetched to speculate that the pattern of fetal growth described above is the result of a similar mechanism operating in humans.

The causes of a disproportionately large placenta are not well understood, but in Preston only 7% of babies born at term to mothers in social classes I and II had placentas that weighed more than 1·5 lb. This compares with 24% for mothers in lower social classes. One factor linking low social class with large placental weight may be poor nutrition. Evidence in support comes from a recent study of 8684 births in Oxford that shows an association between iron deficiency anaemia and increased placental weight (chapter 27).

Studies on the relation between early growth and adult obstructive airways disease have proceeded in parallel with those on cardiovascular disease. There is now strong evidence that obstructive airways disease is associated with retarded growth during the period of rapid lung development in fetal life and infancy, and with acute respiratory infection during infancy (chapter 14).

Conclusions

The results of these studies show that retarded growth in fetal life and infancy is strongly related both to mortality from cardiovascular disease and to adult levels of some of its known risk factors. Any argument concerns the extent to which this relation should be interpreted as being causal. In broad terms there are three possible explanations for our findings. The first is that birth weight is merely a marker for adverse environmental influences that act in later life.[12] Although this interpretation can just be sustained if one is prepared to view the ecological data in isolation, it cannot account for the results of follow up studies of individuals. In Hertfordshire birth weight was not associated with social class, either at birth or currently. The relations with adult risk factors were present within each social class. Further, if a poor early environment caused higher levels of cardiovascular risk factors through the cumulative effect of a variety of adverse influences acting during childhood and adolescence, one would expect these higher levels of risk factors to be associated with shorter adult stature. But the relations we have found between early growth and adult fibrinogen concentrations and blood pressure are independent of adult height.

A second possible explanation for the relation is that genetic influences that first show themselves in early life as growth failure are revealed later in adult life through the occurrence of degenerative disease. The implication here is that the genes that determine low birth weight are the same as, or are closely linked to, the genes that determine cardiovascular disease. This explanation is not likely to be correct because birth weight does not seem to be strongly genetically determined,[13] nor is there much evidence that cardiovascular disease has, in the vast majority of people, a major genetic component.

We think that the relation between impaired growth in early life and risk of adult disease is due to long term effects on physiology and metabolism imposed by an adverse environment during critical periods of development. This conclusion does not imply that the environment in adult life is unimportant, though it may explain why the known adult risk factors predict cardiovascular disease in individuals so poorly. Further work is focusing on the nature and timing of environmental factors that influence the growth of the fetus and infant and programme its metabolism. Laboratory studies that allow direct manipulation of the fetal environment in experimental animals are running in parallel with studies in humans that exploit the ability of ultrasound techniques to examine maternal influences on different aspects of fetal development.

1 Rose G, Marmot MG. Social class and coronary heart disease. *Br Heart J* 1981;**45**:13–9.
2 Rose G. Sick individuals and sick populations. *Int J Epidemiol* 1985;**14**:32–8.
3 Harris GW. Hormonal differentiation of the developing central nervous system with respect to endocrine function. *Philos Trans R Soc Lond [Biol]* 1971;**259**:165–77.
4 Dubos R, Savage D, Schaedler R. Biological Freudianism: lasting effects of early environmental influences. *Pediatrics* 1966;**38**:798–800.
5 Blackwell NM, Blackwell RQ, Yu TTS, Weng YS, Chow BF. Further studies on growth and feed utilization in progeny of underfed mother rats. *J Nutr* 1968;**97**:79–84.
6 Winick M, Noble A. Cellular response in rats during malnutrition at various ages. *J Nutr* 1966;**89**:300–6.
7 Coates PM, Brown SA, Sonaware BR, Koldovsky O. Effect of early nutrition on serum cholesterol levels in adult rats challenged with a high fat diet. *J Nutr* 1983;**113**:1046–50.
8 Mott GE, Lewis DS, McGill HC. Programming of cholesterol metabolism by breast or formula feeding. In: *The childhood environment and adult disease*. Chichester: Wiley, 1991. (Ciba Symposium 156.)
9 Meade TW, North WRS. Population-based distributions of haemostatic variables. *Br Med Bull* 1977;**33**:283–8.
10 Meade TW, Mellows S, Brozovic M, *et al*. Haemostatic function and ischaemic heart disease: principal results of the Northwick Park Heart Study. *Lancet* 1986;**ii**:533–7.
11 Thornberg KL. Fetal response to intrauterine stress. In: *The childhood environment and adult disease*. Chichester: Wiley, 1991. (Ciba Symposium 156.)
12 Ben-Shlomo Y, Davey Smith G. Deprivation in infancy or in adult life: which is more important for mortality risk? *Lancet* 1991;**i**:530–4.
13 Carr-Hill R, Campbell DM, Hall MH, Meredith A. Is birthweight determined genetically? *BMJ* 1987;**295**:687–9.

PART XII
THE FUTURE

30: Ischaemic heart disease in England and Wales around the year 2000

C OSMOND, D J P BARKER

Age and sex specific death rates for 1968–87 in the nine standard regions of England and Wales were used to predict national and regional trends in death rates from ischaemic heart disease until 2007.

There will be a large fall in deaths from ischaemic heart disease, which will be greater in men and women aged under 65. There will, however, be a sharp worsening of the north-south divide. The greatest reduction in any region will be in Wales.

The campaign to change the national diet should therefore give highest priority to the northern regions. Because infant growth is inversely related to adult risk of ischaemic heart disease, the poor growth of young children in some northern areas is a cause for concern.

Introduction

Death rates from ischaemic heart disease are now falling in Britain,[1] but they remain high in comparison with other countries.[2] Future rates can be predicted from recent trends. This prediction must distinguish changes in successive generations from other sources of year to year variation. We present predicted rates for England and Wales, in men and women, in each age group, and within each region, into the next century.

Methods

We abstracted numbers of deaths from ischaemic heart disease (Inter-

325

national Classification of Diseases codes 410–414 in eighth and ninth revisions) and population sizes during 1968–87 for England and Wales in the nine standard regions by age and sex. These data were used to predict future death rates, allowing for cohort (generation) effects. The statistical model used for prediction partitioned the age and sex specific rates for 1968–87 according to age, year of death, and cohort.[3] The year of death and cohort components were extended into the future, and then combined to predict age specific death rates for 1988 to 2007.

We calculated regional rates for deaths in middle age, which is by convention from 45 to 64 years. These were directly standardised to the European standard population,[4] and are presented as mortality ratios based on the figure of 100 for England and Wales.

Results

The figure shows age specific death rates during 1968–87 by year of birth. Rates among men fell progressively at all ages in generations born from 1928 onwards. Similarly among women rates fell in generations born from 1933 onwards. This shows a cohort effect.

Table I shows death rates during 1968–87 and predicted rates for 1988–2007. Rates will fall in both men and women and in each age group. They will fall more in younger than older people. Up to 2003–7 there will be a 43% fall in men aged 45–49 years in relation to 1983–7 rates. The fall at ages 65–69 will be 25%. The corresponding figures for women will be 44% and 18%.

Table II shows observed and predicted mortality ratios by region among middle aged people. There will be a widening in regional differences. The highest death rates will continue to be in the three northern regions, but their ratios to the national average will increase. A large rise in the north west will take the ratio to 137. The ratios in both midland regions will rise to exceed 100. The lowest death rates will continue to be in East Anglia and the two southern regions, but their ratios to the national average will fall. The fall in East Anglia will take the ratio to 70. The position of Wales will improve sharply, the ratio falling from 121 to 90.

Discussion

If the trends over the past 20 years continue there will be a large fall in premature deaths from ischaemic heart disease in England and Wales. The fall at ages over 65 years will be less. There will be a sharp worsening of the north-south divide. Mortality in the three northern and two midland regions will worsen in comparison with East Anglia and the two southern regions. In Wales death rates at younger ages have fallen sharply in successive generations and predict a continuing large fall in premature

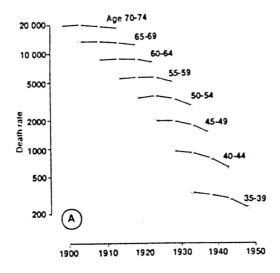

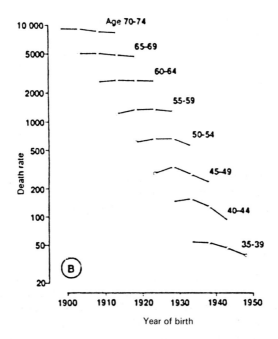

FIG 1—*Age specific death rates (per million person years) from ischaemic heart disease in England and Wales, ages 35–74, 1968–87.* A *men,* B *women*

TABLE I—*Observed and predicted death rates per million years at risk from ischaemic heart disease among men and women aged 35–74 years in England and Wales, 1968 to 2007*

Period	Age group (years)							
	35–39	40–44	45–49	50–54	55–59	60–64	65–69	70–74
	Men							
Observed:								
1968–1972	344	945	1972	3432	5524	8697	13674	19748
1973–1977	326	908	1976	3624	5681	8793	13651	20148
1978–1982	295	793	1765	3435	5657	8771	13094	19507
1983–1987	232	623	1466	2834	5027	8154	12482	18530
Predicted:								
1988–1992	205	563	1281	2592	4583	7923	12607	18393
1993–1997	178	488	1105	2206	4050	7007	11898	18153
1998–2002	153	422	959	1903	3448	6193	10524	17132
2003–2007	133	365	829	1651	2975	5272	9301	15153
	Women							
Observed:								
1968–1972	55	147	290	621	1226	2608	5065	9144
1973–1977	54	157	339	666	1346	2697	5083	9148
1978–1982	47	130	286	670	1371	2683	4915	8680
1983–1987	39	91	235	568	1299	2646	4791	8461
Predicted:								
1988–1992	33	94	192	508	1197	2734	5032	8563
1993–1997	29	78	185	401	1038	2447	5080	8779
1998–2002	25	67	153	385	819	2122	4546	8863
2003–2007	21	58	131	319	787	1674	3942	7932

TABLE II—*Observed and predicted mortality ratios for ischaemic heart disease among men and women aged 45–64 years in the regions of England and Wales, 1968–2007*

Region	Observed in 1968–77	Observed in 1978–87	Predicted for 1988–97	Predicted for 1998–2007
North	121	124	128	128
North West	119	123	127	137
Yorkshire and Humberside	115	116	118	120
East Midlands	97	100	106	115
West Midlands	99	102	107	112
East Anglia	80	76	72	70
South East	87	85	82	80
South West	92	88	83	77
Wales	121	114	107	90

deaths. There may be additional benefits arising from the prevention project Heartbeat Wales.

Studies of both fatal and non-fatal myocardial infarction in the United States of America, Finland, Australia, and New Zealand have shown that death rates are falling and are accompanied by falls in incidence.[5] Except in New Zealand, rates are falling more in younger than older age groups.

A survey of adult diet has shown that dietary fat intake does not differ greatly between one part of England and Wales and another (chapter 8). These findings, based on a study of three towns, were supported by a recent national survey.[6] Nevertheless, because of the greater susceptibility of men and women in the northern and midland regions, however caused, implementation of the recommendations made by the Committee on Medical Aspects of Food Policy is more urgent in those regions. Currently in England only around 25% of men and women aged 35–54 have fat intakes below the recommended 35% of total energy intake, or ratios of polyunsaturated to saturated fatty acids above the recommended 0·45.[7]

The distribution of mortality from ischaemic heart disease throughout England and Wales is closely related to the distribution of neonatal mortality 50 and more years ago (chapter 1). This indication that growth and development during prenatal life and infancy are important risk factors for the disease is supported by the results of a prospective study that showed a strong inverse relation between infant weights and death rates (chapter 13). Given the inverse relation between infant growth and ischaemic heart disease, the current poor growth of young children in the inner city area of Liverpool,[8] and in the other northern towns such as Middlesbrough (Harland E, personal communication), must be a cause for concern. It may foreshadow regional differences in mortality that are even larger than those predicted from recent trends.

1 Registrar General. *Statistical review of England and Wales*. Part 1. Tables, medical. London: HMSO, 1968 and following years.
2 Tunstall-Pedoe H, Smith WCS, Crombie IK. Level and trends of coronary heart disease mortality in Scotland compared with other countries. *Health Bull* 1986;**44**:153–61.
3 Osmond C. Using age, period and cohort models to estimate future mortality rates. *Int J Epidemiol* 1985;**14**:124–9.
4 Breslow NE, Day NE. *The design and analysis of cohort studies*. Lyon: IARC, 1987.
5 Martin CA, Hobbs MST, Armstrong BK, de Kerk NH. Trends in the incidence of myocardial infarction in Western Australia between 1971 and 1982. *Am J Epidemiol* 1989;**129**:655–68.
6 Office of Population Censuses and Surveys. *Dietary and nutritional survey of British adults*. London: HMSO, 1990.
7 Department of Health and Social Security. Report on Health and Social Subjects No 28. *Diet and cardiovascular disease*. London: HMSO, 1984.
8 Hall AJ, Barker DJP, Dangerfield PH, Osmond C, Taylor JF. Small feet and Perthes' disease: a survey in Liverpool. *J Bone Joint Surg* 1988;**70-B**:611–3.

31: Review: rise and fall of Western diseases

D J P BARKER

Nutrition and hygiene during early childhood are important in determining the risk of the diseases which follow industrialisation. We still know little about the processes involved.

The term "Western diseases" is used to describe a group of diseases common in industrialised countries but uncommon elsewhere.[1] These diseases are regarded as a consequence of the environmental changes accompanying industrialisation and prosperity; it is often argued that their prevention depends on a return to practices of the past—for example, resumption of a diet high in complex carbohydrates and low in animal fats.

"Western" characterises only the international distribution of diseases. It does not describe other features of disease distribution in populations. In particular, it does not predict changes in incidence other than the rise with the beginnings of industrialisation.

Two main environmental changes during industrialisation are in hygiene and in diet. Improvements in sanitation and housing lead to falls in mortality from infective diseases, especially among children.[2] Increased intake of total calories, animal fat, fruit and fresh vegetables, vitamins, and minerals leads to better growth and development of children and contributes to the decline of infective diseases such as tuberculosis.

Epidemiological findings suggest that many diseases in industrialised countries fall into one of three groups, which can be shown by data from England and Wales, where numbers and causes of all deaths have been recorded for 140 years. The first group, associated with affluence, includes gall stones, renal stones and cancers of the breast, ovary, and prostate. The incidence of these diseases has risen steeply during this century, particularly in more prosperous areas. The second group, associated with poor living standards, includes chronic bronchitis, stroke, stomach cancer, and rheumatic heart disease. The incidence of these diseases has fallen during the past 50 years as living standards have improved. These diseases are commonest in the least affluent areas and in people with the lowest incomes. The third group is at different times associated with both affluence and poverty, and includes ischaemic heart disease, appendicitis, and duodenal ulcer. The incidence of these diseases rose in the early part of this century, when they were more common among the rich. Subsequently the incidence fell and they are now commoner among poorer people.

The annual death rates from this last group of diseases in England and Wales[3] are shown in fig 1. Together with those in the first group, they can be termed "Western" diseases. Why have they declined when the environmental changes of industrialisation have persisted?

Poliomyelitis was rare in Britain before this century but, as in other countries, it began to appear as hygienic and general living standards improved. This is in contrast to all the other common infective diseases, which were declining at this time. There was a sharp rise in notifications of poliomyelitis after the second world war which persisted until the introduction of large scale immunisation (fig 1). It is now known that the increase in incidence of poliomyelitis resulted from the increasing vulnerability of the central nervous system to poliovirus infection with increasing age. As hygiene, sanitation, and housing improved, the proportion of children escaping infection during the relatively safe period of infancy rose, and the number of cases of paralytic disease at later ages therefore rose in parallel.

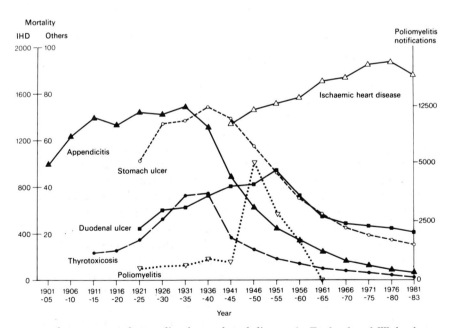

FIG 1—*Average annual mortality from selected diseases in England and Wales from 1901, and numbers of notifications of poliomyelitis in five year periods.*[3] *IHD = ischaemic heart disease.*

331

The outbreaks of appendicitis which have accompanied industrialisation in many parts of the world can similarly be explained as an age dependent consequence of infection.[4] In England and Wales, death rates from appendicitis increased abruptly and steeply from around 1900, and then fell progressively from the 1930s onwards (fig 1). There is strong evidence that this trend reflects changes in incidence of the disease, and similar trends were recorded in other European countries and in the United States. The explanation of these trends is thought to lie in the reduced levels of enteric infection in young children brought about by better hygiene, making them liable to develop appendicitis in response to infections at a later age. With continued improvements in hygiene, exposure to infection throughout childhood and early adult life became more uncommon. Because the appendix seems to be less vulnerable to infection after about 30 years of age, appendicitis declined.

Death rates from duodenal and stomach ulcers rose and fell in a similar way. The distribution of duodenal ulcer with social class was similar to that of appendicitis; while it was increasing it was more common among the rich, but as it declined it became commoner in poorer people. Recent findings of *Campylobacter*-like organisms in peptic ulcers suggest that the disease is spread by an infective agent.[5] The time trends point to age dependent consequences of infection.

The trends in deaths from thyrotoxicosis (fig 1) show another process by which a rise in disease can be followed by a fall. Death rates rose to a peak in the 1930s and thereafter declined. Most deaths from this disease occur in the elderly, among whom toxic multinodular goitre is the usual cause of thyrotoxicosis. Analyses of age specific rates in successive generations show that rates rose progressively in people born after 1836 and reached a peak in those born between 1871 and 1886.[6] This is shown in fig 2, which gives rates in each generation according to their year of birth.

Figure 2 also shows the progressive increase in dietary iodine in Britain during this century, as a consequence of diversification of diet and availability of iodine in many foods including fish, meat, and milk.[7] Iodine deficiency during childhood was widespread among people born in Britain in the 1800s. Successive generations, however, were exposed to more iodine in adult life. There is evidence that people who are iodine deficient in youth are less able to adapt to increased iodine intake in later life and tend to develop thyrotoxicosis.[8] This would explain the rise in deaths from thyrotoxicosis in the early part of this century (fig 1). Successive generations born after 1880 were exposed to more iodine in childhood, which would have lessened their susceptibility to iodine in adult life; accordingly, thyrotoxicosis mortality fell from around 1940 (fig 1). This explanation of the time trends accounts for the apparent paradox that toxic nodular goitre is now common only in those areas of Britain where iodine deficiency used to be prevalent.

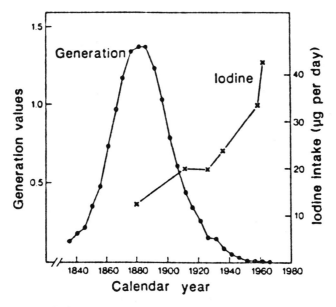

FIG 2—*Relative mortality from thyrotoxicosis in successive generations of women in England and Wales according to year of birth, and estimated per capita daily iodine intake from milk, meat, and fish.*

The essential process thought to underlie the trends of occurrence of toxic nodular goitre is a response to an environmental influence during early life, which has a critical effect on the ability to adapt to subsequent exposure. The same process may determine trends in ischaemic heart disease. Death from ischaemic heart disease was not distinguished from that from other forms of heart disease before 1940, but other evidence shows a steep rise in rates during the first part of the century. From 1940, death rates continued to rise progressively and reached a plateau in the 1970s (fig 1). Since 1980 there has been a small decline. Similar patterns occurred in the United States, Canada, Australia, and New Zealand; initial rises were followed by substantial falls, of around one quarter in the past 20 years in the United States.[9]

Although death from ischaemic heart disease was more common in wealthier people during its steep increase in Britain, it is now more common in less affluent areas and among people with lower incomes. The geographical distribution is the reverse of that for other diseases thought to be caused by the Western diet—gall stones, renal stones, and breast cancer are all more common in more prosperous areas. The geographical distribution of ischaemic heart disease is closely related to that of poor child health and development, indicated by high infant and child mortality about 70 years ago (chapter 1). The aetiology of this disease may therefore depend on two groups of environmental causes: one associated with affluence and likely to be mediated through a high energy, high fat diet; the other acting during childhood and associated with poor living standards. The rise in the disease results from an increase in the first, its fall from reduction in the second.

Further evidence of the effect of this second group of environmental causes is the inverse relation between risk of ischaemic heart disease and height, which is largely determined by growth in childhood. Long term "programming" of lipid metabolism during infancy, in response to infant feeding, is a mechanism for which there is increasing evidence in experimental animals and which could be a link between childhood and ischaemic heart disease. Another link may be the known inverse relation between fetal growth and blood pressure in adult life (chapter 15).

Each of the diseases shown in fig 1 may rise and then fall in response to one environmental change that accompanies industrialisation. Such diseases characterise the change from a mainly rural to a mainly industrial society. Responses to the childhood environment, including age dependent consequences of infection and adaptation to diet during early life, may be important causative factors.

The search for causes of "Western" diseases has concentrated on the adult environment. The importance of the childhood environment in determining responses throughout life may have been underestimated. Models of disease based on the effects of cigarette smoking, an influence in the adult environment which has been intensively studied, may have limited general application. Where differences in individuals' susceptibility to disease cannot be explained by differences in the adult environment, as is the case for ischaemic heart disease, they have often been attributed to genetic causes—especially if the disease has a familial tendency. Part of what is now regarded as the genetic contribution to ischaemic heart disease may turn out to be the effect of the intrauterine or early postnatal environment.

Critical adaptations during early life may determine optimum rates of change within populations. Appendicitis and duodenal ulcer became common at an early stage of improvements in hygiene. The size of epidemics of these diseases may depend on the speed with which hygiene improves throughout the population. The rise of appendicitis in Britain can be linked to the introduction of domestic hot water systems. The introduction of piped water supplies was spread over more than half a century, piped water not reaching some rural areas until after the second world war. Swifter execution of public health reforms begun in the nineteenth century might have reduced the incidence of this disease.

By contrast, critical responses to nutrition in childhood, such as those that occur in toxic nodular goitre and that are suspected in ischaemic heart disease, may limit the extent of dietary change that a generation can be exposed to without adverse effects. It follows that improvements in living standards during early industrialisation should be directed at children. Although the industrial revolution in Britain brought high wages to adults, children continued to grow up undernourished, in large families, and in poor, overcrowded homes.

Steep increases in the incidence of "Western" diseases regularly follow industrialisation in the developing world. Among people of Chinese origin, improvements in hygiene may occur without changes in the traditional diet. Elsewhere, as in the slums of many cities in the developing world, diet changes but poor hygiene persists. If more was known about the processes by which the environment in early life influences adult health, the hygienic and nutritional benefits which will accompany industrial development might be maximised, and the rise in incidence of "Western" disease minimised.

1 Trowell HC, Burkitt DP. *Western diseases: their emergence and prevention*. London: Arnold, 1981.
2 McKeown T, Lowe CR. *An introduction to social medicine*. Oxford: Blackwell Scientific, 1974.
3 *Registrar general's statistical review of England and Wales*. Part 1. Tables, medical. London: HMSO, 1901 and following years.
4 Barker DJP, Osmond C, Golding J, Wadsworth MEJ. Acute appendicitis and bathrooms in three samples of British children. *BMJ* 1988;**296**:956–8.
5 Marshall B, McGechie D, Rogers P, Clancy R. Pyloric campylobacter infection and gastroduodenal disease. *Med J Aust* 1985;**142**:439–44.
6 Phillips DIW, Barker DJP, Winter PD, Osmond C. Mortality from thyrotoxicosis in England and Wales and its association with the previous prevalence of endemic goitre. *J Epidemiol Community Health* 1983;**37**:305–9.
7 Greaves JP, Hollingsworth DF. Trends in food consumption in the United Kingdom. *World Rev Nutr Diet* 1966;**6**:34–89.
8 Barker DJP, Phillips DIW. Current incidence of thyrotoxicosis and past prevalence of goitre in 12 British towns. *Lancet* 1984;**i**:567–70.
9 Pisa Z, Uemura K. Trends of mortality from ischaemic heart disease and other cardiovascular diseases in 27 countries, 1968–1977. *World Health Stat Q* 1982;**35**:11–47.

Index